2005 YEAR BOOK OF ONCOLOGY®

The 2005 Year Book Series

Year Book of Allergy, Asthma, and Clinical Immunology™: Drs Rosenwasser, Boguniewicz, Milgrom, Routes, and Weber

Year Book of Anesthesiology and Pain Management™: Drs Chestnut, Abram, Black, Gravlee, Mathru, Lee, and Roizen

Year Book of Cardiology®: Drs Gersh, Cheitlin, Graham, Kaplan, Sundt, and Waldo

Year Book of Critical Care Medicine®: Drs Dellinger, Parrillo, Balk, Bekes, Dorman, and Dries

Year Book of Dentistry®: Drs Zakariasen, Horswell, McIntyre, Scott, and Zakariasen Victoroff

Year Book of Dermatology and Dermatologic Surgery™: Drs Thiers and Lang

Year Book of Diagnostic Radiology®: Drs Osborn, Birdwell, Dalinka, Gardiner, Levy, Maynard, Oestreich, and Rosado de Christenson

Year Book of Emergency Medicine®: Drs Burdick, Cydulka, Hamilton, Handly, Quintana, and Werner

Year Book of Endocrinology®: Drs Mazzaferri, Bessesen, Howard, Kannan, Kennedy, Leahy, Meikle, Molitch, Rogol, and Rubin

Year Book of Family Practice®: Drs Bowman, Apgar, Bouchard, Dexter, Miser, Neill, and Scherger

Year Book of Gastroenterology™: Drs Lichtenstein, Burke, Dempsey, Drebin, Ginsberg, Katzka, Kochman, Morris, Nunes, Shah, and Stein

Year Book of Hand and Upper Limb Surgery®: Drs Berger and Ladd

Year Book of Medicine®: Drs Barkin, Frishman, Klahr, Loehrer, Mazzaferri, Phillips, Pillinger, and Snydman

Year Book of Neonatal and Perinatal Medicine®: Drs Fanaroff, Maisels, and Stevenson

Year Book of Neurology and Neurosurgery®: Drs Gibbs and Verma

Year Book of Nuclear Medicine®: Drs Coleman, Blaufox, Royal, Strauss, and Zubal

Year Book of Obstetrics, Gynecology, and Women's Health®: Dr Shulman

Year Book of Oncology®: Drs Loehrer, Arceci, Glatstein, Gordon, Hanna, Morrow, and Thigpen

Year Book of Ophthalmology®: Drs Rapuano, Cohen, Eagle, Grossman, Hammersmith, Myers, Nelson, Penne, Sergott, Shields, Tipperman, and Vander

Year Book of Orthopedics®: Drs Morrey, Beauchamp, Peterson, Swiontkowski, Trigg, and Yaszemski

Year Book of Otolaryngology-Head and Neck Surgery®: Drs Paparella, Otto, and Keefe

Year Book of Pathology and Laboratory Medicine®: Drs Raab, Grzybicki, Bejarano, Bissell, and Stanley

Year Book of Pediatrics®: Dr Stockman

Year Book of Plastic and Aesthetic Surgery™: Drs Miller, Bartlett, Garner, McKinney, Ruberg, Salisbury, and Smith

Year Book of Psychiatry and Applied Mental Health®: Drs Talbott, Ballenger, Buckley, Frances, Jensen, and Markowitz

Year Book of Pulmonary Disease®: Drs Phillips, Barker, Dunlap, Lewis, Maurer, and Willsie

Year Book of Rheumatology, Arthritis, and Musculoskeletal Disease™: Drs Panush, Hadler, Hellmann, Hochberg, Lahita, and Seibold

Year Book of Sports Medicine®: Drs Shephard, Alexander, Cantu, Feldman, McCrory, Nieman, Rowland, Sanborn, and Shrier

Year Book of Surgery®: Drs Copeland, Bland, Cerfolio, Daly, Eberlein, Fahey, Mozingo, Pruett, and Seeger

Year Book of Urology®: Drs Andriole and Coplen

Year Book of Vascular Surgery®: Dr Moneta

2005

The Year Book of ONCOLOGY®

Editor-in-Chief

Patrick J. Loehrer, Sr, MD

Bruce Kenneth Wiseman Professor of Medicine; Director, Division of Hematology-Oncology, Indiana University School of Medicine, Indianapolis, Indiana

ELSEVIER
MOSBY

Vice President, Continuity Publishing: Timothy M. Griswold
Managing Editor: David Orzechowski
Developmental Editor: Dana M. Lamparello
Senior Manager, Continuity Production: Idelle L. Winer
Senior Issue Manager: Pat Costigan
Senior Illustrations and Permissions Coordinator: Chidi M. Nwaseki

2005 EDITION

Printed in the United States of America
Composition by Thomas Technology Solutions, Inc
Printing/binding by Sheridan Books, Inc.

Editorial Office:
Elsevier
Suite 1800
1600 John F. Kennedy Blvd
Philadelphia, PA 19103-2899

International Standard Serial Number: 1040-1741
International Standard Book Number: 0-323-02112-3

Associate Editors

Robert J. Arceci, MD, PhD
Professor of Pediatrics and Oncology, Director and King Fahd Professor of Pediatric Oncology, Sidney Kimmel Comprehensive Cancer Center at Johns Hopkins University, Baltimore, Maryland

Eli Glatstein, MD
Morton Kligerman Professor of Radiation Oncology, Department of Radiation Oncology, University of Pennsylvania, Philadelphia, Pennsylvania

Michael S. Gordon, MD
Associate Professor of Medicine, University of Arizona College of Medicine; Associate Director, Arizona Cancer Center—Greater Phoenix Area, Scottsdale, Arizona

Nasser H. Hanna, MD
Assistant Professor of Medicine, Indiana University, Indianapolis, Indiana

Monica Morrow, MD
Professor of Surgery, Temple University School of Medicine; Chairman, Department of Surgical Oncology; G. Willing Pepper Chair in Cancer Research, Fox Chase Cancer Center, Philadelphia, Pennsylvania

James Tate Thigpen, MD
Professor of Medicine and Director, Division of Oncology, University of Mississippi Medical Center, Jackson, Mississippi

Table of Contents

Journals Represented

Journals represented in this YEAR BOOK are listed below.

American Journal of Clinical Oncology
American Journal of Neuroradiology
American Journal of Obstetrics and Gynecology
American Journal of Roentgenology
Annals of Oncology
Annals of Plastic Surgery
Annals of Surgery
Annals of Surgical Oncology
Archives of Otolaryngology-Head and Neck Surgery
Archives of Surgery
Blood
Bone Marrow Transplantation
British Journal of Cancer
British Journal of Plastic Surgery
Cancer
Cancer Research
Clinical Cancer Research
Clinical Radiology
Diseases of the Colon and Rectum
European Journal of Cancer
European Journal of Nuclear Medicine and Molecular Imaging
European Journal of Surgical Oncology (London)
European Urology
Gastroenterology
Gynecologic Oncology
Intensive Care Medicine
International Journal of Cancer
Journal of Clinical Investigation
Journal of Clinical Oncology
Journal of General Internal Medicine
Journal of Oral and Maxillofacial Surgery
Journal of Pathology
Journal of Pediatric Surgery
Journal of Thoracic and Cardiovascular Surgery
Journal of Urology
Journal of the American College of Surgeons
Journal of the American Medical Association
Journal of the National Cancer Institute
Lancet
Lung Cancer
Mayo Clinic Proceedings
Molecular Cancer Therapeutics
Neuro-Oncology
New England Journal of Medicine
Proceedings of the National Academy of Sciences
Radiology
Science
The Oncologist
Urology

World Journal of Surgery

Standard Abbreviations

The following terms are abbreviated in this edition: acquired immunodeficiency syndrome (AIDS), cardiopulmonary resuscitation (CPR), central nervous system (CNS), cerebrospinal fluid (CSF), computed tomography (CT), deoxyribonucleic acid (DNA), electrocardiography (ECG), health maintenance organization (HMO), human immunodeficiency virus (HIV), intensive care unit (ICU), intramuscular (IM), intravenous (IV), magnetic resonance (MR) imaging (MRI), ribonucleic acid (RNA), ultrasound (US), and ultraviolet (UV).

Note

The Year Book of Oncology is a literature survey service providing abstracts of articles published in the professional literature. Every effort is made to assure the accuracy of the information presented in these pages. Neither the editors nor the publisher of the Year Book of Oncology can be responsible for errors in the original materials. The editors' comments are their own opinions. Mention of specific products within this publication does not constitute endorsement.

To facilitate the use of the Year Book of Oncology as a reference tool, all illustrations and tables included in this publication are now identified as they appear in the original article. This change is meant to help the reader recognize that any illustration or table appearing in the Year Book of Oncology may be only one of many in the original article. For this reason, figure and table numbers will often appear to be out of sequence within the Year Book of Oncology.

Introduction

This past year has been an exciting and interesting year in the field of oncology. Cancer dates back to the times of the pharaohs; it is only in the last few decades that we have truly begun to understand the molecular forces behind the development and treatment of neoplastic diseases. With the burgeoning of technology, our capability of screening patients has exploded beyond the simple Papanicolaou (Pap) smear and mammogram to an era of virtual colonoscopies, MRI of the breast, and proteomics. How to best implement this new technology is unclear; it is clearly a challenge for the future to identify those at high risk to minimize the total cost burden for our society while maximizing the therapy to impact.

Similarly, the discovery of the molecular changes surrounding cancer has led to the discovery of targeted compounds. A number of these have emerged in the clinical arena and include lymphoma, breast cancer, and now colon cancer. Many more are to come. The impact of novel therapies in metastatic colon cancer has dramatically changed the prognosis of patients with stage IV disease over the past two decades.

I wish to deeply thank our co-editors for doing an outstanding job of selecting some of the most interesting and diverse articles in the field of oncology, and these involve both pediatric and adult patients. More importantly, I also wish to thank them for their candid comments that illuminate these articles and help put them into perspective.

Finally, I would like to dedicate this issue to one of our finest friends and colleagues, Dr Daniel C. Ihde, who recently passed away. Dan was a quiet man with a brilliant intellect and incredibly dry wit. It was his honest and insightful approach that served as a role model for many of us.

Patrick J. Loehrer, Sr, MD

1 Etiology, Epidemiology, and Carcinogenesis

Enthusiasm for Cancer Screening in the United States

Schwartz LM, Woloshin S, Fowler FJ Jr, et al (VA Outcomes Group, White River Junction, Vt; Dartmouth Med School, Hanover, NH; Univ of Massachusetts, Boston)

JAMA 291:71-78, 2004 1–1

Introduction.—There is a growing recognition in the medical community that cancer screening is a 2-edged sword. Some persons benefit from early detection and others may be treated for cancer unnecessarily. To understand the issues facing public health officials who hope to bring balanced information to the public concerning cancer screening, a national telephone survey was conducted during 2001 and 2002 to explore general beliefs regarding early detection, personal commitment to screening, screening as an obligation, attitudes toward false-positive results, and desire for total-body CT screening.

Methods.—The 500 survey participants were women aged 40 years or older and men aged 50 years or older without a history of cancer. The primary outcome measures were responses to a survey with 5 modules: a general screening module (eg, value of early detection, total-body CT), and 4 screening test modules; the 4 were Papanicolaou test, mammography, prostate-specific antigen test, and sigmoidoscopy or colonoscopy.

Findings.—Most adults (87%) regarded routine screening as almost always a good idea and thought that finding cancer early saves lives (74%, most or all of the time). Less than one third thought there was a time when they would stop undergoing routine screening. A substantial proportion considered that an 80-year-old who chose not to be tested was irresponsible (ranging from 41% for mammography to 32% for colonoscopy). Thirty-eight percent of respondents had experienced at least 1 false-positive screening test; more than 40% characterized that experience as "very scary" or the "scariest time of my life." Yet 98% reported that they were glad they underwent the initial screening test.

Most participants had a strong desire to know about the presence of cancer, regardless of its implications. Two thirds indicated that they would like to be tested for cancer even if nothing could be done, and 56% reported that they would want to be screened for "pseudodisease" (cancers growing so slowly that they would never cause problems during the person's lifetime, even if untreated). Rather than receive $1000 cash, 73% indicated they would prefer to receive a total-body CT scan.

Conclusion.—Public enthusiasm concerning cancer screening is not dampened by false-positive test results or the possibility that testing could lead to unnecessary treatment. This enthusiasm could place the public at risk of overtesting and overtreatment.

► The subject of screening for cancer is surprisingly controversial among physicians. There are issues of efficacy and cost that are not easily answered. However, as this article shows, the enthusiasm for screening for cancer within the general public is exceptionally high. The issues of efficacy and cost do not seem to seep into the public's point of view. It is this euphoric affection for cancer screening that seems to make total-body CT scanning for screening appealing to the public. It is interesting to note just how supportive of screening the public actually is. This is even without issues of efficacy or cost being considered.

In the same issue of *JAMA* is a commentary by Merenstein on his personal experience as a resident in dealing with the science of screening, which turned out to be in conflict with public attitudes.[1] It is a kind of an eye-popping experience that is worth the reader's attention. The essential point is that no matter how solid scientific evidence may be, there is a tremendous amount of bias in the lay public. If this conflict ever gets involved in a court case, all bets are off.

E. Glatstein, MD

Reference

1. Merenstein D: Winners and losers. *JAMA* 291:15-16, 2004.

► This study is both encouraging and discouraging. First, it is encouraging that a high percentage of the public support cancer screening. It is discouraging, though, in that patients are not so discriminating. Many people would undergo screening for diseases in which there is no known treatment or controversial at best. With the rising costs of health care, it is the responsibility of the medical community to educate the public and to channel enthusiasm for cancer screening into appropriate areas.

P. J. Loehrer, Sr, MD

Racial and Ethnic Disparities in Cancer Screening: The Importance of Foreign Birth as a Barrier to Care

Goel MS, Wee CC, McCarthy EP, et al (Harvard Med School, Boston)

J Gen Intern Med 18:1028-1035, 2003 1–2

Background.—Racial and ethnic subgroups largely composed of foreign-born persons have been shown to have lower rates of cancer screening than white Americans. However, little is known about whether these disparities are related primarily to the race/ethnicity or birthplace of these persons. Whether foreign birthplace can explain some of the racial/ethnic disparities observed in cancer screening was determined.

Methods.—This cross-sectional study used 1998 data from the National Health Interview Survey. The main outcome measures were completion of cervical, breast, or colorectal cancer screening.

Results.—Of the 98,785 respondents, 15% were foreign born. After adjustment for sociodemographic characteristics and illness burden, black respondents were as or more likely to report cancer screening than white respondents. However, Hispanic and Asian-American and Pacific Islander (AAPI) respondents were significantly less likely to report screening for most cancers. When race/ethnicity and birthplace were considered together, US-born Hispanic and AAPI respondents were as likely to report cancer screening as US-born whites; however, foreign-born white, Hispanic, and AAPI respondents were less likely than US-born whites to report Pap smears (Tables 4 and 5). Foreign-born Hispanic and AAPI respondents were also less likely to report fecal occult blood testing and sigmoidoscopy. In addition, foreign-born AAPI respondents were less likely to report mammography. Adjust-

TABLE 4.—Multivariable Analysis of Relation Between Combined Birthplace and Race/Ethnicity and Screening for Cervical, Breast, and Colorectal Cancer*†

	Pap Smear, $N = 10,486$ AOR (95% CI)	Mammogram, $N = 4,597$ AOR (95% CI)	Fecal Occult Blood Test, $N = 9,823$ AOR (95% CI)	Sigmoidoscopy, $N = 9,968$ AOR (95% CI)
U.S.-born				
White	1.00	1.00	1.00	1.00
Black	2.44 (1.81 to 3.28)‡	1.18 (0.91 to 1.53)	1.05 (0.86 to 1.28)	1.15 (0.92 to 1.43)
Hispanic	0.94 (0.74 to 1.20)	1.17 (0.76 to 1.80)	0.77 (0.56 to 1.05)	0.85 (0.64 to 1.13)
AAPI	1.57 (0.62 to 4.02)	0.50 (0.17 to 1.47)	1.36 (0.73 to 2.54)	0.85 (0.45 to 1.60)
Foreign-born				
White	0.58 (0.41 to 0.82)‡	0.86 (0.60 to 1.23)	0.83 (0.64 to 1.07)	0.98 (0.75 to 1.28)
Black	1.05 (0.49 to 2.24)	1.62 (0.53 to 4.99)	0.40 (0.18 to 0.88)‡	0.48 (0.21 to 1.09)
Hispanic	0.65 (0.53 to 0.79)‡	0.84 (0.58 to 1.22)	0.72 (0.53 to 0.98)‡	0.70 (0.51 to 0.97)‡
AAPI	0.28 (0.19 to 0.39)‡	0.49 (0.28 to 0.86)‡	0.61 (0.39 to 0.96)‡	0.63 (0.40 to 0.99)‡

*Analysis adjusted for sociodemographic characteristics (age, marital status, region of residence, education, income) and illness burden (self-reported health status, smoking, concurrent illnesses, body mass index, hospitalizations in past year).

†Unadjusted odds ratios did not differ substantially from the adjusted odds ratios presented in this table.

‡$P \leq .05$.

Abbreviations: AOR, Adjusted odds ratio; *CI*, confidence interval.

TABLE 5.—Multivariable Analysis of Relation Between Birthplace and Screening Among Hispanic and AAPI Respondents

	Pap Smear, Odds Ratio (95% CI)	Mammogram, Odds Ratio (95% CI)	Fecal Occult Blood Test Odds Ratio (95% CI)	Sigmoidoscopy, Odds Ratio (95% CI)
U.S.-born Hispanics	1.00	1.00	1.00	1.00
Foreign-born Hispanics				
Unadjusted model	0.65 (0.50 to 0.83)*	0.64 (0.42 to 0.99)*	0.81 (0.54 to 1.21)	0.69 (0.48 to 1.01)*
Partially adjusted†	0.69 (0.52 to 0.91)*	0.72 (0.41 to 1.24)	0.94 (0.62 to 1.42)	0.83 (0.54 to 1.25)
Fully adjusted‡	0.96 (0.69 to 1.33)	1.21 (0.61 to 2.41)	1.05 (0.68 to 1.64)	0.89 (0.59 to 1.37)
U.S.-born AAPIs	1.00	1.00	1.00	1.00
Foreign-born AAPIs				
Unadjusted model	0.16 (0.07 to 0.39)*	0.65 (0.20 to 2.07)	0.40 (0.18 to 0.88)*	0.66 (0.30 to 1.44)
Partially adjusted†	0.18 (0.07 to 0.47)*	0.98 (0.30 to 3.20)	0.45 (0.21 to 0.98)*	0.74 (0.34 to 1.58)
Fully adjusted‡	0.24 (0.07 to 0.79)*	1.70 (0.64 to 4.48)	0.62 (0.29 to 1.33)	0.96 (0.44 to 2.09)

*$P \leq .05$.

†Analysis adjusted for sociodemographic characteristics (age, marital status, region of residence, education, income) and illness burden (self-reported health status, smoking, concurrent illnesses, body mass index, hospitalizations in past year).

‡Additionally adjusted for access to care (number of office visits in past year, type of health insurance, usual source of care).

Abbreviation: CI, Confidence interval.

(Courtesy of Goel MS, Wee CC, McCarthy EP, et al: Racial and ethnic disparities in cancer screening: The importance of foreign birth as a barrier to care. *J Gen Intern Med* 18:1028-1035, 2003. Reprinted by permission of Blackwell Publishing.)

ment for access to care partially attenuated disparities among foreign-born respondents.

Conclusions.—Some disparities in cancer screening that have been attributed to race or ethnicity may be explained by foreign birthplace, which is an important barrier to cancer screening, even after adjustment for other factors. These disparities may be improved somewhat by increasing access to health care, but further study is needed to identify other barriers to screening among foreign-born persons in the United States.

▶ This article states what may seem obvious. Foreign-born individuals are less likely to seek preventative health care screening compared with individuals born in the United States. It should be noted that those foreign-born whites do less well than US-born whites, implying that it is more than racial issues, but language and other cultural factors, that may cause health disparities.

P. J. Loehrer, Sr, MD

Hospital Volume and Operative Mortality in Cancer Surgery: A National Study

Finlayson EVA, Goodney PP, Birkmeyer JD (Dept of Veterans Affairs Med Ctr, White River Junction, Vt)

Arch Surg 138:721-725, 2003 1–3

Introduction.—Several trials have reported that high-volume hospitals achieve lower operative mortality with selected high-risk procedures. The relative importance of volume in cancer surgery is disputed. The surgical mortality was assessed for 8 different cancer resections (colectomy, gastrectomy, esophagectomy, pancreatic resection, nephrectomy, cystectomy, pulmonary lobectomy, and pneumonectomy) in the United States population to better quantify the impact of hospital volume.

Methods.—Data from the all-payer Nationwide Inpatient Sample for 1995 through 1997 were used to assess mortality among the 8 cancer resections in 195,152 cases. After separating patients into 3 evenly sized volume groups based on hospital procedure (low, medium, and high), regression techniques were used to describe relationships between hospital volume and in-hospital mortality, with adjustment for patient characteristics.

Results.—Trends toward lower surgical risks at high-volume hospitals were seen for 7 of the 8 procedures. Differences between low- and high-volume hospitals were statistically significant for 3 surgeries (esophagectomy, 15.0% and 6.5%; pancreatic resection, 13.1% and 2.5%; and pulmonary lobectomy, 10.1% and 8.9%, respectively). They were not statistically significant, but absolute differences in mortality between low- and high-volume hospitals were greater than 1% for gastrectomy, 8.7% and 6.9%; cystectomy, 3.6% and 2.5%; and pneumonectomy, 10.6% and 8.9%, respectively. The mortality reductions for both nephrectomy and colectomy were small. Generally, in terms of absolute differences in mortality, the effect of volume was greatest among elderly patients.

Conclusion.—Surgical mortality diminishes with increasing hospital volume for several cancer resections. Volumes may be most important in older patients and those who are at higher risk.

▶ Multiple studies have reported a decrease in operative mortality for complex surgical procedures for the treatment of cancer, such as esophagectomy and pancreatectomy, when they are performed in high-volume hospitals or by high-volume surgeons. Similar trends are noted for less complex resections, although the small absolute differences in survival do not always reach statistical significance. Since it is not feasible that the majority of cancer surgeries be performed in high-volume hospitals, it is time to take the next step and define the processes of care that differ between high- and low-volume hospitals. This task will be more readily accomplished by studying common cancers, which will allow an adequate number of cases to be sampled in a relatively brief time period.

M. Morrow, MD

American Society of Clinical Oncology Technology Assessment: Chemotherapy Sensitivity and Resistance Assays

Schrag D, for the ASCO Working Group on Chemotherapy Sensitivity and Resistance Assays (American Society of Clinical Oncology, Alexandria, Va)

J Clin Oncol 22:3631-3638, 2004 1–4

Background.—Chemotherapy and resistance assays (CSRAs) may enable clinicians to select cancer treatments that are based on the responsiveness of individual tumors as determined by in vitro assays. A technology assessment of CSRAs was developed to better define the role of these tests in routine oncology practice.

Methods and Findings.—The technology assessment was developed by a working group established by the American Society of Clinical Oncology (ASCO). Independent criteria were listed for selecting articles for inclusion, and a structured data abstraction tool was created to facilitate review. In a literature search, 12 articles were identified. The evidence base was judged to be insufficient to support the routine clinical use of any CSRA.

Conclusions.—This ASCO Working Group does not recommend the use of CSRAs outside of clinical trials to select chemotherapeutic agents for individual patients. Clinicians' chemotherapy recommendations should be based on published reports of clinical trials and a patient's health status and treatment preferences. Participation in clinical trials that evaluate CSRAs remains a priority.

Chemotherapy Sensitivity and Resistance Assays: A Systematic Review

Samson DJ, Seidenfeld J, Ziegler K, et al (Blue Cross and Blue Shield Association Technology Evaluation Ctr, Washington, DC)

J Clin Oncol 22:3618-3630, 2004 1–5

Background.—In vitro chemotherapy sensitivity and resistance assays (CSRAs) demonstrate whether a tumor tissue sample responds when exposed to selected chemotherapeutic agents in laboratory conditions. Evidence comparing CSRA-guided therapy with empiric chemotherapy was assessed.

Methods.—The literature was reviewed for studies comparing patients treated contemporaneously by assay-guided chemotherapy and empiric therapy. Studies were chosen by using predetermined selection criteria.

Findings.—Ten studies plus 1 retrospective study involving a total of 7 different CSRAs were analyzed. Patients were randomly assigned to assay-guided or empiric treatment in only 2 studies. In 5 of the 9 nonrandomized studies, response rates were significantly higher among patients receiving assay-guided treatment than among those treated empirically. One of the 2 randomized studies reported a higher response rate in the assay-guided patients. In another 4 studies, response rates favored assay-guided treatment but did not reach statistical significance. Two nonrandomized studies reported significantly improved overall survival associated with assay-guided treatment. In 1 randomized study, the cross-over design made determining whether survival differed between groups difficult. The other randomized study reported no between-group difference in survival. In 6 studies, baseline patient characteristics were not reported. Adverse events data were described in only 1 study.

Conclusions.—Studies have reported higher response rates associated with assay-guided chemotherapy, yet the differences found may have been due to bias or confounding factors in these studies. Little evidence is available on survival. The relative efficacies of assay-guided therapy and empiric treatment have yet to be established. More prospective randomized studies are needed.

▶ Chemotherapy sensitivity and resistance assays have been used in various means over the past 20 to 30 years. This has an extreme appeal to the public and physicians in that theoretically individualized treatment can be determined with the use of these assays in a matter similar to bacterial cultures sensitivity to antibiotics. Indeed, a cottage industry has developed for this approach. These 2 articles (Abstracts 1–4 and 1–5) offer independent reviews by the American Society of Clinical Oncology and by Blue Cross and Blue Shield, which come to similar conclusions. It is just too soon to embrace this technology. Perhaps the greatest concern is for those patients with curable malignancies who are treated with alternative regimens based on these assays. We have seen examples of this at Indiana University including a patient with good risk testicular cancer. There is perhaps no greater warning for those who use this technology than caveat emptor.

P. J. Loehrer, Sr, MD

Effect of a Computer-Based Decision Aid on Knowledge, Perceptions, and Intentions About Genetic Testing for Breast Cancer Susceptibility: A Randomized Controlled Trial

Green MJ, Peterson SK, Baker MW, et al (Penn State Univ, Hershey; Univ of Texas, Houston; Lehigh Valley Hosp, Allentown, Pa; et al)

JAMA 292:442-452, 2004 1–6

Background.—Genetic testing has become widely available in recent years for determining inherited cancer predisposition. As the availability of and demand for genetic testing for hereditary cancers increases, alternative or adjunct educational methods for traditional genetic counseling will be needed. The effectiveness of a computer-based decision aid was compared with standard genetic counseling for educating women about *BRCA1* and *BRCA2* genetic testing.

Methods.—This randomized controlled trial was conducted from May 2000 to September 2002 at outpatient clinics in 6 medical centers. A total of 211 women with personal or family histories of breast cancer were enrolled and received either standard one-on-one genetic counseling (105 patients) or education by a computer program followed by genetic counseling (106 patients). The main outcome measures were participants' knowledge, risk perception, intention to undergo genetic testing, decisional conflict, satisfaction with decision, anxiety, and satisfaction with the intervention. Counselor group measures were administered at baseline and after counseling. Computer group measures were administered at baseline, after computer use, and after counseling. Testing decisions were assessed at 1 and 6 months. Outcomes were analyzed as high versus low risk of carrying a *BRCA1* or *BCRA2* mutation.

Results.—Both groups had comparable demographics, prior computer experience, medical literacy, and baseline knowledge of breast cancer and genetic testing; both counseling and computer use were rated highly. Both groups demonstrated increases in knowledge scores regardless of risk status; however, the change in knowledge was greater in the computer group than in the counselor group among women at low risk of carrying a mutation. There was a significant decrease in the perception of absolute risk of breast cancer after either intervention in all participants. The intention to undergo testing decreased significantly after either intervention among low-risk but not high-risk women. The counselor group had lower mean scores on a decisional conflict scale, and in lower-risk women, higher mean scores on a satisfaction-with-decision scale. The mean state anxiety scores were reduced by counseling but were within normal ranges for both groups at baseline and after either intervention, regardless of risk status.

Conclusions.—An interactive computer program was shown to be more effective than standard genetic counseling for increasing knowledge of breast cancer and genetic testing among women at low risk of carrying a *BRCA1* or *BRCA2* mutation. However, genetic counseling was shown to be more effective than the computer program at reducing women's anxiety and facilitating more accurate perceptions of risk. It is suggested that the computer program has the potential to stand alone as an education intervention for low-risk women but should be used as a supplement to genetic counseling for persons at high risk.

▶ One of the greatest obstacles for screening is the physician's failing to order the appropriate tests. With the increased use of genetics to identify high-risk populations, cancer screening is becoming more of targeted intervention. Unfortunately, a great deal of time can be spent with individual patients explaining the risks, benefits, and limitations of screening. This report reflects methods to shortcut the time demands while still enhancing the knowledge base of patients who have *BRCA1* and *BRAC2* mutations. In the end, a genetics counselor is still important with respect to reducing anxiety and characterizing complex problems. But it is clear that using computer-based education materials should have a favorable impact on enhancing the knowledge base and hopefully compliance to screening in a subset of motivated patients.

P. J. Loehrer, Sr, MD

2 Breast Cancer

Miscellaneous Topics

Factors Contributing to Mammography Failure in Women Aged 40-49 Years

Buist DSM, Porter PL, Lehman C, et al (Group Health Cooperative, Seattle; Univ of Washington, Seattle; Fred Hutchinson Cancer Research Ctr, Seattle; et al)

J Natl Cancer Inst 96:1432-1440, 2004 2–1

Introduction.—Younger women (aged 40-49 years) have lower mammographic sensitivity (ie, higher proportion of cancers identified after a negative mammogram) compared with older women (≥50 years old). The effect of tumor growth rate, breast density, mammographic image quality, and breast cancer risk factors on mammographic sensitivity was examined in younger and older women.

Methods.—A total of 576 women diagnosed with invasive breast cancer between 1988 and 1993 were evaluated. Of these, 73 were 40 to 49 years of age and 503 were 50 years of age or older. Interval cancers were considered those cancers diagnosed within 12 or 24 months after a negative screening mammogram and before a subsequent mammogram. Tumor growth rate was evaluated by mitotic figure count and Ki-67 positivity. The primary outcome measures were percentage of women with interval cancer by age, odds ratio (OR) of interval cancer by age, and excess odds (ie, the percentage of the OR for age that was explained by individual covariates).

Results.—Interval cancers were observed in 27.7% of younger women and 13.9% of older women within 12 months (OR, 2.36; 95% confidence interval [CI], 1.14-4.77), 52.1% of younger women, and 24.7% of older women within 24 months (OR, 3.58; 95% CI, 2.15-5.97). Greater breast density explained 67.6% of the diminished mammographic sensitivity in younger women at 12 months; rapid tumor growth explained 30.6% and breast density explained 37.6% of diminished sensitivity in younger women at 24 months.

Conclusion.—Breast density greatly explained reduced mammographic sensitivity at 12 months; rapid tumor growth contributed to diminished mammographic sensitivity at 24 months. A 12-month versus a 24-month mammography screening interval may therefore decrease the adverse impact of faster growing tumors on mammographic sensitivity in younger women.

► The use of screening mammography in women aged 40 to 49 years has been the subject of great controversy. This study examines factors responsible for the decreased sensitivity of detection in younger women. Both rapid tumor growth and breast density were responsible for decreased sensitivity. While breast density is not a modifiable factor, more frequent screening intervals may be useful in women with rapidly growing tumors. This study supports the use of annual rather than every other year screening intervals in women younger than 50 years.

M. Morrow, MD

Efficacy of MRI and Mammography for Breast-Cancer Screening in Women With a Familial or Genetic Predisposition

Klijn M, for the Magnetic Resonance Imaging Screening Study Group (Erasmus Med Ctr, Rotterdam, The Netherlands; et al)

N Engl J Med 351:427-437, 2004 2–2

Introduction.—The value of regular screening for breast cancer in women with a genetic or familial predisposition to breast cancer is not known. The efficacy of MRI versus mammography was examined in women with a familial or genetic predisposition.

Methods.—Women with a cumulative lifetime risk of breast cancer of 15% or more were screened every 6 months via clinical breast examination and once yearly by mammography and MRI; readings were independent. The characteristics of the cancers that were identified were compared with those of 2 different age-matched control groups.

Results.—A total of 1909 eligible women were screened, including 358 carriers of germ-line mutations. During a median follow-up of 2.9 years, 51 tumors (44 invasive cancers, 6 ductal carcinomas in situ, and 1 lymphoma) and 1 lobular carcinoma in situ were identified. The sensitivities of clinical breast examination, mammography, and MRI for identifying invasive breast cancer were 17.9%, 33.3%, and 79.5%, respectively; specificity values were 98.1%, 95.0%, and 89.8%, respectively. The overall discriminating capacity of MRI was significantly better than that of mammography ($P < .05$). The proportion of invasive tumors 10 mm or less in diameter was significantly greater in the surveillance group than in either control group (43.2%, 14.0% [$P < .001$], and 12.5% ($P = .04$], respectively). The combined incidence of positive axillary nodes and micrometastases in invasive cancers was 21.4% versus 52.4% ($P < .001$) and 56.4% ($P = .001$) in the control groups.

Conclusion.—MRI seems to be more sensitive than mammography in identifying tumors in women with an inherited susceptibility to breast cancer.

► This study evaluated the relative merits of MRI and mammography as screening techniques for 1909 patients at high risk (15% or more lifetime) for breast cancer. MRI appears to be superior in regard to the proportion of invasive tumors 10 mm or less (43% vs either 14% or 12%) and to the incidence of positive axillary nodes or micrometastases (21% vs either 52% or 56%). This advantage was bought at the price of twice as many unneeded additional examinations and 3 times as many unneeded biopsies. MRI should certainly not replace mammography as the screening tool of choice without further study to confirm or refute these results and to examine further the problem of increased unneeded procedures.

J. T. Thigpen, MD

Clinicopathologic Factors Predicting Involvement of Nonsentinel Axillary Nodes in Women With Breast Cancer
Hwang RF, Krishnamurthy S, Hunt KK, et al (Univ of Texas, Houston)
Ann Surg Oncol 10:248-254, 2003 2–3

Introduction.—Sentinel lymph node (SLN) biopsy has become an important tool for determining involvement of the axillary lymph nodes in patients with breast cancer, yet it is not clear which patients need completion axillary lymph node dissection. Various clinicopathologic characteristics were analyzed in cases of SLN-positive breast cancers to ascertain factors that may help predict involvement of nonsentinel axillary lymph nodes (NSLNs).

Methods.—The medical records of all patients with invasive breast cancer who underwent SLN biopsy between 1993 and August 2001 were reviewed. Multivariate analysis was used to identify clinicopathologic characteristics that predicted involvement of NSLNs in patients who were SLN-positive.

Results.—A total of 131 patients with positive SLNs underwent completion axillary lymph node dissection. Multivariate analysis showed that primary tumors larger than 2 cm (P = .009), SLN metastasis over 2 mm (P = .24), and lymphovascular invasion (P = .28) were independent predictors of positive NSLNs (Table 3). The number of SLNs harvested was a significant negative predictor (P = .04) of NSLNs. With this model, based on the presence of these factors, the positive predictive value was 100% for a score of 4.

TABLE 3.—Independent Predictors of Positive Nonsentinel Axial Lymph Nodes According to Multivariate Analysis

Characteristic	Odds Ratio	95% Confidence Interval	*P* Value	β Coefficient
Tumor size >2 cm	4.1	1.42-11.89	.009	1.41
Number of SLNs removed ≥3	.19	.04-.93	.04	−2.40
Largest SLN metastasis >2 mm	6.0	1.26-28.70	.024	1.80
Presence of lymphovascular invasion	3.7	1.15-11.70	.028	1.30

Abbreviation: SLN, Sentinel lymph node.
(Courtesy of Hwang RF, Krishnamurthy S, Hunt KK, et al: Clinicopathologic factors predicting involvement of nonsentinel axillary nodes in women with breast cancer. *Ann Surg Oncol* 10(3):248-254, 2003.)

Conclusion.—The likelihood of positive NSLNs is associated with primary tumor size, size of the largest SLN metastasis, and the presence of lymphovascular invasion. A scoring system incorporating these features may help ascertain which patients could benefit from additional axillary surgery.

▶ The need for completion axillary dissection after a positive SLN biopsy remains controversial. For many years, axillary surgery has been considered a staging procedure, and patients with metastases to the SLN have clearly been staged as node-positive. Potential benefits of completion axillary dissection include improved definition of prognosis, maintenance of local control in the axilla, and perhaps improvements in survival. These benefits only apply to patients with additional nodal metastases, so a reliable method of identifying patients with a very low risk of additional axillary nodal involvement would allow them to avoid the morbidity of axillary dissection. Other studies have identified patients with T1a tumors with SLN metastases less than 2 mm in size[1] or these characteristics and the absence of lymphovascular invasion[2] as the only group with a very low risk of NSLN metastases.

The importance of these factors is confirmed in the work of Hwang et al, but they have developed a model which also includes the number of SLNs removed to increase the size of the low-risk group. However, even with this 4 factor model, only 24% of patients could be classified as low risk, even though 40.5% had no additional nodal metastases. For most patients, the question of the need for axillary dissection after a positive SLN biopsy will have to be answered by the outcome of the American College of Surgeons Oncology Group Z11 trial.

M. Morrow, MD

References

1. Chu KU, Turner RR, Hansen NM, et al: Do all patients with sentinel node metastases from breast carcinoma need complete axillary dissection? *Ann Surg* 229:536-541, 1999.
2. Weiser MR, Montgomery LL, Tan LK, et al: Lymphovascular invasion enhances the prediction of non-sentinel node metastases in breast cancer patients with positive sentinel nodes. *Ann Surg Oncol* 8:145-149, 2001.

Obesity Influences Outcome of Sentinel Lymph Node Biopsy in Early-Stage Breast Cancer

Derossis AM, Fey JV, Cody HS III, et al (Mem Sloan-Kettering Cancer Ctr, New York)

J Am Coll Surg 197:896-901, 2003 2–4

Background.—The use of sentinel lymph node (SLN) biopsy is quickly becoming the standard of care for staging of the axilla in patients with early breast cancer. SLN biopsy, like any newly emerging technique, has undergone evaluation to determine the proper application of this technique in the clinical setting. A previous study has evaluated the success of SLN biopsy by extensively examining tumor characteristics, tumor location, and method of isotope injection. Increasing body mass with age has been shown to be inversely related to the success of SLN biopsy. This relationship is important because a proportion of SLN biopsy patients are both overweight and age 65 years or older. The success of SLN biopsy in relation to body mass index (BMI) and age was evaluated.

Methods.—Mapping successes and failures were reviewed in 2495 SLN biopsy procedures performed between September 1996 and June 2001. Clinical stage T1 N0, T2 N0, and T3 N0 breast cancer cases were included in this study. A technique that combined radioisotope and blue dye was used for detection of SLNs. Failure was defined as the inability to identify any nodes with either blue dye or in vivo counts. BMI was determined for each patient, and cases were stratified by BMI and age.

Results.—There were 62 failures and 2433 successful mappings among the 2495 cases, for a failure rate of 2.48%. The mean age, weight, and BMI were significantly higher in the failure group. An inverse relationship was identified between the success of SLN biopsy and BMI. Stratification of patient age (<50 vs ≥50 years) showed that this inverse relationship was more pronounced among the patients age 50 years or older. On multivariate analysis it was shown that age and BMI were predictive of SLN mapping success, but weight alone was not a statistically significant factor.

Conclusions.—Increasing age and BMI are not contraindications for SLN biopsy. Instead, surgeons should be cognizant of the finding that increasing body mass and age are potential risk factors for a failed procedure, which would require a completion axillary node dissection for staging.

► With refinements in the sentinel node technique, a sentinel node can be identified by experienced surgeons in more than 95% of patients. This large study identifies age older than 50 years and increased BMI as predictors of a higher rate of failure of lymphatic mapping. The higher rate of failure in older women with higher BMI is of concern, because this group is at increased risk for the development of lymphedema after axillary dissection.[1] Older age and obesity are not contraindications to SLN biopsy, because a SLN can be identified in the majority of these women. Evaluation of technical modifications such as injection of a larger volume of blue dye or radioisotope, or allowing a longer migration time, would be worthwhile for this subset of patients.

M. Morrow, MD

Reference

1. Petrek JA, Senie RT, Peters M, et al: Lymphedema in a cohort of breast carcinoma survivors 20 years after diagnosis. *Cancer* 92:1368-1377, 2001.

Validation of Subareolar and Periareolar Injection Techniques for Breast Sentinel Lymph Node Biopsy

Chagpar A, for the University of Louisville Breast Cancer Sentinel Lymph Node Study Group (Univ of Louisville, Ky; Univ of Texas, Galveston; Mem Sloan-Kettering Cancer Ctr, New York; et al)

Arch Surg 139:614-620, 2004 2–5

Introduction.—Sentinel lymph node (SLN) biopsy has become increasingly popular in the management of breast cancer, but questions exist regarding the optimal injection technique. Whether subareolar or periareolar injection of radioactive technetium sulfur colloid is equivalent to other injection techniques for breast cancer SLN biopsy was examined in 3961 patients with clinical stage I and II breast cancer in a prospective, multicenter clinical trial.

Methods.—Attempted SLN biopsy followed by completion axillary dissection was performed in all patients. Injection technique was ascertained by the preference of every participating surgeon. Most surgeons had little or no experience with SLN before participation in this trial. The primary outcome measures were SLN identification and false-negative rates.

Results.—All 3961 participants underwent SLN biopsy with blue dye alone or radioactive colloid plus blue dye. Both the subareolar and periareolar radioactive colloid injection techniques were linked with SLN identification rates of 99.2% and 95.6%, respectively. The identification rates were significantly higher for these 2 techniques than for peritumoral injection of radioactive colloid (91.1%) or the use of blue dye alone (88.5%) ($P < .001$). The false-negative rates were similar for all SLN techniques. Multivariate analysis revealed that type of injection, patient age, and tumor palpability were statistically significant factors that affect the SLN identification rate (Table 4).

TABLE 4.—Multivariate Analysis of Factors That Affect the Sentinel Lymph Node Identification Rate

Factor	*P* Value	Odds Ratio (95% CI)
Age	<.001	0.979 (0.968-0.990)
Injection type	<.001	
(compared with peritumoral)		
Dermal	<.001	3.812 (2.482-5.854)
Subdermal	<.001	2.222 (1.483-3.331)
Subareolar	.007	14.856 (2.057-107.299)
Periareolar	.04	2.214 (1.056-4.639)
Blue dye only	.14	0.747 (0.505-1.105)
Palpable tumor	.005	1.529 (1.140-2.052)
Tumor size	.53	1.042 (0.915-1.186)
Histologic findings	.58	
(compared with ductal)		
Lobular	.36	1.275 (0.757-2.146)
Other	.55	1.167 (0.703-1.935)

Abbreviation: CI, Confidence interval.

Conclusion.—The results of this study support the use of subareolar and periareolar injections for sentinel node identification.

▶ The original premise of lymphatic mapping and SLN biopsy was that each individual tumor had a unique pathway of lymphatic drainage that could be identified by peritumoral injection of radioisotope or blue dye. Subsequent studies have suggested that the skin envelope, subareolar plexus, and breast parenchyma share a common lymphatic drainage in the majority of cases. This large clinical study confirms that injection of the mapping agent into the rich lymphatic network of the subareolar space facilitates SLN identification compared with peritumoral injection and does not alter false-negative rates.

M. Morrow, MD

Prospective Multicenter Study of Axillary Nodal Staging by Positron Emission Tomography in Breast Cancer: A Report of the Staging Breast Cancer With PET Study Group

Wahl RL, Siegel BA, Coleman RE, et al (Johns Hopkins Univ, Baltimore, Md; Univ of Michigan, Ann Arbor; Washington Univ, St Louis; et al)

J Clin Oncol 22:277-285, 2004 2–6

Introduction.—Early clinical trials have shown that essentially all primary breast cancers and most nonnodal soft tissue metastases can be identified by ^{18}F-labeled 2-fluoro-2-deoxy-D-glucose (FDG) positron emission tomography (PET). More recent trials have demonstrated that smaller primary breast lesions can escape detection by using FDG-PET. This probably reflects resolution and sensitivity limitations of the current scanning systems. The accuracy of FDG-PET in identifying axillary nodal metastases was evaluated in women with primary breast cancer in a prospective multicenter trial.

Methods.—A total of 360 women with newly diagnosed invasive breast cancer underwent FDG-PET. The images were blindly interpreted by 3 experienced nuclear medicine physicians for abnormally increased axillary FDG uptake. The imaging findings from 308 assessable axillae were compared with axillary node pathology findings.

Results.—For identifying axillary nodal metastasis, the mean estimated area under the receiver operator curve was 0.74 (range, 0.70-0.76) for the 3 readers. The mean (and range) sensitivity, specificity, and positive and negative predictive values across the 3 readers for PET were 61% (54%-67%), 80% (79%-81%), 62% (60%-64%), and 79% (76%-81%), respectively (Table 3). False-negative axillae on PET had significantly smaller and fewer tumor-positive lymph nodes (2.7%) than true-positive axillae (5.1; P < .005). Semiquantitative analysis of axillary FDG uptake revealed that a nodal standardized uptake value (lean body mass) over 1.8 had a positive predictive value of 90% and a sensitivity of 32%. The detection of 2 or more intense foci of tracer uptake in the axilla was highly predictive of axillary metastasis (78% 83% positive predictive value), albeit insensitive (27%).

TABLE 3.—Sensitivity, Specificity, Predictive Values, and Likelihood Ratios for Three Readers, for the Combined Data Set

Reader	Sensitivity		Specificity		PPV		NPV		LR+		LR−	
	Value	95% CI	Value	95% CI	Value	95% CI	Value	95% CI	Value	95% CI	Value	95% CI
1	0.62	0.53 to 0.71	0.81	0.75 to 0.86	0.64	0.54 to 0.73	0.80	0.73 to 0.85	3.25	2.36 to 4.48	0.47	0.36 to 0.6
2	0.67	0.57 to 0.76	0.79	0.73 to 0.84	0.63	0.54 to 0.72	0.81	0.75 to 0.87	3.17	2.35 to 4.28	0.42	0.32 to 0.55
3	0.54	0.44 to 0.63	0.81	0.74 to 0.86	0.60	0.50 to 0.70	0.76	0.69 to 0.82	2.76	1.97 to 3.85	0.58	0.46 to 0.71

Abbreviations: CI, Confidence interval; *PPV*, positive predictive value; *NPV*, negative predictive value; *LR+*, likelihood ratio for a positive reading; *LR−*, likelihood ratio for a negative reading.

(Courtesy of Wahl RL, Siegel BA, Coleman RE, et al: Prospective multicenter study of axillary nodal staging by positron emission tomography in breast cancer: A report of the Staging Breast Cancer with PET Study Group. *J Clin Oncol* 22(2):277-285, 2004. Reprinted with permission from the American Society of Clinical Oncology.)

Conclusion.—FDG-PET has moderate accuracy for identifying axillary metastases, but it often fails to discern axillae with small and few nodal metastases. It is recommended that FDG-PET not be used routinely in axillary staging of patients with newly diagnosed breast cancer.

► Axillary dissection is associated with significant short- and long-term morbidity, so the identification of alternative staging techniques would be a clinical advance. This study demonstrates that FDG-PET is not a satisfactory technique for identifying small-axillary node metastases, with a false negative rate of 77%. This is not surprising since the current spatial resolution of PET for breast cancer is approximately 5mm.[1] The availability of sentinel node biopsy, a procedure which identifies axillary metastases with the same frequency as axillary dissection and with considerably lower morbidity,[2-3] has removed much of the impetus for an imaging procedure to stage the axilla. In addition the relatively low specificity of PET in this study (80%) should serve as a cautionary note for physicians considering upstaging patients and denying them potentially curative surgery solely on the basis of PET findings.

M. Morrow, MD

References

1. Raylman RR, Kison,PV, Wahl RL: Capabilities of two and three-dimensional FDG-PET for detecting small lesions and lymph nodes in the upper torso: A dynamic phantom study. *Eur J Nuc Med* 26:39-45, 1999.
2. Veronesi U, Paganelli G, Viale G, et a:. A randomized comparison of sentinel node biopsy with routine axillary dissection in breast cancer. *N Engl J Med* 349:546-553, 2003.
3. Mansel RE, Goyal A, Fallowfield L, et al: Sentinel node biopsy in breast cancer: The latest results of the randomized multicenter ALMANAC Trial. *Proc Am Soc Clin Oncol* 23:4 (#506), 2004.

A Randomized Comparison of Sentinel-Node Biopsy With Routine Axillary Dissection in Breast Cancer

Veronesi U, Paganelli G, Viale G, et al (European Inst of Oncology, Milan, Italy; Univ of Milan, Italy)

N Engl J Med 349:546-553, 2003 2–7

Background.—Numerous studies have demonstrated the accuracy of sentinel lymph node status as a predictor of the status of axillary lymph nodes in breast cancer. However, the safety and efficacy of sentinel-node biopsy require validation. The safety and efficacy of sentinel-node biopsy, followed by routine axillary dissection was compared with that of sentinel-node biopsy, followed by axillary dissection only if the sentinel node was found to be positive on intraoperative histologic examination.

Methods.—A total of 516 patients with primary breast cancer were randomly assigned to either sentinel-node biopsy and total axillary dissection (the axillary-dissection group) or sentinel-node biopsy, followed by axillary

TABLE 3.—Side Effects in the 2 Study Groups

Side Effect	Axillary-Dissection Group (N=100)		Sentinel-Node Group (N=100)	
	No. of Patients			
	6 Mo	24 Mo	6 Mo	24 Mo
Axillary pain*				
No	9	61	84	92
Yes, sporadic	72	34	14	7
Yes, continuous	19	5	2	1
Numbness or paresthesias on operated side†				
No	15	32	98	99
Yes	85	68	2	1
Arm mobility‡				
80-100%	73	79	100	100
60-79%	22	18	0	0
40-59%	5	2	0	0
20-39%	0	1	0	0
<20%	0	0	0	0
Aesthetic appearance of axillary scar§				
Good	91	85	98	100
Bad	9	15	2	0
Arm swelling (difference in circumference)¶				
No difference	31	25	89	93
<1 cm	44	38	11	6
1-2 cm	17	25	0	1
>2 cm	8	12	0	0

*Postoperative axillary pain was evaluated as continuous (lasting >50% of the day), sporadic, or absent.

†Numbness and paresthesias were assessed by comparing skin sensitivity on the inner and outer upper arms, axillae, and chest wall on the operated side with that on the untreated side. Sensitivity was recorded as either the presence or absence of numbness.

‡Arm mobility was judged by asking the patient to assign the restriction in motion in the operated arm a value on a scale of 0% (severe restriction) to 100% (no restriction).

§The appearance of the axillary scar was judged by asking the patient simply to say whether the result was good or bad.

¶Arm swelling and edema were assessed by comparing the circumference (in centimeters) of the treated arm 15 cm above the lateral epicondyle with that of the untreated arm.

(Reprinted by permission of *The New England Journal of Medicine* from Veronesi U, Paganelli G, Viale G, et al: A randomized comparison of sentinel-node biopsy with routine axillary dissection in breast cancer. *N Engl J Med* 349:546-553, 2003.)

dissection only if the sentinel node contained metastases (the sentinel-node group). Tumors in all patients were no larger than 2 cm in diameter.

Findings.—The number of sentinel nodes found was the same in both groups. A sentinel node was positive in 32.3% of patients in the axillary-dissection group and in 35.5% of the patients in the sentinel-node group. The overall accuracy of the sentinel-node status was 96.9% in the axillary-dissection group; the sensitivity was 91.2% and the specificity was 100%. Patients who underwent only sentinel-node biopsy had less pain and better arm mobility than did patients who underwent axillary dissection (Table 3).

Fifteen adverse events associated with breast cancer occurred in the axillary-dissection group compared with 10 adverse events in the sentinel-node group. No overt axillary metastasis was found during follow-up among the 167 patients who did not undergo axillary dissection. The overall survival rate was no different for those who had axillary dissection and those who did not.

Conclusion.—Sentinel-node biopsy is a safe and accurate method for screening the axillary nodes for metastasis in women with a small (2 cm or smaller) cancer of the breast.

▶ For women undergoing breast conserving therapy, axillary dissection accounts for the majority of the short- and long-term morbidity of breast cancer surgery. Multiple prospective studies have demonstrated that the sentinel-node concept is applicable in breast cancer, and that the sentinel-node reliability predicts the status of the remaining axillary nodes in more than 90% of patients. This randomized study confirms that nodal metastases are identified at the same rate with sentinel-node biopsy and axillary dissection. After a median follow-up of 46 months, no isolated axillary recurrences were observed in the sentinel-node biopsy group, consistent with other reports indicating that the incidence of axillary failure after sentinel-node biopsy alone is lower than the false-negative rate of sentinel-node biopsy, followed by axillary dissection.[1] Finally, this trial provides convincing documentation that sentinel-node biopsy has significantly fewer sequelae than axillary dissection, and that significant differences in pain, numbness, and lymphedema persist 2 years after surgery. This study clearly supports the use of sentinel-node biopsy rather than axillary dissection for staging of clinically node-negative breast cancer when the procedure is performed by a surgeon experienced with sentinel-node techniques.

M. Morrow, MD

Reference

1. Grube B, Rose C, Giuliano A: Local management of invasive breast cancer: *Axilla Diseases of the Breast*, ed 3, Harris JR, Lippman ME, Morrow M, et al (eds). Lippincott Williams and Wilkins, Philadelphia, 2004, pp 745-784.

The Accuracy of Sentinel Lymph Node Biopsy in Multicentric and Multifocal Invasive Breast Cancers

Tousimis E, Van Zee KJ, Fey JV, et al (Mem Sloan-Kettering Cancer Ctr, New York)

J Am Coll Surg 197:529-535, 2003 2–8

Background.—The pathologic status of the axillary lymph nodes is still the most important prognostic indicator in breast cancer and continues to guide adjuvant therapy. Sentinel lymph node biopsy (SLNB) has been shown to be an accurate alternative to complete axillary lymph node dissection (ALND) for patients with clinically node-negative breast cancer. However, multicentric (MC) and multifocal (MF) invasive breast cancers have been viewed as relative contraindications to SLNB. The accuracy of SLNB in patients with MC and MF invasive breast cancer was evaluated.

Methods.—From September 1996 to August 2001, 3501 patients with clinically node-negative breast cancer underwent SLNB with both blue dye and radioisotope at 1 institution. A total of 70 patients had MC or MF invasive breast cancer, a successful SLNB, and mastectomy for local control. All the patients had 10 or more axillary nodes excised (including the SLN) in a planned ALND. Patients were excluded from the analysis if they had MC or MF in situ carcinoma; breast conservation therapy; previous breast irradiation, ALND, or SLNB; recurrent breast cancer; neoadjuvant chemotherapy; or ALND solely on the basis of intraoperative diagnosis of disease in the SLN.

Findings.—Thirty-eight of the 70 patients in this study were found to have axillary metastases (54%). The SLNB had an accuracy of 96%, a sensitivity of 92%, and a false-negative rate of 8%. All the patients with inaccurate results on SLNB had a dominant invasive tumor larger than 5 cm in diameter, and 1 patient had palpable axillary disease intraoperatively. The SLN was the only site of axillary metastasis in 37% of patients. A comparison of these findings with those of published SLNB validation studies found no statistically significant differences in accuracy, sensitivity, or false-negative rate.

Conclusions.—The accuracy of SLNB for patients with MC or MF disease was found to be comparable with that in published validation studies, most of which involved single-site invasive breast cancers. Patients with MC or MF disease and a dominant T3 tumor (larger than 5 cm) or axillary disease that is palpable during surgery should undergo concurrent formal ALND. These retrospective findings suggest that SLNB may be a reliable alternative to conventional ALND for selected patients with MC or MF disease.

▶ When lymphatic mapping for breast carcinoma was initially developed, each tumor was thought to have a unique pathway of lymphatic drainage, raising concerns that the SLN technique might not be applicable in MC carcinoma. Subsequent studies have shown that the majority of the breast lymph drains into a subareolar collecting system before passing to the axilla.[1] This observation addresses most of the theoretical objections to SLNB in MC carcinoma. In this study, Tousimis and coauthors confirm that the SLN accurately predicts the status of the remaining axillary nodes in patients with MC carcinoma. Another small study has previously suggested that lymphatic mapping is accurate in MC carcinoma,[2] and this should no longer be considered a contraindication to SLNB. The tracer can be injected into the subareolar plexus, or separate peritumoral injections can be carried out.

M. Morrow, MD

References

1. Borgstein PJ, Meijer S, Pijpers RJ, et al: Functional lymphatic anatomy for sentinel node biopsy in breast cancer: Echos from the past and the periareolar blue methos. *Ann Surg* 232:81-99, 2000.

2. Fernandez K, Swanson M, Verbanac K, et al: Is sentinel lymphadenectomy accurate in multifocal and multicentri breast cancer [abstract]. *Ann Surg Oncol* 9:S16-S17, 2002.

Association of Frequency and Duration of Aspirin Use and Hormone Receptor Status With Breast Cancer Risk

Terry MB, Gammon MD, Zhang FF, et al (Columbia Univ, New York; Univ of North Carolina, Chapel Hill; Mt Sinai School of Medicine, New York; et al)
JAMA 291:2433-2440, 2004 2–9

Introduction.—The use of aspirin and additional nonsteroidal anti-inflammatory drugs (NSAIDs) has been linked with a reduction in the risk of several cancers, including breast cancer. The NSAIDs inhibit cyclo-oxygenase activity and thus decrease prostaglandin synthesis. Prostaglandins stimulate aromatase expression and therefore stimulate the biosynthesis of estrogen.

Given the significance of estrogen in the pathogenesis of breast cancer, the ability of aspirin and other NSAIDs to protect against breast cancer may vary according to hormone receptor status. A population-based case-control investigation of women with breast cancer was conducted to (1) ascertain the relationship between the incidence and duration of use of aspirin and other NSAIDs and breast cancer risk, and (2) investigate whether any observed relationship is more pronounced in women with hormone receptor–positive breast cancer.

Methods.—In-person interviews were performed during 1996 and 1997 in 1442 case subjects and 1420 control subjects. The primary outcome measure was incident invasion and in situ breast cancer by aspirin and NSAID use and hormone receptor status.

Results.—Ever use of aspirin or NSAIDs at least once a week for 6 months or longer was described for 301 case subjects (20.9%) and 245 control subjects (24.3%) (odds ratio [OR], 0.80; 95% confidence interval [CI], 0.66-0.97 for ever versus nonusers). The inverse correlation was more pronounced in frequent users (7 tablets or more per week) (OR, 0.72; 95% CI, 0.58-0.90). The results for ibuprofen, which was used by fewer participants on a regular basis, were usually weaker (OR, 0.78; 95% CI, 0.55-1.10 for less than 3/wk vs OR, 0.92; 95% CI, 0.70-1.22 for 3 times a week or greater).

The use of acetaminophen (which does not inhibit prostaglandin synthesis, was not correlated with a decrease in the incidence of breast cancer. The decrease in risk with aspirin use was observed among participants with hormone receptor–positive tumors (OR, 0.74; 95% CI, 0.60-0.93). This was not observed in women with hormone receptor–negative tumors (OR, 0.97; 95% CI, 0.67-1.40).

Conclusion.—These data add to the growing evidence that advocates the regular use of aspirin and other NSAIDs (which may operate through inhibition of estrogen biosynthesis) as effective chemopreventive agents for breast cancer.

▶ Epidemiologic evidence that NSAIDS reduce the risk of colorectal neoplasms has led to investigations of their effects on other tumor types. Studies in breast cancer have suggested a 20% to 40% reduction in risk with NSAID use.[1-3] This lesser effect has been attributed to less frequent overexpression of cyclo-oxygenase (COX) in human breast cancer than is observed in colorectal cancer.[4] The study by Terry et al is the first to examine the effect of NSAIDS on the risk of cancer by hormone receptor status and suggests that NSAIDS are effective in reducing the risk of hormone dependent (any positive receptor), but not hormone independent (both estrogen and progesterone receptor negative), breast cancers.

This finding was most evident in postmenopausal women. While the inhibition of prostaglandin-driven synthesis of estrogen and progesterone by NSAIDS provides a biologically plausible explanation for these results, they are somewhat at odds with the observation that COX overexpression in human breast cancer is most frequent in hormone receptor–negative tumors.[5] The low cost of NSAIDS and benefits in reducing the risk of cardiovascular disease make their suitability as chemopreventive agents worthy of future studies. In addition, the possible synergy between NSAIDS and aromatase inhibitors for breast cancer treatment is being examined in clinical trials.

M. Morrow, MD

References

1. Schreinmachers DM, Everson RB: Aspirin use and lung, colon, and breast cancer incidence in a prospective study. *Epidemiology* 5:138-146, 1994.
2. Johnson TW, Anderson KE, Lazovich D, et al: Association of aspirin and nonsteroidal anti-inflammatory drug use with breast cancer. *Cancer Epidemiol Biomarkers Prev* 11:1586-1591, 2002.
3. Harris RE, Chlebowski RT, Jackson RD, et al: Breast cancer and nonsteroidal anti-inflammatory drugs: Prospective results from the Women's Health Institute Initiative. *Cancer Res* 63:6096-6101, 2003.
4. Ristimaki A, Sivula A, Lundin J, et al: Prognostic significance of elevated cyclooxygenose-2 expression in breast cancer. *Cancer Res* 62:632-635, 2002.
5. Goss PE: Breast cancer prevention—Clinical trials strategies involving aromatase inhibitors. *J Steroid Biochem Mol Biol* 86:487-493, 2003.

▶ This case-control study examines the use of aspirin or other NSAID (ever-use at least once per week for 6 months or longer) among 1442 cases and 1420 control subjects as it relates to the risk of developing breast cancer. The data demonstrate a hazard rate of 0.80 in ever-users compared with nonusers, a significant reduction in breast cancer risk. This reduction was seen only in regard to the risk of developing hormone-receptor-positive breast cancer. This is further, albeit not definitive, evidence for NSAIDs as effective chemopreventive agents for breast cancer.

J. T. Thigpen, MD

Contralateral Breast Cancer in *BRCA1* and *BRCA2* Mutation Carriers

Metcalfe K, Lynch HT, Ghadirian P, et al (Univ of Toronto; Toronto Sunnybrook Regional Cancer Centre; Centre Hospitalier de Université de Montreal (CHUM), Canada; et al)

J Clin Oncol 22:2328-2335, 2004 2–10

Introduction.—Women who carry a germline mutation in either the *BRCA1* or *BRCA2* gene may opt for contralateral mastectomy as an initial preventive measure. It is not known to what degree the risk of contralateral breast cancer varies with age or whether the risk is equivalent among carriers of *BRCA1* versus *BRCA2* mutations. The risk of contralateral breast cancer in *BRCA1* and *BRCA2* carriers was examined after diagnosis, along with which factors are predictive of the risk of a second primary breast cancer.

Methods.—A total of 491 women with stage I or stage II breast cancer for whom a BRCA1 or BRCA2 mutation had been identified in the family were followed up from initial diagnosis of cancer until contralateral mastectomy, contralateral breast cancer, or last follow-up.

Results.—The overall actuarial risk of contralateral breast cancer was 29.5% at 10 years. Factors predictive of a decreased risk included: the presence of a *BRCA2* mutation (vs *BRCA1* mutation: hazard ratio [HR], 0.73; 95% confidence interval [CI], 0.47-1.15); age 50 years or older at first diagnosis (vs ≤49 years; HR, 0.63; 95% CI, 0.36-1.10); use of tamoxifen (HR, 0.59; 95% CI, 0.35-1.01); and history of oophorectomy (HR, 0.44; 95% CI, 0.21-0.91). The effect of oophorectomy was especially strong in women first diagnosed before age 49 years (HR, 0.24; 95% CI, 0.07-0.77). For women who did not have an oophorectomy or did not take tamoxifen, the 10-year risk of contralateral cancer was 43.4% for BRCA1 carriers and 34.6% for BRCA2 carriers.

Conclusion.—The risk of contralateral breast cancer in women with a BRCA mutation is approximately 40% at 10 years; this is decreased in women who take tamoxifen or undergo an oophorectomy.

▶ This study defines the risk of developing a contralateral breast cancer in 491 women with stage I or II breast cancer for whom a *BRCA1* or *BRCA2* mutation had been identified in the family. The authors report the actuarial risk of contralateral breast cancer was nearly 30% at 10 years, with a slightly higher risk in women with *BRCA2* ($P = .10$). Undergoing a prophylactic oophorectomy significantly reduced the risk of developing contralateral breast cancer (HR = 0.44, $P = .03$), while age and having received chemotherapy or radiation therapy had no impact. Women receiving tamoxifen also had a trend toward a reduced incidence of contralateral breast cancer (HR = 0.59, $P = .12$). These findings have important implications for preventing a contralateral breast cancer in women who have the *BRCA1* or *BRCA2* mutation.

N. H. Hanna, MD

Use of Genetic Testing and Prophylactic Mastectomy and Oophorectomy in Women With Breast or Ovarian Cancer From Families With a *BRCA1* or *BRCA2* Mutation

Meijers-Heijboer H, Brekelmans CTM, Menke-Pluymers M, et al (Rotterdam Family Cancer Clinic, The Netherlands; Daniel den Hoed Cancer Ctr, Rotterdam, The Netherlands)

J Clin Oncol 21:1675-1681, 2003 2–11

Introduction.—Women with *BRCA1/BRCA2* mutations are at increased risk for contralateral breast cancer, ipsilateral events, and ovarian cancer. Genetic testing can provide these individuals with information for personal health management and treatment decisions, along with information regarding the cancer risks for their children and other relatives. The use of genetic testing, prophylactic mastectomy, and oophorectomy was evaluated in women with breast and/or ovarian cancer from a consecutive series of 112 families with a *BRCA1* or *BRCA2* mutation.

The incidence of prophylactic bilateral and contralateral mastectomy and prophylactic oophorectomy was assessed in women who carried a BRCA1/ BRCA2 mutation and who had no metastatic disease at the time of the genetic test disclosure. Predictors for genetic test uptake and prophylactic surgery were evaluated using both univariate and multivariate analyses.

Results.—A total of 192 of 220 women (87%) with primary tumors underwent genetic testing. Of these, 11 (6%) appeared not to carry the family-specific *BRAC1/BRCA2* mutation. Genetic testing was performed significantly more in women younger than 50 years of age ($P = .04$) and in women with multiple primary tumors ($P = .02$). Among eligible women, 35 of 101 (35%) requested bilateral or contralateral mastectomy; 47 of 95 (49%) asked for oophorectomy. Women younger than 50 years and those who had their first tumor after the initial identification of a *BRCA1/BRCA2* mutation in the family were significantly (both $P = .01$) more likely to chose prophylactic bilateral or contralateral mastectomy (Table 2).

Conclusion.—The patient demand for *BRCA1/BRCA2* testing was high, as was prophylactic surgery in women with breast and/or ovarian cancer who are from high-risk families.

▶ This study clearly indicates that a very large number of women diagnosed with breast or ovarian cancer are willing to undergo genetic testing, either to inform their own treatment decisions or to assist family members. The 87% uptake rate for genetic testing in women affected with breast or ovarian cancer reported in this study is considerably higher than rates reported for unaffected individuals. This suggests a window of opportunity around the time of cancer diagnosis for increasing patient utilization of genetic counseling services. The results of genetic testing appeared to influence patients' therapeutic decisions, with 35% of women opting for prophylactic mastectomy and 49% for prophylactic oophorectomy.

Unfortunately, the 4 to 6 weeks that it takes to obtain the results of genetic testing in the United States is longer than many newly diagnosed breast can-

TABLE 2.—Predictive Factors for Prophylactic Mastectomy

Variable	Subgroup	With PM No.	With PM %	Univariate OR	95% CI	*P*	Multivariate OR*	95% CI	*P*
Age, years	< 50	27 of 58	47	1.00			1.00		
	≥ 50	8 of 43	19	0.26		.005	0.27	0.10 to 0.73	.01
Parenthood	No children	4 of 14	29	1.00					
	Children	31 of 87	36	1.38	0.40 to 4.78	.61			
DNA diagnosis	After cancer	29 of 93	31	1.00			1.00		
	Before cancer	6 of 8	75	6.62	1.26 to 34.8	.03	8.91	1.55 to 51.2	.01
Tumor stage breast cancer	I	13 of 24	54	1.00					
	II/III	19 of 57	33	0.42	0.16 to 1.12	.08			
	Unknown	2 of 10	20	—					
Time interval, years‡	0 to 2	3 of 20	40	1.00					
	≥ 2	21 of 73	29	0.61	0.22 to 1.69	.34			
Type of cancer‡	Breast cancer	34 of 91	37	1.00					
	Ovarian cancer	1 of 6	17	0.33	0.04 to 2.99	.033			
Bilateral breast cancer in family	Yes	24 of 58	41	1.00					
	No	11 of 43	26	0.49	0.21 to 1.15	.10			

*Included were all variables with univariate $P < .01$; only the variables that remained significant in the final model are shown in the table.
†Time between (last) cancer diagnosis and personal DNA diagnosis.
‡Excluding 4 women with both breast cancer and ovarian cancer.
Abbreviations: PM, Prophylactic mastectomy; *OR*, odds ratio; *CI*, confidence interval.
(Courtesy of Meijers-Heijboer H, Brekelmans CTM, Menke-Pluymers M, et al: Use of genetic testing and prophylactic mastectomy and oophorectomy in women with breast or ovarian cancer from families with a *BRCA1* or *BRCA2* mutation. *J Clin Oncol* 21(9):1675-1681, 2003. Reprinted with permission from the American Society of Clinical Oncology.)

cer patients are willing to wait to make a decision about local therapy. In cases where family history is not highly suggestive of a mutation, we perform breast-conserving surgery and have the patient undergo genetic testing during the time she is receiving adjuvant chemotherapy. If the test results indicate a mutation, she can make a decision about whether she wishes to proceed with bilateral mastectomy before beginning breast irradiation.

M. Morrow, MD

Gene Expression Profiles of Primary Breast Tumors Maintained in Distant Metastases

Weigelt B, Glas AM, Wessels LFA, et al (The Netherlands Cancer Institute, Plesmanlaan, Amsterdam; Delft Univ of Technology, The Netherlands)
Proc Natl Acad Sci U S A 100:15901-15905, 2003 2–12

Background.—How cancer cells acquire their metastatic ability has been debated for decades. Some authorities propose that metastases are derived from distinct subpopulations of tumor cells in the primary site with greater metastatic potential, whereas others suggest that metastases originate from a random fraction of tumor cells. If the latter view is correct, and the capacity to metastasize is acquired relatively early in multistep tumorigenesis, a metastasis might be expected to be genetically similar or even identical to that of the primary tumor of origin. This hypothesis was tested.

Methods and Findings.—Tumor samples from 8 patients with breast cancer and a surgically removed distant metastasis were obtained from 1 center's fresh-frozen tissue bank. Metastases were found in the ovary, lymph node, lung, or arm. The interval to metastases detection ranged from 1.6 to 15 years. Gene expression profiling revealed a striking similarity between distant metastases and the primary breast tumor in the same patient. Genetic similarity was supported by unsupervised hierarchical clustering, multidimensional scaling, and permutation testing. Comparison of significantly expressed genes within a pair also demonstrated genetic similarity between metastasis and primary tumor in a patient.

Conclusions.—Gene expression profiles of primary breast tumors are maintained in their distant metastases. This finding was apparent even in patients in whom metastases developed after a long interval. Thus, the metastatic capacity of breast cancer appears to be an inherent feature rather than one based on clonal selection.

▶ While some cancers remain confined to their sites of origin for many years, prior to metastasizing, other tumors metastasize early in their natural history. The inherent features of individual tumors that predispose them to develop early versus late metastases and the biologic differences in primary tumors versus their metastatic deposits is not well characterized. In this article by Weigelt et al, hierarchical clustering, multidimensional scaling, and permutation testing, reveal genetic similarities between primary breast cancers and their metastasis, suggesting an inherent capability of cancer cells within primary tumors to metastasize. This understanding has the potential to allow us to study organ-confined primary tumors (of breast and other sites) to predict their capability of metastasis and direct the need for additional therapies.

N. H. Hanna, MD

HER-2 Testing in Breast Cancer Using Parallel Tissue-Based Methods

Yaziji H, Goldstein LC, Barry TS, et al (Univ of Washington, Seattle)

JAMA 291:1972-1977, 2004 2–13

Introduction.—Testing for the human epidermal growth factor receptor 2 (HER-2) oncogene in breast cancer has increased due to its role as a prognostic and predictive factor. Some support gene testing by means of fluorescence in situ hybridization (FISH) versus protein testing by immunohistochemistry (IHC) as the technique that most accurately assesses and predicts response to the anti–HER-2 antibody, trastuzumab. Critical examination of FISH as a screening method has not been done and was performed to ascertain the correlation between FISH and IHC results by determining HER-2/*neu* gene status on tumor sections with indeterminate IHC result (2+ score), verify gene amplification on tumor sections with positive results (3+ score), and validate gene status on tumor sections with negative results (0 or 1+ score).

Methods.—A quality control and quality assurance program for HER-2 testing by FISH used tumor specimens from 2963 patients (median age, 56 years) with breast cancer received from 135 hospitals and cancer centers in 29 states. It was conducted at a reference laboratory from January 1, 1999, to May 15, 2003. All tests assessed by FISH were parallel-tested with IHC. With FISH as the presumed standard testing method, the positive and negative predictive values and sensitivity and specificity of IHC were determined and acted as the primary outcome measures.

Results.—A total of 3260 clinical HER-2 tests by FISH were conducted on 2963 serially referred breast cancer specimens. Of these, 2933 tests were successful. A total of 2913 breast cancer specimens underwent both FISH and IHC testing. With FISH as the standard testing method, the positive predictive value of positive IHC score (3+) was 91.6% and the negative predictive value of negative IHC score (0 or 1+) was 97.2%.

The sensitivity of IHC tests, including tumor sections with scores of 2+ or 3+, was 92.6%; the specificity of IHC tests with scores of 3+ was 98.8%. Compared to IHC tests, the FISH test had a significantly higher failure rate (5.0% vs 0.08%), higher reagent costs ($140 vs $10), longer testing times (36 hour vs 4 hours), and interpretation times (7 minutes vs 45 seconds).

Conclusion.—A testing algorithm for HER-2 determination is most efficient with IHC as the method of choice, with FISH being performed for cancers with indeterminate results (2+ score).

▶ The clinical success of molecular targeting as a strategy for cancer treatment is dependent upon reliable, cost effective identification of patients with the abnormality of interest. This has resulted in a new interest in quality control standards for procedures such as IHC, which are routinely performed in pathology laboratories. This study demonstrates that with appropriate quality control procedures, very high concordance rates can be achieved between IHC and FISH for detection of HER2 abnormalities, suggesting that FISH is not necessary for routine screening purposes.

This is important, since FISH is substantially more expensive, time consuming, and associated with a higher failure rate than IHC. Limitation of the use of FISH to cases where IHC results are indeterminate (2+ staining) resulted in the need for FISH in only 15% of cases in this study. This report also emphasizes the need for clinicians to ensure that appropriate quality control measures are in place in the laboratories handling their clinical specimens.

M. Morrow, MD

Decongestive Lymphatic Therapy for Patients With Breast Carcinoma–Associated Lymphedema: A Randomized, Prospective Study of a Role for Adjunctive Intermittent Pneumatic Compression

Szuba A, Achalu R, Rockson SG (Stanford Univ, Calif)

Cancer 95:2260-2267, 2002 2–14

Introduction.—Disruption of the lymphatic circulation during axillary lymph node dissection, with or without radiation therapy, is the most frequent cause of lymphedema in developed countries. Prospective investigation of the safety and efficacy of intermittent pneumatic compression (IPC) in the adjunctive treatment of patients with breast carcinoma-associated upper extremity lymphedema is needed and was therefore examined with the use of compression bandaging and manual lymphatic massage.

Methods.—IPC was evaluated as a component of the initial therapeutic regimen for 23 patients who had not previously been treated for cancer-associated lymphedema. Patients were randomly assigned to treatment with either decongestive lymphatic therapy (DLT) alone or DLT with daily adjunctive IPC. Patients with stable, treated breast carcinoma–related lymphedema were also evaluated during the maintenance phase of therapy.

In a separate trial, 27 patients were randomly assigned to treatment with either DLT alone or DLT coupled with daily IPC. In both trials, objective evaluation included serial measurement of volume by water displacement, tissue tonometry to evaluate elasticity of the skin, and goniometry to determine joint mobility.

Results.—During initial treatment, the addition of IPC to standard DLT produced an additional mean volume decrease (45.3% vs 26%; $P < .05$). During maintenance DLT alone, there was a mean increase in volume (32.7 mL vs 115.2 mL). In the DLT and IPC group, there was a mean volume decrease (89.5 mL vs 195 mL; $P < .05$). In both trials, IPC was well tolerated without identifiable adverse effects on skin elasticity or joint range of motion.

Conclusion.—When IPC is used adjunctively with other, established elements of DLT, it allows enhanced therapeutic response. It is well tolerated and remarkably free of complications.

▶ In spite of a greater awareness of the risk of lymphedema after axillary dissection and technical modifications of the surgical procedure, lymphedema remains a major cause of postoperative morbidity after axillary surgery. In a recent randomized trial comparing axillary dissection and sentinel node biopsy, Veronesi et al[1] reported that 75% of patients undergoing axillary dissection had a measurable difference in arm circumference at 24 months, although it was greater than 2 cm in only 12%. The therapy of lymphedema has been frustrating since the problem cannot be cured.

Limited randomized data documenting the effectiveness of lymphedema therapy have been available until relatively recently. This study contributes to that literature by documenting that the addition of IPC to DLT, either at the time of presentation with new lymphedema or during maintenance therapy, significantly reduces the volume of lymphedema. The availability of an effective intervention for lymphedema management highlights the importance of prompt referral to a trained therapist when symptoms develop.

M. Morrow, MD

Reference

1. Veronesi U, Paganelli G, Viale G, et al: A randomized comparison of sentinel node biopsy with routine axillary dissection in breast cancer. *N Eng J Med* 349:546-553, 2003.

Bone Mineral Density Among Premenopausal Women With Early Breast Cancer in a Randomized Trial of Adjuvant Endocrine Therapy

Sverrisdóttir Á, Fornander T, Jacobsson H, et al (Karolinska Inst, Stockholm, Sweden; Univ Hosp, Stockholm, Sweden)

J Clin Oncol 22:3694-3699, 2004 2–15

Introduction.—Early results of trials with luteinizing hormone-releasing hormone (LHRH) analogs in the adjuvant setting have reported significant benefits in prolonged disease-free survival and improved survival with 2 years of treatment, regardless of other systemic treatments. The effects of 2 years of treatment with an LHRH agonist alone or in combination with tamoxifen or tamoxifen alone on bone mineral density (BMD) were examined in 89 women from 2 centers participating in a randomized, multicenter trial of 3 different endocrine approaches in the adjuvant setting (Zoladex in Premenopausal Patients Trial).

Methods.—Participants were randomly assigned to receive the LHRH agonist goserelin with or without tamoxifen, tamoxifen alone, or no endocrine therapy. Treatment was administered for 2 years. Total body BMD was determined before initiation of treatment and at 12, 24, and 36 months.

Results.—After 2 years of treatment, significant loss of BMD (mean change, −5%; $P < .001$) was observed in women receiving goserelin alone. The combined goserelin and tamoxifen treatment, along with tamoxifen treatment alone, resulted in a lesser yet statistically significant reduction in BMD (mean change, −1.4%; $P = .02$; and −1.5%; $P < .001$). At 1 year after cessation of treatment, the goserelin group alone had a partial recovery from bone loss (mean change, 1.5%; $P = .02$).

Conclusion.—Two years of ovarian ablation from goserelin treatment produced a significant reduction in BMD; there was partial recovery from the bone loss 1 year after the end of treatment. The addition of tamoxifen appears to partially counteract the demineralization effects of goserelin.

▶ The improvement in disease-free survival in postmenopausal women seen with the use of aromatase inhibitors compared with tamoxifen has prompted interest in complete ovarian suppression in premenopausal women. However, as adjuvant therapy is used in women at lower risk of relapse from breast cancer, a thorough evaluation of the risks and benefits of treatment becomes particularly important. This study documents that the use of an LHRH agonist in premenopausal women is associated with significant BMD loss during 2 years of treatment that is partially ameliorated with tamoxifen. One year after treatment, some recovery of BMD was seen, but whether levels return to baseline is uncertain. This study has important implications regarding the need to monitor BMD in premenopausal patients treated with LHRH agonists, particularly when used with aromatase inhibitors.

M. Morrow, MD

Synergistic Interactions Between Tamoxifen and Trastuzumab (Herceptin)

Argiris A, Wang C-X, Whalen SG, et al (Yale Univ, New Haven, Conn)

Clin Cancer Res 10:1409-1420, 2004 2–16

Introduction.—The HER-2/*neu* and estrogen receptor (ER) are important in the biology of breast carcinoma; both are validated therapeutic targets. Extensive interactions between the signaling pathways of these receptors have been observed, indicating that targeting both receptors simultaneously may have a dramatic effect on the biology of breast cancer. The combined effect of antiestrogen and anti-HER-2/*neu* treatment in vitro was examined by using 2 clinically useful drugs in the treatment of breast cancer, tamoxifen and trastuzumab (Herceptin).

Methods.—ER-positive, HER-2/*neu*-overexpressing BT-474 human breast carcinoma cells were cultured in the presence of Herceptin, tamoxifen, or both. The effects on cell growth, cell cycle distribution, clonogenicity, survival, and the level and activity of HER-2/*neu* were evaluated.

Results.—The combination of tamoxifen and Herceptin resulted in synergistic growth inhibition and enhancement of cell accumulation in the G_0-G_1 phase of the cell cycle, with a reduction in cells in S phase. Clonogenicity was inhibited in the presence of each drug; this was compounded by the combination of both drugs. Prior exposure to drugs did not affect subsequent clonogenicity in drug-free media; neither drug nor the combination of both drugs induced apoptosis. Herceptin, and not tamoxifen, inhibited signaling by HER-2/*neu*.

Conclusion.—The combination of tamoxifen and Herceptin results in synergistic growth inhibition and enhancement of G_0-G_1 cell cycle accumulation. In vitro, the individual drugs or combination causes a cytostatic effect. It appears that combination inhibition of ER and HER-2/*neu* signaling may represent a powerful approach in the treatment of breast cancer.

Mechanisms of Tamoxifen Resistance: Increased Estrogen Receptor-HER2/neu Cross-Talk in ER/HER2–Positive Breast Cancer

Shou J, Massarweh S, Osborne CK, et al (Baylor College of Medicine, Houston; AstraZeneca, Cheshire, England; Imperial College of Science, Technology & Medicine, London)

J Natl Cancer Inst 96:926-935, 2004 2–17

Introduction.—Patients receiving adjuvant tamoxifen whose tumors express high levels of both HER2/neu (HER2) and the estrogen receptor (ER) coactivator AIB1 commonly have tamoxifen resistance. A breast cancer model system with high expression of AIB1 and HER2 was used to assess the possible mechanism underlying this resistance.

Methods.—MCF-7 breast cancer cells, which express high levels of AIB1, and a tamoxifen-resistant derivative cell line engineered to overexpress HER2 (MCF-7/HER2-18) underwent treatment with estrogen, tamoxifen, epidermal growth factor (EGF), or heregulin in the absence or presence of the EGF receptor (EGFR) tyrosine kinase inhibitor gefitinib. Phosphorylation of signaling intermediates were evaluated by immunoblotting; ER transcriptional activity by reporter gene constructs; and immunoblot analysis of endogenous gene products, promoter assembly by chromatin immunoprecipitation assay, and tumor cell growth in vitro by anchorage-independent colony formation and in vivo by using xenografts in nude mice.

Results.—MCF-7/HER2-18 tumors were completely growth inhibited by estrogen deprivation; they were growth stimulated by tamoxifen. Molecular cross-talk between ER and HER2 pathways was intensified in MCF-7/HER-2 cells versus MCF-7 cells, with cross-phosphorylation and activation of both ER and EGFR/HER2 receptors, signaling molecules AKT and ERK 1,2 mitogen-activated protein kinase, and AIB1 itself with both estrogen and tamoxifen treatment. Tamoxifen recruited coactivator complexes (ER, AIB1, CBP, p300) to the ER-regulated pS2 gene promoter in MCF-7/HER2-18 cells, along with corepressor complexes (NCoR, histone deacetylase 3) in MCF-7 cells. Gefitinib pretreatment blocked receptor cross-talk, reestablished corepressor complexes with tamoxifen-bound ER on target gene promoters, eradicated tamoxifen's agonist effects, and restored anti-tumor activity both in vitro and in vivo in MCF-7/HER2-18 cells.

Conclusion.—Tamoxifen acts as an estrogen antagonist in breast cancer cells that express high levels of AIB1 and HER2, resulting in de novo resistance. The ability of gefitinib to eliminate cross-talk and restore the antitumor effects of tamoxifen needs to be further evaluated.

▶ There has been much discussion about the role of tamoxifen therapy in patients who overexpress HER2/neu. In an early randomized trial examining the efficacy of tamoxifen in HER2/neu-negative and HER2/neu-positive breast cancer patients, there was a suggestion that patients who were positive for ER and progesterone receptor and also positive for HER2/neu did worse with tamoxifen than with no tamoxifen.[1] Although subsequent trials have suggested a benefit, that benefit appears to be reduced. Studies of the interaction between the ER and HER2 pathways in response to tamoxifen treatment have followed. The article by Argiris et al (Abstract 2–16) reports that the combination of tamoxifen and trastuzumab results in synergistic growth inhibition and accumulation of cells in G_0-G_1 in a human breast cancer cell line positive for ER and overexpressing HER2/neu and that lesser degrees of these effects are seen with either agent alone. The article by Shou et al (Abstract 2–17) suggests that, in patients with tumors positive for ER and overexpressing HER2/neu, molecular cross-talk between the ER and HER2 pathways is increased with tamoxifen and that concomitant treatment with gefitinib eliminates the cross-talk and restores the antitumor effects of tamoxifen. These 2 studies provide additional light on the issue of tamoxifen and the HER2 pathway and also identify some interesting interactions between tamoxifen therapy and 2 biologic agents, trastuzumab and gefitinib. Both suggest some potentially interesting future clinical trials.

J. T. Thigpen, MD

Reference

1. Bianco AR, De Laurentis M, Carlomagno C, et al: 20-year update of the Naples GUN Trial of adjuvant breast cancer therapy: Evidence of an interaction between c-erb B-2 expression and tamoxifen efficacy. *Proc Annu Meet Am Soc Clin Oncol* 17:97a, 1998 (abstract).

Early Stage and Adjuvant Therapy

Intramammary Lymph Node Metastases Are an Independent Predictor of Poor Outcome in Patients With Breast Carcinoma

Shen J, Hunt KK, Mirza NQ, et al (Univ of Texas, Houston)
Cancer 101:1330-1337, 2004 2–18

Background.—Stage II breast carcinoma is defined as intramammary lymph node (intraMLN) metastases, even without axillary lymph node involvement. However, the clinical significance of intraMLN metastases is not well understood. The clinical relevance of intraMLN metastases and the relation between such metastases and outcome were determined in women with breast carcinoma.

Methods.—One hundred thirty intraMLN specimens associated with primary breast malignancy obtained between 1983 and 2003 were analyzed. Patient age ranged from 27 to 84 years. Median patient follow-up was 36 months.

Findings.—In 18% of the patients, intraMLNs were preoperatively identified by mammography or sonography. In the remaining women, intraMLNs were found on pathologic evaluation of surgical breast specimens. Twenty-eight percent of the overall group had intraMLN metastases. Eighty-one percent of women with intraMLN also had axillary metastases. In 5%, isolated intraMLN metastases were identified (Table 2). According to univariate analysis, patients with intraMLN metastases had a lower 5-year disease-free survival rate (54% and 89%, respectively), disease-specific survival (66% and 90%, respectively), and overall survival (64% and 88%, respectively). In a multivariate analysis, intraMLN involvement independently predicted decreased disease-free survival, disease-specific sur-

TABLE 2.—Incidence of Intramammary Lymph Node Metastases (n = 130)

Disease Feature	No. With IntraMLN Metastases (%)	*P* Value
Tumor diameter (cm)		NS
≤ 1	6 (19)	
> 1	30 (30)	
Tumor status		0.02
T1	7 (16)	
T2	18 (40)	
T3	3 (38)	
T4	8 (53)	
Tumor grade		NS
I	3 (20)	
II	13 (21)	
III	20 (38)	
Lymphovascular invasion		<0.001
Present	24 (53)	
Absent	12 (14)	
Tumor location		NS
Upper outer quadrant	23 (30)	
Other	13 (25)	
AxLN status[a]		<0.001
Negative	6 (11)	
Positive	29 (46)	
Pathologic LN status[a]		<0.001
pN0	6 (11)	
pN1 (1-3 positive AxLNs)	16 (41)	
pN2 (4-9 positive AxLNs)	7 (47)	
pN3 (≥ 10 positive AxLNs)	6 (67)	

Abbreviations: NS, Not significant; *AxLN*, axillary lymph node; *LN*, lymph node.

[a]Axillary lymph node dissection was not performed in 1 patient who had intramammary lymph node metastases.

(Courtesy of Shen J, Hunt KK, Mirza NQ, et al: Intramammary lymph node metastases are an independent predictor of poor outcome in patients with breast carcinoma. *Cancer* 101:1330-1337, 2004. Copyright 2004 American Cancer Society. Reprinted by permission of Wiley-Liss, Inc, a subsidiary of John Wiley & Sons, Inc.)

vival, and overall survival, with hazard ratios of 2.33, 5.32, and 3.22, respectively.

Conclusions.—The presence of intraMLN metastases independently predicts poor outcome in women with breast carcinoma. The finding of an intraMLN on preoperative imaging merits further histopathologic evaluation. Detecting malignant intraMLNs on lymphatic mapping may be useful for identifying high-risk patients requiring further assessment of the axillary lymph nodes, despite otherwise clinically negative axillary findings.

▶ Improvements in breast imaging and the adoption of lymphatic mapping and sentinel node biopsy have resulted in more frequent identification of intramammary lymph node metastases. The prognostic significance of these metastases has been unclear. This study documents that intraMLNs are usually associated with axillary nodal metastases. The poorer prognosis seen in patients with both axillary and intramammary metastases is reflective of an increased tumor burden, just as the combination of metastases to both the axillary and internal mammary nodes is associated with a poorer prognosis than metastases to either basin alone. However, the difference in 4-year disease-free survival observed between patients with only axillary metastases (84%) and those with only intramammary metastases (40%) is most likely due to the small number of patients in the latter group (n = 6) and is insufficient evidence for aggressive treatment for patients with intraMLNs. Disease in the intramammary nodes is a reflection of the continuum of nodal involvement and warrants the same systemic therapy that would be used in a patient with an equivalent number of axillary nodes involved with metastatic disease.

M. Morrow, MD

Skin-Sparing Mastectomy With Conservation of the Nipple-Areola Complex and Autologous Reconstruction is an Oncologically Safe Procedure

Gerber B, Krause A, Reimer T, et al (Univ of Rostock, Germany)
Ann Surg 238:120-127, 2003 2–19

Introduction.—Skin-sparing mastectomy (SSM) involves removal of the breast, nipple-areolar complex (NAC), previous biopsy incisions, and skin overlying superficial tumors. The preservation of the native skin envelope facilitates performance of immediate breast reconstruction. The risk of involvement of the NAC in patients with breast cancer may be overestimated. The first ever results regarding SSM with and without conservation of the NAC were reported.

Methods.—Between 1994 and 2000, 286 selected patients with an indication for modified radical mastectomy (MRM) and tumor margins of over 2 cm from the nipple were offered the alternative of an SSM. Follow-up data were available for 112 patients with SSM and 134 with MRM. Immediate reconstruction was performed with the use of a latissimus dorsi flap or a transverse rectus abdominis myocutaneous flap. The mean follow-up was 59 months (range, 18-92 months).

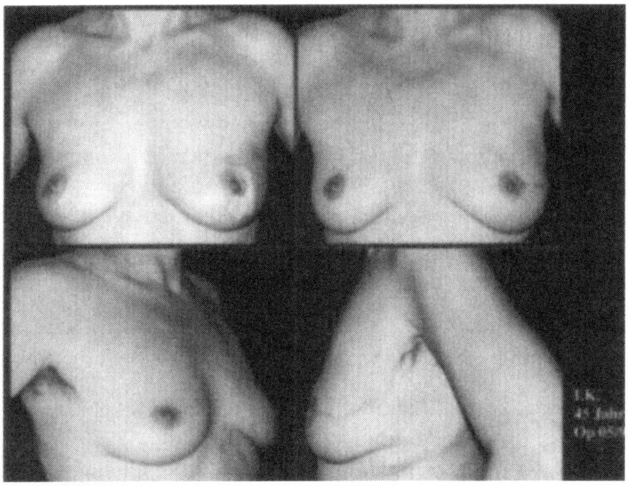

FIGURE 4.—A 40-year-old patient with breast cancer pT2 (21 mm, m) N1 (3/22) MO, RO, and skin-sparing mastectomy with nipple-areola complex conservation and latissimus dorsi flap reconstruction 6 months after surgery. (Courtesy of Gerber B, Krause A, Reimer T, et al: Skin-sparing mastectomy with conservation of the nipple-areola complex and autologous reconstruction is an oncologically safe procedure. *Ann Surg* 238(1):120-127, 2003.)

Results.—Patients who underwent SSM were significantly younger than those who underwent MRM. Otherwise, the 2 groups were similar concerning clinical data, tumor parameters, adjuvant treatment, and overall complications. After intraoperative frozen sections of the NAC-ground, the NAC could be conserved in 61 (54.5%) patients. It was resected in 51 (45.5%) patients in the SSM group. The esthetic results after SSM were rated as excellent or good in 91.1% (102/112) of patients. They were significantly better after preservation of the NAC (P = .001) (Fig 4). There were 6 (5.4%) recurrences in 112 patients with SSM versus 11 (8.2%) after MRM. One recurrence in a conserved nipple was treated by wide excision of the nipple with conservation of the areola. This patient remained free of disease at 52 months' follow-up.

Conclusion.—In patients who are candidates for a mastectomy and have tumors distant from the nipple, SSM with intraperative frozen section of the NAC group provided the opportunity for NAC conservation without increasing the risk of locally recurrent disease.

▶ Changes in our understanding of the biology of breast cancer have dramatically changed the approach to breast reconstruction. The recognition that treatment of stage I and II breast carcinoma did not necessitate removal of large pieces of normal skin resulted in SSM. Removal of the NAC has continued to be regarded as an oncologic necessity, due to the absence of subcutaneous fat beneath these structures. Preservation of the NAC necessitates leaving some breast tissue in place to provide a blood supply. The study of Gerber et al suggests that in a carefully selected group of patients, preservation of the NAC can be accomplished with good cosmetic results and a very small risk of local failure in the preserved nipple.

Questions that remain to be answered about this approach include its applicability to the universe of women undergoing mastectomy, since extensive intraductal carcinoma alone, or in conjunction with an invasive tumor, is a common indication for mastectomy. In addition, more details regarding sensation, pigmentation, and symmetry with the contralateral nipple are needed. Finally, although partial necrosis of the nipple occurred in only 10% of the cases in this series—all of which were reconstructed with autologous tissue—it remains to be seen if a higher rate of necrosis will occur after reconstruction with expanders or implants.

M. Morrow, MD

Uncontrolled Local Disease After Salvage Treatment for Ipsilateral Breast Tumour Recurrence

Dalberg K, Liedberg A, Johansson U, et al (Uppsala Univ Hosp, Stockholm; Karolinska Hosp, Stockholm; Svdersjukhuset, Stockholm)

Eur J Surg Oncol 29:143-154, 2003 2–20

Background.—Breast-conserving surgery and irradiation for stage I or II breast cancer has been shown to as effective as mastectomy in terms of overall survival and local control. The ipsilateral breast tumor recurrence (IBTR) rate at 5 years has varied from 2% to 36%, mainly because of the use or nonuse of radiotherapy. Other variables affecting the rate of IBTR are surgical technique, adjuvant systemic radiotherapy, and patient selection. Uncontrolled local disease (ULD) also has a significant effect on quality of life through symptoms such as ulceration, bleeding, and pain. Although not life-threatening in the short term, the psychological effects of watching a tumor growing at the surface of the body can be devastating. The outcome after treatment of IBTR and the risk of ULD in an effort to identify risk factors for ULD were analyzed.

Methods.—A group of 307 patients with subsequent IBTR was identified from a cohort of 5502 patients treated for stage I-II invasive breast cancer with breast-conserving surgery from 1976 to 1998 in Stockholm. Most of these patients (219) had received postoperative radiotherapy; 26% received adjuvant tamoxifen for 2 or 5 years; and 9% received adjuvant polychemotherapy. The median length of follow-up was 11 years (range, 2-23 years). Fifty patents had ULD develop. Multivariate linear logistic regression was used to identify prognostic factors for ULD.

Findings.—The cumulative incidence of ULD at 5 years after the diagnosis of IBTR was 13%. Five independent risk factors for ULD were identified: nonsurgical treatment of IBTR, the appearance of disseminated disease concurrent with IBTR, the presence of axillary lymph node metastases at primary breast conservation, an interval of less than 3 years between breast conservation and IBTR, and no adjuvant endocrine therapy. Most (88%) of the patients were treated with salvage mastectomy (207 patients) or reexcision (62 patients). The cumulative incidence of ULD at 5 years after salvage mastectomy was 10% and that after salvage reexcision was 16%,

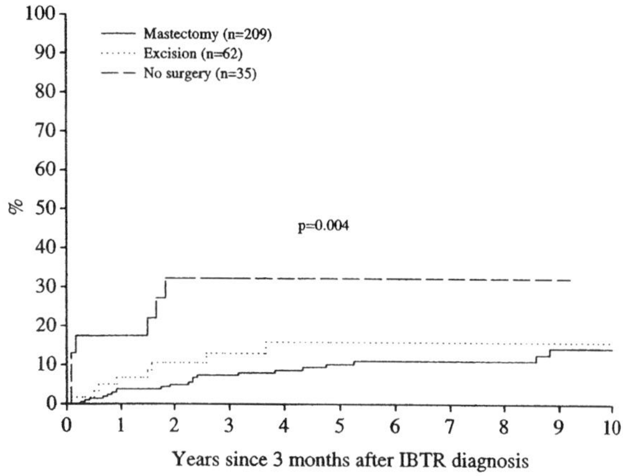

FIGURE 1.—Cumulative incidence of ULD after IBTR. (Courtesy of Dalberg K, Liedberg A, Johansson U, et al: Uncontrolled local disease after salvage treatment for ipsilateral breast tumour recurrence. *Eur J Surg Oncol* 29:143-154, 2003.)

compared with 32% among patients treated nonsurgically (Fig 1). After IBTR, the 5-year overall survival rate among patients with local control was 78% compared with 21% among patients with ULD.

Conclusions.—The occurrence of ULD after breast-conserving surgery is rare but can have devastating effects on the patient's quality of life. Primary postoperative radiotherapy reduces the risk of IBTR and thus is recommended as part of the primary treatment to avoid both IBTR and ULD. Adjuvant therapy in addition to radiotherapy reduces the risk of IBTR and thus the risk of subsequent ULD. Patients with IBTR, regardless of the presence or absence of concurrent distant metastases, should undergo salvage surgery whenever possible, because salvage surgery provides better local control than salvage systemic therapy only does.

▶ Improvements in patient selection, breast imaging, and pathologic evaluation of lumpectomy specimens of resection, coupled with the increased use of adjuvant systemic therapy have made local failure after breast conserving therapy an infrequent occurrence. The majority of local failures can be salvaged with completion mastectomy, so uncontrolled local recurrence is rare. However, the significant morbidity of ULD makes avoidance of this problem extremely important. In this study, 13% of 307 patients treated for IBTR had ULD at 5 years. Many of the predictors of ULD are related to poor prognosis of the primary breast cancer and include a short disease-free interval after initial surgery, axillary lymph node metastases at initial presentation, and the concurrent appearance of local and distant recurrence. These factors are not modifiable. However, nonsurgical treatment of the initial breast recurrence was the strongest predictor of ULD, and treatment with re-excision was associated with more ULD than was seen after mastectomy. These results emphasize that local recurrence after breast conservation is a surgical disease that should be treated with mastectomy. Equally important is the prevention of any local failure after initial breast conserving therapy. The routine use of breast irradiation is the most effective way to do this, and education of patients regarding the consequences of inadequate local therapy should be carried out before the final selection of surgical treatment.

M. Morrow, MD

Immediate Endoscopic Latissimus Dorsi Flap: Risk or Benefit in Reconstructing Partial Mastectomy Defects

Losken A, Schaefer TG, Carlson GW, et al (Emory Univ, Atlanta, Ga)
Ann Plast Surg 53:1-5, 2004 2–21

Background.—The management of breast cancer has evolved from radical surgical procedures to more conservative resection in conjunction with radiation therapy. Breast conservation therapy (BCT) is now the preferred therapeutic approach for women with early stage breast cancer. As a result, the partial mastectomy defect is now a common entity. A number of reconstructive options have been proposed in select patients after BCT in an effort to maintain esthetic results. Experience with endoscopic-assisted harvest of the latissimus dorsi muscle for reconstruction of partial mastectomy defects, with a focus on the indications, patient selection, technique, complications, recurrence, and long-term outcome was reviewed.

Methods.—A total of 39 women with early stage breast cancer were treated with BCT and simultaneous endoscope-assisted latissimus muscle transfer at the time of resection. The average duration of follow-up was 3.7 years. Patient demographics and tumor characteristics were included in the analysis.

Results.—Donor site morbidity occurred in 12 patients (31%). Tumor recurrence occurred in 6 patients (15%) after lumpectomy and latissimus reconstruction. Local recurrence developed in 2 patients, and 4 patients had distant recurrence. There was no evidence of disease in 33 patients (85%) at long-term follow-up. Lumpectomy and latissimus flap transfer was the definitive reconstructive procedure used in 33 of the 39 patients (85%). Patients who subsequently required completion mastectomy were easily reconstructed with a TRAM flap or implants.

Conclusions.—There has been a shift away from immediate simultaneous reconstruction for the management of partial mastectomy defects on the basis of concerns regarding the appropriateness this approach from an oncologic and reconstructive perspective. The use of rigorous patient selection, confirmation of negative margins, and possibly delaying of the latissimus flap transfer will maximize the benefits of this reconstructive modality while limiting the risks associated with immediate reconstruction of partial mastectomy defects.

► Women with T2 breast carcinomas are significantly less likely to undergo BCT than their counterparts with T1 tumors, in part because of the difficulty of resecting larger tumors and maintaining a good cosmetic result.[1] One strategy to increase the use of BCT is neoadjuvant chemotherapy. Randomized trials have demonstrated a statistically significant increase in BCT with this approach,[2] although the absolute increase in the use of BCT in the National Surgical Adjuvant Breast and Bowel project B18 study was only 7%.[2] In general, 25% to 33% of women who are not initially candidates for BCT because of large, localized primary tumors can be converted with this approach. Preoperative chemotherapy is most effective in high-grade, hormone receptor negative tumors without an extensive intraductal component. In addition, some patients are reluctant to undergo preoperative chemotherapy even when they are advised that chemotherapy will be part of postoperative treatment. An alternative approach to increasing the use of BCT is partial breast reconstruction with a latissimus flap. The placement of the flap does not interfere with the mammographic detection of local recurrence. Although the latissimus reconstructions in this study were performed at the time of lumpectomy, I have found that a 2-stage procedure is a more prudent approach. Lumpectomy and sentinel node biopsy are performed as the first stage of the procedure. This ensures negative margins before positioning of the flap. If axillary dissection is required, it is performed at the same procedure as the flap because the latissimus muscle is tunnelled into the breast through an axillary incision.

M. Morrow, MD

References

1. Morrow M, Bucci C, Rademaker A: Medical contraindications are not a major factor in the underutilization of breast conserving therapy. *J Am Coll Surg* 186:269-274, 1998.
2. Fisher B, Brown A, Maumonas E, et al: Effect of preoperative chemotherapy on local regional disease in women with operable breast cancer: Findings from National Surgical Adjuvant Breast and Bowel Project B-18. *J Clin Oncol* 15:2483-2493, 1997.

Acute Toxicity of High–Dose-Rate Intracavitary Brachytherapy With the MammoSite Applicator in Patients With Early-Stage Breast Cancer

Richards GM, Berson AM, Rescigno J, et al (St Vincent's Comprehensive Cancer Ctr, New York; New York Med College, Valhalla, NY)

Ann Surg Oncol 11:739-746, 2004 2–22

Background.—There is overwhelming evidence to support the use of breast conservation therapy, yet studies have indicated that 50% or greater of patients with early stage breast cancer continue to undergo mastectomy. However, medical contraindications are not the major factors driving the high rate of mastectomies. Factors related to the nature of external beam radiotherapy and the standard treatment regimen (5 weeks of daily treatment followed by up to 2 weeks of boost therapy to the tumor bed) have a substantial effect on the choice of treatment. These disadvantages have prompted the development of accelerated regimens of partial-breast radiotherapy, including interstitial brachytherapy. However, this approach can be technically challenging and is not widely available. Whether intracavitary brachytherapy with the MammoSite applicator (Proxima Therapeutics, Alpharetta, Ga) as the only radiation treatment in breast-conserving therapy is a viable alternative for women with early stage breast cancer was determined.

Methods.—A total of 31 patients with 32 stage I or II breast carcinomas underwent breast-conserving therapy, including lumpectomy with negative margins, sentinel node biopsy, or axillary dissection, followed by brachytherapy with the MammoSite applicator. Acute radiation skin complications were graded on the day of radiotherapy completion and again at 2, 4, 6, and 12 weeks after radiation treatment. Cosmesis was graded on the Harvard Scale at all follow-up time points.

Results.—The median follow up was 11 months, with a range of 4 to 15 months. Of the 31 patients treated with the MammoSite device, 27 were treated with this device as the sole method of radiotherapy. There were no cases of acute toxicity during the 5 days of treatment. No mild acute skin reactions occurred in 19 patients (68%), and bright erythema and patchy moist desquamation developed in 25% of these patient. Confluent moist desquamation developed in 2 patients (7%) within the first 4 weeks (grade 3), and this desquamation healed by week 12. All the skin reactions were localized to the area overlying the balloon. Infection developed in 5 of 32 (16%) breasts with implants. Cosmesis was good to excellent in 86% of cases.

Conclusions.—The use of high-dose-rate intracavitary brachytherapy resulted in mild acute skin toxicities in most patients in this study. The infection rate was higher than in prior studies that used interstitial brachytherapy. The intracavitary brachytherapy catheter was well tolerated, and cosmesis was good to excellent in most patients. These findings are supportive of further investigation of breast brachytherapy with this intracavitary system.

► The need for 6 weeks of external beam irradiation (RT) after lumpectomy is thought to cause some women to opt for mastectomy as a surgical alternative. There has been significant interest in identifying patients who do not require postlumpectomy irradiation and in the development of alternative techniques to deliver radiotherapy in a shorter time interval. Intracavitary radiotherapy with the MammoSite device has been enthusiastically embraced as a simple and widely applicable technique for partial breast irradiation. This method of treatment has not been compared with traditional external beam whole breast RT in a randomized trial. The study of Richards et al demonstrates that although acute skin reactions were limited, 16% of patients had infections develop and the majority of these required drainage. This is higher than would be anticipated. Interestingly, cosmetic outcome was graded as excellent or good in 86% of patients after a median follow-up of 11 months. In a report of patients treated with external beam RT at the Joint Center for Radiotherapy between 1982 and 1985, 94% of patients had an excellent or good cosmetic outcome[1] after 67 months of follow-up. This early report of the results with the MammoSite device may actually underestimate the incidence of fair or poor cosmetic results because cosmesis does not stabilize until 3 years after treatment with external beam RT.[2] Most importantly, this study demonstrates the importance of controlled trials to assess the relative value of treatment techniques. Radiation with the MammoSite device is undoubtedly more convenient. It has not yet been proven to provide local control equivalent to that seen with whole breast RT, and this small study does not provide convincing evidence of improved cosmesis. Until the results of randomized trials are available, this technique should be considered experimental.

M. Morrow, MD

References

1. de la Rochefordiere A, Abner AL, Silver B, et al: Are cosmetic results following conservative surgery and radiation therapy for early breast cancer dependent on technique? *Int J Rad Oncol Biol Phys* 23:925-931, 1992.
2. Rose MA, Olivotto I, Cady B, et al: Conservative surgery and radiation therapy for early breast cancer: Long-term cosmetic results. *Arch Surg* 124:153-157, 1989.

Retrospective Study of Women Presenting With Axillary Metastases From Occult Breast Carcinoma

Blanchard DK, Farley DR (Mayo Clinic, Rochester, Minn)
World J Surg 28:535-539, 2004 2–23

Background.—Palpable axillary lymphadenopathy is usually associated with benign disorders but can be an indication of underlying advanced malignancy. Axillary metastasis is the only initial clinical manifestation of breast cancer in less than 1% of the patients diagnosed. The Mayo Clinic experience with women with occult breast cancer with axillary metastases was reported.

Methods.—Of 66 women diagnosed as having axillary metastases from an unknown primary tumor at the Mayo Clinic between 1975 and 1998, 44 underwent axillary biopsy for a palpable mass. Thirty-five had histologic evidence of metastatic carcinoma of primary breast cancer origin. The workup, identification, treatment, and outcomes of these 35 women were analyzed.

Findings.—All 35 patients had a palpable axillary nodule but no dominant breast mass, normal mammograms, and normal chest radiographs. In all women, histologic analysis of the axillary node indicated probable breast cancer. Long-term follow-up data were available on 33 women followed up for a mean 71.5 months. Fifty-one percent of the patients underwent mastectomy as part of their primary treatment. A primary breast tumor was found in 33% of these patients. Of the 17 women undergoing mastectomy for whom follow-up data were available, 6 had a recurrence (35%) and 4 died of their disease (24%). Of the 17 women not undergoing mastectomy, follow-up data in 12 of 16 showed disease recurrence (75%), and 11 died from breast cancer (69%) (Fig 1).

Conclusions.—Despite extensive clinical and radiologic assessment at the Mayo Clinic, no primary tumor was found initially in 35 women with axil-

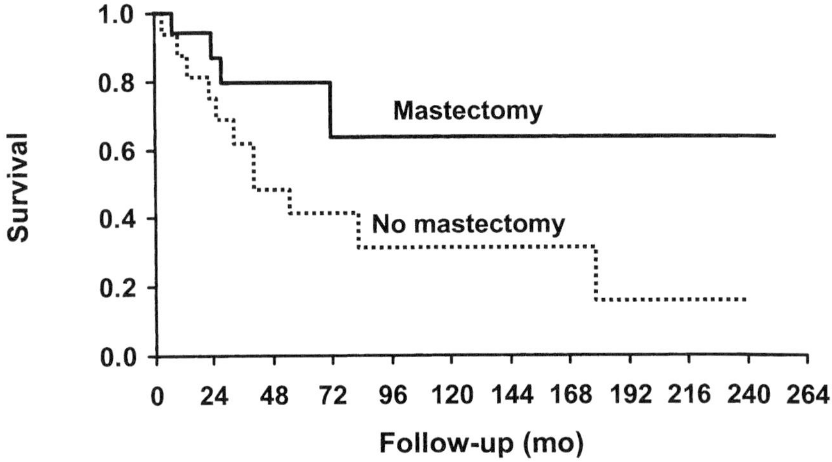

FIGURE 1.—Survival of patients with axillary metastases from an occult primary tumor. Mastectomy (n = 17) vs no mastectomy (n = 16); *P* = .047. (Courtesy of Blanchard DK, Farley DR: Retrospective study of women presenting with axillary metastases from occult breast carcinoma. *World J Surg* 28:535-539, 2004. Copyright 2004 Springer-Verlag.)

lary metastases from a presumed occult breast carcinoma. Women undergoing aggressive surgical intervention ultimately fared significantly better than those who did not undergo mastectomy.

▶ Carcinoma of the breast presenting as axillary nodal metastases with an occult primary tumor is an infrequent problem. In older studies, large areas of cancer were often identified after histologic examination of the breast, leading to a recommendation for routine management by mastectomy. The availability of high-quality mammography, US, and most recently MRI has made large unidentified areas of cancer much less common, and in many mastectomy specimens no tumor can be identified. This has given rise to the concept of breast preservation as an appropriate management strategy. This study compares outcomes for women treated with and without mastectomy and finds a significant survival benefit for those treated by mastectomy. This is alarming, but it is noteworthy that of the 16 patients who did not have mastectomy, 8 had no additional treatment at all and of the remaining 8, not all received both chemotherapy and irradiation. It is clear that if the breast is left untreated, approximately 42% of patients will develop a detectable breast tumor, and this is not an appropriate approach.[1]

However, other studies examining the use of irradiation to the whole breast in this setting report survival rates comparable to those seen after mastectomy, and this is an appropriate alternative approach when a careful clinical exam and imaging studies fail to reveal a breast primary.[2,3]

M. Morrow, MD

References

1. Fourquet A, Meunier M, Campana F: Occult primary cancer with axillary metastases, in Harris JR, Lippman ME, Morrow M, et al (eds): *Diseases of the Breast*, ed 3. Philadelphia, Lippincott Williams & Wilkins, 2004, p 1047.
2. Baron PL, Moore MP, Kinne DW, et al: Occult breast cancer presenting with axillary metastases: Updated management. *Arch Surg* 125:210-214, 1990.
3. Ellerbroek N, Holmes F, Singletary SE, et al: Treatment of patients with isolated axillary nodal metastases from an occult primary carcinoma consistent with breast origin. *Cancer* 66:1461-1467, 1990.

Limited-Field Radiation Therapy in the Management of Early-Stage Breast Cancer

Vicini FA, Kestin L, Chen P, et al (William Beaumont Hosp, Royal Oak, Mich)
J Natl Cancer Inst 95:1205-1211, 2003 2–24

Background.—Several phase III trials have demonstrated equivalent long-term survival after breast conservation surgery plus radiation therapy versus after mastectomy for the management of early stage breast cancer. However, these studies have not included information on the optimal volume of breast tissue requiring postlumpectomy radiation therapy. The 5-year results of the experience of a single institution with radiation therapy limited to the region of the tumor bed in selected patients treated with breast-conserving therapy was examined. Outcomes after this treatment were compared with outcomes after breast conserving therapy with whole-breast radiation therapy.

Methods.—The study group consisted of 199 patients with early stage breast cancer who underwent breast-conserving therapy and limited-field, interstitial brachytherapy. Potential differences in local recurrence rates on the basis of the volume of breast tissue irradiated were compared by matching these patients with another 199 patients who underwent whole-breast radiation therapy on the basis of tumor size, lymph-node status, patient age, margins of excision, estrogen-receptor status, and use of adjuvant tamoxifen therapy. Local-regional control and disease-free and overall survival rates were analyzed with the Kaplan-Meier method, and the statistical significance of differences between treatment groups was calculated with log-rank tests.

Findings.—The median follow-up time for surviving patients was 65 months (range 12-115 months). Five ipsilateral breast failures appeared in the limited-field radiation group. The cumulative incidence of local recurrence was 1% (95% CI 0%-2.8%). Matched-pair analysis showed that the rate of local recurrence was not statistically significantly different between the limited-field group (1%, 95% CI 0%-2.8%) and the whole-breast group (1%, 95% CI 0%-2.4%).

Conclusion.—Limited-field radiation therapy delivered to the tumor bed region provides 5-year local control rates comparable to those achieved with whole-breast radiation therapy for selected patients.

▶ Over the last few years, there has been the development of "limited field radiation therapy" or partial breast radiation therapy in the management of patients with early stage breast cancer. The techniques for this will vary, sometimes using interstitial brachytherapy, which has a significant track record, and sometimes using the "mammosite," which is a balloon placed into the tumor cavity at the time of excision and filled with radioactive isotope to deliver an intense but relatively concentrated dose of radiation around the cavity left behind by the surgical procedure. This is a very thorough review of the experience from 1 of the major institutions carrying out such treatment.

Undoubtedly, there are patients who are served well by this treatment. Many of these will be patients who live long distances away from radiotherapeutic facilities and simply are unable to spend the long period required for optimal treatment with classic external beam to the whole breast. On the other hand, one has to remember exactly why these patients are treated with definitive radiation therapy rather than a mastectomy. It is about cosmesis. The sine qua non for long-term radiation effect is cell atrophy and cell death, presumably coming from apoptosis induced by radiation treatment. It may take 10 years before that becomes evident. If only part of the breast is irradiated, one can anticipate dimpling of the skin and subcutaneous tissue as though a divot had been removed. If the cosmesis is not very good, patients will be disenchanted with radiation treatment, because the removal of the breast is far quicker than anything that can be done with radiation.

The other issue to focus on explicitly is the fact that local control with classic external beam is referring to the entire breast; whereas, local control for partial breast irradiation is talking only about the area that is irradiated. Thus, there is a significant semantic problem with interpreting the literature on this point, and it bears close watching. After all, whatever the factors are that may have resulted in a breast cancer developing, they are still operating despite treatment.

Obviously, the key to the use of this treatment and its successful outcome is careful patient selection. The smaller the lesion, the more sense it makes. In today's world where there are many patients who are diagnosed radiologically without having a palpable mass, this will probably prove to be useful treatment. Of course, the data need to be generated first. When this is applied to lesions that are physically measurable, this may not be the way to go.

E. Glatstein, MD

Her2/neu Expression Predicts the Response to Antiaromatase Neoadjuvant Therapy in Primary Breast Cancer: Subgroup Analysis From Celecoxib Antiaromatase Neoadjuvant Trial

Zhu L, Chow LWC, Loo WTY, et al (Univ of Hong Kong; Tokyo Metropolitan Komagome Hosp)

Clin Cancer Res 10:4639-4644, 2004 2–25

Introduction.—Several trials have suggested that Her2/neu has an important role in neoadjuvant endocrine therapy. The level of Her2/neu expression in advanced breast cancer was evaluated to ascertain if it changes after antiaromatase neoadjuvant treatment. The association between Her2/neu expression and response to this treatment approach was also examined.

Methods.—Thirty-six postmenopausal women with hormonal receptor–positive primary breast cancer underwent 3 monthly cycles of neoadjuvant endocrine therapy with either Aromasin (25 mg daily) or Femara (2.5 mg daily). Immunohistochemistry and fluorescence in situ hybridization (FISH) for Her2/neu were performed both on pretreatment biopsies and surgical tumors.

Results.—By using immunohistochemistry, 5 (13.9%) of 26 patients had Her2/neu overexpression after treatment compared with 16 (44.4%) of 36 before treatment. There was no change in 21 (58.3%) patients; through FISH, there was a change from amplification to no amplification in 15 (41.7%) patients. Treatment response rates were 75% and 35%, respectively, for Her2/neu-positive and Her2/neu-negative tumors (P = .017) while FISH was performed. The response rate was also significantly affected by the reduction in Her2/neu status after treatment; 73% of tumors demonstrated reduced Her2/neu expression and 38% showed no change in Her2/neu expression (P = .037).

Conclusion.—By using both immunohistochemistry and FISH, advanced breast cancers demonstrate statistical evidence of reducing the incidence of Her2/neu expression after antiaromatase neoadjuvant treatment. It is possible that Her2/neu expression and its change during treatment may be predictive markers for this therapy approach.

Letrozole Inhibits Tumor Proliferation More Effectively Than Tamoxifen Independent of HER1/2 Expression Status

Ellis MJ, Coop A, Singh B, et al (Duke Univ, Durham, NC; Lombardi Cancer Ctr, Washington, DC; Instituto Valenciano de Oncologia, Valencia, Spain; et al)

Cancer Res 63:6523-6531, 2003 2–26

Introduction.—The biologic basis for the efficacy of breast cancer endocrine treatment is complex and includes induction of G_1-S phase cell cycle arrest, apoptosis, and alterations in gene expression associated with inactivation of estrogen receptor (ER)–dependent transcription. The biologic basis for the superior efficacy of neoadjuvant letrozole versus tamoxifen in postmenopausal women was assessed by analyzing tumor proliferation and expression of estrogen-regulated genes before and after initiation of therapy.

Methods.—Tumor samples were obtained at baseline and completion of treatment from 185 patients participating in a double-blind, randomized, phase III trial of neoadjuvant endocrine therapy. The paired specimens were simultaneously examined for Ki67, ER, progesterone receptor (PgR), trefoil factor 1 (PS2), HER1 (epidermal growth factor receptor), and HER2 (ErbB2 or *neu*) by semiquantitative immunohistochemistry.

Results.—The treatment-induced decrease in geometric mean Ki67 was significantly greater with letrozole than with tamoxifen (67% vs 75%; $P = .0009$). Differences in the average Ki67 reduction were especially substantial for ER-positive tumors that overexpressed HER1 or HER2 (88% vs 45%; $P = .0018$). Twenty-three (25%) of 92 tumors and 14 (15%) of 93 tumors treated with tamoxifen versus letrozole demonstrated a paradoxic increase in Ki67; most cases were HER1/2 negative. Letrozole, not tamoxifen, significantly diminished expression of the estrogen-regulated proteins PgR and trefoil factor 1, regardless of HER1/2 status ($P < .0001$). ER downregulation occurred with both agents; levels dropped more with tamoxifen than with letrozole ($P < .0001$).

Conclusion.—Letrozole inhibited tumor proliferation to a greater extent than did tamoxifen. The molecular basis for this advantage seems complex; it includes possible tamoxifen agonist effects on the cell cycle in both HER1/2-positive and HER1/2-negative tumors. A pattern of continued proliferation despite appropriate downregulation of PgR expression with estrogen deprivation or tamoxifen was also observed. It appears that estrogen regulation of proliferation and PgR expression may be dissociated in endocrine therapy–resistant cells.

A Randomized Trial of Exemestane After Two to Three Years of Tamoxifen Therapy in Postmenopausal Women With Primary Breast Cancer

Coombes RC, for the Intergroup Exemestane Study (Imperial College, London; et al)

N Engl J Med 350:1081-1092, 2004 2–27

Background.—Tamoxifen reduces the risk of recurrence of estrogen receptor–positive breast cancer for 5 years after surgery by 47% and reduces the risk of death by 26%. However, some patients relapse despite tamoxifen treatment. Several trials have confirmed the superiority of aromatase inhibitors over progestin in these patients. The results were reported of a second planned interim analysis of the Intergroup Exemestane Study (IES), which investigated whether exemestane given to postmenopausal women who remained recurrence free after receiving adjuvant tamoxifen therapy for 2 to 3 years for primary breast cancer could prolong disease-free survival compared with continued tamoxifen study.

Methods.—A double-blind randomized trial was conducted in patients with histologically confirmed and completely resected unilateral invasive estrogen-positive breast carcinoma. All the patients were postmenopausal and had received adjuvant tamoxifen therapy for at least 2 years but not more than 3 years and 1 month. The patients were then randomly assigned to an additional 2 to 3 years of tamoxifen therapy (2362 patients) or 2 to 3 years of exemestane therapy (2380 patients).

Results.—After a median follow-up of 30.6 months, 449 first events were reported, including 183 in the exemestane group and 266 in the tamoxifen group. The unadjusted hazard ratio in the exemestane group compared with the tamoxifen group was 0.68, representing a 32% reduction in risk and corresponding to an absolute benefit in terms of disease-free survival of 4.7% at 3 years after randomization. The overall survival rate was not significantly different between the 2 groups. Severe toxic effects of exemestane were rare. Contralateral breast cancer developed in 20 patients in the tamoxifen group and in 9 patients in the exemestane group.

Conclusions.—This analysis found significant improvement in disease-free survival with exemestane therapy after 2 to 3 years of tamoxifen therapy compared with the standard 5 years of tamoxifen treatment.

▶ Continuing the theme of the interaction between HER2 status and response to hormonal therapy, Zhu et al (Abstract 2–25) studied HER2/neu overexpression before and after neoadjuvant treatment for 3 months with either exemestane or letrozole. There was a significant drop in HER2 overexpression by immunohistochemistry (11 of 16 reverted to negative) and by FISH (15 of 16 reverted to no amplification, and no patients negative initially became positive). These data suggest that antiaromatase therapy can inhibit overexpression of HER2/neu and can induce a high response rate in HER2-positive tumors (75% compared with 35% in HER2-negative tumors). Ellis et al (Abstract 2–26) examined 185 tumor samples from before and after neoadjuvant treatment with either tamoxifen or letrozole and identified a significantly greater reduction in Ki67 with letrozole, particularly in ER-positive tumors that overexpressed either HER1 or HER2. Other molecular effects studied favored letrozole as well. These 2 studies provide a molecular basis for regarding antiaromatase therapy as potentially superior to tamoxifen. The study of Coombes et al (Abstract 2–27) puts this information into practice in a randomized trial comparing exemestane to tamoxifen given after 2 to 3 years of tamoxifen adjuvant therapy in 4742 postmenopausal women. Exemestane achieved a 32% reduction in risk of recurrence without, as yet, a significant difference in overall survival (only 199 events for survival at the time of the report). There was also a significant reduction in the incidence of contralateral breast cancers with letrozole.

The data from these 3 trials, when combined with other reports of superiority of antiaromatase therapy in postmenopausal women, make a strong case for antiaromatase therapy as the first hormonal treatment of choice in postmenopausal women.

J. T. Thigpen, MD

Tamoxifen With or Without Breast Irradiation in Women 50 Years of Age or Older With Early Breast Cancer

Fyles AW, McCready DR, Manchul LA, et al (Univ of Toronto; British Columbia Cancer Agency, Vancouver, Canada)
N Engl J Med 351:963-976, 2004 2–28

Background.—Previous research has suggested that the risk of local relapse declines after 50 years of age in women who have had lumpectomy and irradiation. The role of adjuvant radiation therapy in women aged 50 years or older who had early breast cancer was investigated by comparing the patients treated with tamoxifen plus breast irradiation and those treated with tamoxifen alone.

Methods.—Seven hundred sixty-nine women with early breast cancer were enrolled in a randomized study between 1992 and 2000. All had tumors with a diameter of 5 cm or less. Three hundred eighty-six were assigned to breast irradiation plus tamoxifen, and 383 were assigned to tamoxifen alone. The patients were followed up for 5.6 years.

Findings.—The 5-year local relapse rates in the tamoxifen-only group and the tamoxifen plus radiation group were 7.7% and 0.6%. The corresponding 5-year disease-free survival rates were 84% and 91%, respectively. A subgroup analysis of 611 women with T1, receptor-positive tumors showed a benefit with radiotherapy; the 5-year local relapse rates were 0.4% in the combined therapy group and 5.9% in the monotherapy group. Overall, significant differences were observed in the axillary relapse rate at 5 years: 2.5% in patients receiving tamoxifen only and 0.5% in patients receiving tamoxifen plus irradiation. However, the rates of distant relapse and overall survival did not differ significantly.

Conclusions.—Adding radiation therapy to tamoxifen therapy appears to significantly reduce the local relapse rate in women aged 50 years or older with T1 or T2 node-negative breast cancer. In the current series of older women who had had lumpectomy, the local relapse rate at 5 years was only 0.6% in those receiving tamoxifen plus radiation therapy compared with 7.7% in those receiving tamoxifen alone.

Lumpectomy Plus Tamoxifen With or Without Irradiation in Women 70 Years of Age or Older With Early Breast Cancer

Hughes KS, for the Cancer and Leukemia Group B, Radiation Therapy Oncology Group, and Eastern Cooperative Oncology Group (Massachusetts Gen Hosp, Boston; et al)
N Engl J Med 351:971-984, 2004 2–29

Background.—Whether lumpectomy plus tamoxifen is as effective as lumpectomy followed by tamoxifen plus radiation therapy to treat early breast cancer in women aged 70 years or older is unclear. Whether women in this age group with early, estrogen-receptor-positive breast cancer can be treated safely with tamoxifen alone instead of irradiation plus tamoxifen was investigated.

Methods.—Six hundred thirty-six women aged 70 years or older with clinical stage I, estrogen-receptor-positive breast carcinoma were enrolled in the study between 1994 and 1999. By random assignment, 317 received tamoxifen plus radiation therapy after lumpectomy and 319 received tamoxifen alone after lumpectomy.

Findings.—The groups differed significantly only in the rate of local or regional recurrence at 5 years: 1% in women given combined therapy and 4% in those given tamoxifen alone. The groups did not differ in rates of mastectomy for local recurrence, distant metastases, or 5-year overall survival. Patient and physician assessment of cosmetic results and adverse events rated tamoxifen alone as superior to tamoxifen plus irradiation.

Conclusions.—Lumpectomy followed by tamoxifen alone appears to be a feasible alternative to adjuvant therapy with tamoxifen plus radiation therapy in women aged 70 years or older with early, estrogen-receptor-positive breast cancer. Patients and clinicians need to weigh the slightly increased risk of local recurrence against the adverse effects of irradiation. The needs of the patient should be considered in making treatment decisions.

▶ The need for 6 weeks of external beam radiotherapy (RT) after breast-conserving surgery is a major drawback to the procedure for some women. This is particularly true for older women with decreased mobility or the inability to obtain transportation. The studies by Fyles et al (Abstract 2–28) and Hughes et al (Abstract 2–29) address the issue of whether tamoxifen can substitute for RT in women with estrogen-receptor-positive breast carcinomas. Both studies confirm what was previously demonstrated in the National Surgical Adjuvant Breast and Bowel Project B21 study: local control is maximized with the use of both RT and tamoxifen.[1] However, for some subsets of women, the absolute benefit of RT is small. In the study of Hughes et al, which was restricted to women aged 70 years and older, the rate of locoregional recurrence at 5 years was 4% after tamoxifen alone and 1% after tamoxifen plus RT. In a planned subset analysis of 611 women of all ages with the same tumor characteristics in the Fyles et al study, the local recurrence rate at 5 years was reduced from 5.9% to 0.4% with the addition of RT. These studies clearly suggest that the omission of RT for older women with stage I breast cancer is a consideration.

Several caveats apply to this observation. First, the follow-up interval of both studies is relatively short. In the Fyles et al study, the local recurrence rate increased from 7.7% at 5 years to 17.6% at 8 years.[1] In the United States, the life expectancy of a 70-year-old women is approximately 14.3 years, a significant time period at risk for local recurrence. Although no survival differences were observed between treatment groups, local recurrence is a psychologically morbid occurrence. In the Hughes et al study, as in other trials of conservative surgery without RT, 50% of patients with local recurrence were treated with mastectomy, indicating that further breast preservation is not desired or is not possible in a significant number of patients.[2]

Finally, for the subset of women with tumors less than 1 cm in size and negative nodes, tamoxifen is an optional treatment. It is worth considering whether trading 6 weeks of RT for 5 years of tamoxifen improves the risk/benefit ratio of treatment. RT is well tolerated in older women, and the side effects, primarily related to cosmesis and fatigue, are maximal in the early posttreatment period.[3] Tamoxifen, although also well tolerated, does have potentially life-threatening side effects, such as an increased risk of thrombosis and an increased risk of endometrial carcinoma.

In the end, the decision to use RT after lumpectomy in older women with small, estrogen-receptor-positive breast cancers is a highly individual one that will depend on the presence of comorbid conditions, the anticipated life span, and a woman's attitude toward small risks and benefits of treatment. These studies provide important information on the risk of local recurrence after excision alone in a well-characterized population and indicate that excision alone is a viable option for some women.

M. Morrow, MD

References

1. Fisher B, Bryant J, Dignam JJ, et al: Tamoxifen, radiation therapy, or both for prevention of ipsilateral breast tumor recurrence after lumpectomy in women with invasive breast cancers of 1 cm or less. *J Clin Oncol* 20:4141-4149, 2002.
2. Morrow M, Harris JR, Schnitt S: Local control following breast conserving surgery for invasive cancer: Results of clinical trials. *J Natl Cancer Inst* 87:1669-1673, 1995.
3. Toonkel LJ, Fix I, Jacobson LH, et al: Management of elderly patients with primary breast cancer. *Int J Radiol Oncol Biol Phys* 14:677-681, 1998.

Benefit and Projected Cost-Effectiveness of Anastrozole Versus Tamoxifen as Initial Adjuvant Therapy for Patients With Early-Stage Estrogen Receptor–Positive Breast Cancer

Hillner BE (Virginia Commonwealth Univ, Richmond)

Cancer 101:1311-1322, 2004 2–30

Background.—The largest subgroup of patients with breast cancer are women with estrogen receptor (ER)–positive disease of postmenopausal onset who receive tamoxifen as standard adjuvant therapy. Anastrozole has been found to significantly decrease breast cancer recurrence rate; however, it does not appear to increase survival rates at 4 years. The disease-free survival (DFS) rate and potential survival benefits associated with anastrozole use were investigated.

Methods.—In a computer simulation model, the outcomes of 64-year-old women with ER-positive breast cancer subsequently given anastrozole or tamoxifen for 5 years were estimated. Data from an ongoing randomized study were used to determine daily recurrence risks and the relative risks correlated with various treatment-related events. End points were recurrence-free survival, anticipated survival resulting from an anastrozole-induced reduction in systemic disease recurrence rates, and survival adjusted for quality of life and hip fracture risk for 4, 12, and 20 years.

TABLE 4.—Baseline Results in Anastrozole Arm and Baseline Differences Between Anastrozole Arm and Tamoxifen Arm[a]

	Projection Horizon (Yrs)			
	4	8	12	20
Endpoint 1: DFS[b]				
DFS (%)	88.1	73.7	59.0	29.5
Increase in DFS (%)	1.8	3.4	4.1	3.4
Median increase in DFS duration (days)	14	47	88	161
Cost per yr of DFS gained ($)	167,500	60,700	32,800	16,700
Endpoint 2: Projected survival[c]				
Death rate (%)	5.8	16.3	28.9	58.2
Increase in overall survival (%)	0.4	1.1	1.6	1.8
Median increase in survival (days)	2	11	26	60
Increase in cost ($)	6353	7264	6907	6699
Cost per life yr gained ($)	1,112,000	235,400	96,000	40,600
Endpoint 3: Projected survival with quality-of-life adjustments for nonfatal outcomes and for projected differences in hip fracture risk				
Median increase in quality-adjusted survival (days)	4	14	26	45
Cost per QALY gained ($)	533,000	201,800	111,300	75,900

Abbreviation: QALY Quality-adjusted life-years.

[a]Benefit estimates are rounded to the nearest whole day, and cost estimates are rounded to the nearest $100. Benefits and costs were discounted at a rate of 3% per year. Patients were aged 64 years at baseline.

[b]Freedom from contralateral breast cancer, local recurrence, systemic recurrence, or death from any cause.

[c]For anastrozole arm, overall survival projection included a survival benefit associated with an observed reduction in risk of systemic recurrence.

(Courtesy of Hillner BE: Benefit and projected cost-effectiveness of anastrozole versus tamoxifen as initial adjuvant therapy for patients with early-stage estrogen receptor–positive breast cancer. *Cancer* 101:1311-1322, 2004. Copyright 2004 American Cancer Society. Reprinted by permission of Wiley-Liss, Inc, a subsidiary of John Wiley & Sons, Inc.)

Findings.—The projected 4-year DFS benefit associated with anastrozole was 14 days, with an incremental cost effectiveness (ICE) of $167,500 per year (Table 4). Projected into the future by 12 and 20 years, DFS benefit rose to 2.9 and 5.3 months, respectively. The corresponding overall survival benefits were 0.9 and 2 months, respectively, with ICE declining to less than $100,000 per life-year when the projection horizon surpassed 12 years. Including quality-of-life weightings for nonfatal outcomes modestly favored anastrozole in the short term. However, if anastrozole use correlated with an increased risk of hip fracture, the long-term benefit related to anastrozole declined by approximately 25%.

Conclusions.—Adjuvant anastrozole was projected to lead to marked improvements in DFS for patients with breast cancer. If this DFS benefit were to result in a survival benefit, the ICE of anastrozole use would be acceptable for patients expected to live for more than 12 years.

▶ The Arimidex, Tamoxifen Alone or in Combination (ATAC) trial has demonstrated a small but statistically significant disease-free survival benefit for anastrozole compared with tamoxifen at 4 years.[1] Toxicities vary between the 2 drugs, and anastrozole is significantly more expensive than tamoxifen. This has engendered considerable controversy regarding which agent is the adjuvant treatment of choice for postmenopausal women with hormone-sensitive breast cancer. This model demonstrates the extremely modest benefits associated with anastrozole therapy and the associated costs. After 4 years of treatment the median increase in quality-adjusted survival with anastrozole is only 4 days, at a cost of $533,000 per quality-adjusted life-years gained. After 12 years, this increases to 26 days, at a cost of $111,300 per life-year. If agents to prevent bone fracture are used in conjunction with anastrozole, costs increase. This study provides clinicians with food for thought about the costs to society of new treatments and emphasizes the importance of appropriate patient selection for costly therapies with significant but small benefits.

M. Morrow, MD

Reference

1. Baum M, Buzdar A, Cuzick J, et al: Anastrozole alone or in combination with tamoxifen versus tamoxifen alone for adjuvant treatment of postmenopausal women with early stage breast cancer: Results of the ATAC (Arimidex, Tamoxifen Alone or in Combination) trial efficacy and safety update analyses. *Cancer* 98:1802-1810, 2003.

Advanced

Intravenous Iron Optimizes the Response to Recombinant Human Erythropoietin in Cancer Patients With Chemotherapy-Related Anemia: A Multicenter, Open-Label, Randomized Trial

Auerbach M, Ballard H, Trout JR, et al (Averbach Hematology-Oncology, Baltimore, Md; New York Univ; Rutgers Univ, New Brunswick, NJ; et al)

J Clin Oncol 22:1301-1307, 2004 2–31

Background.—Mild to moderate anemia occurs in up to 75% of cancer patients receiving chemotherapy, radiation therapy, or both. This anemia is marked by serum erythropoietin levels elevated above normal but not to the degree seen in iron-deficiency anemia and hemolytic anemia. Administration of recombinant human erythropoietin alfa (rHuEPO) has been shown to increase hemoglobin (Hb) levels in anemic cancer patients. As a result, transfusion requirements are decreased and quality of life (QOL) is improved. However, these responses are slow to develop, and 30% to 50% of cancer patients do not achieve a meaningful response. IV iron supplementation has been used successfully in patients with chronic kidney disease to improve the Hb response to rHuEPO therapy. Administration of IV iron to cancer patients has been avoided because of the risk of anaphylaxis associated with iron dextran, which is a rare event. The effect of combined rHuEPO and iron therapy and the optimal route of iron administration (oral or IV) for cancer patients with chemotherapy-related anemia were evaluated.

Methods.—The 157 participants had Hb levels of 105 g/L or less, and serum ferritin levels of 450 pmol/L or less, or serum ferritin levels of 675 pmol/L or less with transferrin saturation of 19% or less. All participants received rHuEPO 40,000 U once a week subcutaneously. They were randomly assigned to receive no iron (36 patients), oral iron 325 mg twice a day

(43 patients), iron dextran repeated 100 mg IV bolus (37 patients), or iron dextran total dose infusion (TDI; 41 patients). QOL and Hb determinations were obtained at baseline and weekly thereafter.

Results.—A total of 132 patients completed at least 6 weeks of therapy or all bolus treatments. All treatment groups had significant increases in Hb levels from baseline. The mean increases were 9 g/L with no iron, 15 g/L with oral iron, 25 g/L with IV bolus iron, and 24 g/L with TDI iron. Both IV iron groups had significantly higher mean Hb increases than the no-iron or oral iron groups. Hb responses were independent of baseline transferrin saturation levels, chemotherapy toxicity, cancer diagnosis, and disease response. A significantly higher percentage of patients receiving IV iron had a hematopoietic response than in the oral and no-iron groups. Of the TDI and IV bolus groups, 68% had a hematopoietic response; 25% of the no-iron and 36% of the oral iron groups responded. The IV iron groups had improved energy, activity, and QOL measures. The no-iron group had a slight decrease in activity, and the oral iron group had a small change in activity and overall QOL. Increased Hb levels correlated significantly with improved energy, activity, and overall QOL. When iron was given with rHuEPO, improved Hb levels were achieved after a mean of 6 weeks rather than the 8 weeks or more usually required. Adverse events developed in 7 patients, with 3 in the TDI group, 3 in the bolus group, and 1 in the oral iron group. Twenty-two patients had a clinically significant decline in Hb level after having treatment and were classified as treatment failures. These patients were given transfusions (19 patients) or parenteral iron therapy (3 patients).

Conclusions.—Hb levels were increased with rHuEPO therapy with or without iron supplementation, producing better QOL. IV iron plus rHuEPO therapy produced significantly greater Hb increases than oral iron supplements plus rHuEPO. The response to rHuEPO was achieved in 6 weeks rather than the 8 weeks usually required.

► Erythropoietin is widely used to raise Hb levels to above 12 g/dL in order to minimize fatigue and to improve the QOL of patients. This role is supported by extensive studies (phase I-II, phase III, and phase IV trials). More recently, reports that suggest a survival benefit associated with Hb levels above 12 g/dL during chemoradiation have emerged in cancers of the cervix and the head and neck. A study by Bottini et al[1] evaluated 144 patients treated with neoadjuvant therapy for breast carcinoma to determine whether Hb level during chemotherapy (CMF or epirubicin) related to outcome. Their observations are similar to the reports in carcinomas of the cervix and head and neck. Hb levels above 12.5 g/dL were associated with a better survival in a multivariate analysis that accounted for other significant prognostic factors. Although not definitive by any means, this adds one more piece of supporting evidence for maintaining Hb levels above 12 g/dL during chemotherapy, radiotherapy, or both.

Of related interest is this report of Auerbach et al, which shows that the magnitude and rate of Hb increase and QOL improvement can be enhanced by the concurrent use of IV iron.

J. T. Thigpen, MD

Reference

1. Bottini A, Berruti A, Brizzi MP, et al: Pretreatment haemoglobin levels significantly predict the tumour response to primary chemotherapy in human breast cancer. *Br J Cancer* 89:977-982, 2003. (2004 YEAR BOOK OF ONCOLOGY, p 366.)

Multicenter Randomized Trial Comparing Sequential With Concomitant Administration of Doxorubicin and Docetaxel as First-Line Treatment of Metastatic Breast Cancer: A Spanish Breast Cancer Research Group (GEICAM-9903) Phase III Study

Alba E, Martín M, Ramos M, et al (Complejo Hospitalario Virgen de la Victoria, Málaga, Spain; Hosp Universitario San Carlos, Spain; Centro Oncológico Regional, La Coruña; et al)

J Clin Oncol 22:2587-2593, 2004 2–32

Introduction.—The sequential administration of doxorubicin and docetaxel (A→T) may preserve antitumor efficacy and decrease the incidence and severity of toxicity in patients with metastatic breast cancer. This randomized, multicenter, phase III trial is the first known to assess whether A→T decreases the incidence of hematologic toxicity, particularly the incidence of febrile neutropenia versus concomitant administration (AT) in patients with metastatic breast cancer.

Methods.—A total of 144 patients with metastatic breast cancer were randomly assigned to receive either 3 cycles of doxorubicin 75 mg/m^2 every 21 days followed by 3 cycles of docetaxel 100 mg/m^2 every 21 days (A→T) or 6 cycles of AT 50 mg/m^2 every 21 days. Patients who had prior anthracycline treatment received 2 cycles of doxorubicin followed by 4 cycles of docetaxel (A→T) or 3 cycles of AT followed by 3 cycles of docetaxel 100 mg/m^2 every 21 days.

Results.—Febrile neutropenia occurred less frequently in the A→T arm (29.3% of patients; 6.9% of cycles) compared with the AT arm (47.8% of patients; 14.8% of cycles; $P = .02$ and $P = .004$, respectively). Asthenia, diarrhea, and fever were more common in the AT than in the A→T arm. Overall response rates were 61% (95% confidence interval, 50%-72%) and 51% (95% confidence interval, 39%-63%) in the A→T and AT arms. Median duration of response was 8.7 months and 7.6 months in the A→T and AT arms, respectively; median time to progression was 10.5 and 9.2 months, respectively; and median overall survival was 22.3 months and 21.8 months, respectively (P = not significant).

Conclusion.—The A→T arm significantly diminished febrile neutropenia compared with AT in patients with metastatic breast cancer and maintains comparable antitumoral efficacy; it may be a valid treatment option in this patient population.

Failure of Higher-Dose Paclitaxel to Improve Outcome in Patients With Metastatic Breast Cancer: Cancer and Leukemia Group B Trial 9342

Winer EP, Berry DA, Woolf S, et al (Dana-Farber/Partners Cancer Care, Boston; State Univ of New York, Syracuse; Mount Sinai School of Medicine, New York; et al)

J Clin Oncol 22:2061-2068, 2004 2–33

Introduction.—Several trials have compared various doses and schedules of paclitaxel. The Cancer and Leukemia Group B Protocol 9342 was initiated to ascertain the optimal dose of paclitaxel administered as a 3-hour infusion every 3 weeks to women with metastatic breast cancer.

Methods.—A total of 474 women with metastatic breast cancer who had received 1 or no prior chemotherapy regimens were randomly assigned to 1 of 3 paclitaxel dosing regimens: 175 mg/m^2, 210 mg/m^2, or 250 mg/m^2. Each regimen was administered as a 3-hour infusion every 3 weeks. Women completed self-administered quality of life and symptom assessment questionnaires at baseline and after 3 treatment cycles.

Results.—No evidence of a significant dose-response relation was seen over the dose range evaluated. Treatment response rates were 23%, 26%, and 21%, respectively, for the 175, 210, and 250 mg/m^2 regimens. A marginally significant correlation (P = .04) was observed between dose and time to progression. In multivariate analysis, the difference was less apparent. No statistically significant difference was observed in survival. Neurotoxicity and hematologic toxicity were more severe with the higher dose arms. Quality of life was similar for the 3 treatment arms.

Conclusion.—Higher doses of paclitaxel administered as a 3-hour infusion to women with metastatic breast cancer did not enhance response rate, survival, or quality of life. There was a slight improvement in time to progression with higher dose therapy; this was offset by greater toxicity. When a 3-hour infusion of paclitaxel is administered every 3 weeks, the 175 mg/m^2 dose is optimal.

High-Dose Chemotherapy With Autologous Hematopoietic Stem-Cell Support Compared With Standard-Dose Chemotherapy in Breast Cancer Patients With 10 or More Positive Lymph Nodes: First Results of a Randomized Trial

Zander AR, Kröger N, Schmoor C, et al (Univ Hosp Hamburg-Eppendorf, Germany; Albertinen-Hospital, Hamburg, Germany; Univ Hosp, Freiburg, Germany; et al)

J Clin Oncol 22:2273-2283, 2004 2–34

Introduction.—The role of high-dose chemotherapy (HD-CT) in breast cancer remains controversial, and the optimal regimen needs to be defined. The therapeutic effect of HD-CT followed by autologous hematopoietic stem cell support was compared in a randomized trial with that of standard-dose chemotherapy (SD-CT) in patients with primary breast cancer and 10 or more positive axillary lymph nodes.

Methods.—A total of 307 patients were randomly assigned to receive (after 4 IV cycles of epirubicin 90 mg/m^2 and cyclophosphamide 600 mg/m^2 every 21 days) either HD-CT of cyclophosphamide 1500 mg/m^2, thiotepa 150 mg/m^2, and mitoxantrone 10 mg/m^2 IV for 4 consecutive days followed by stem cell support; or SD-CT in 3 cycles of cyclophosphamide 500 mg/m^2, methotrexate 30 mg/m^2, and fluorouracil 600 mg/m^2 IV on days 1 and 8, every 28 days. The major end point was event-free survival.

Results.—At a median follow-up of 3.8 years, there were 144 events in terms of event-free survival (HD-CT, 63 events; SD-CT, 81 events). The first event of failure (HD-CT vs SD-CT) was an isolated locoregional recurrence (9 vs 11 cases), a distant failure (52 vs 68 cases), and death without recurrence (2 vs 2). The estimated relative risk of HD-CT compared with SD-CT was 0.75 (95% confidence interval, 0.54-1.06; $P = .095$). Overall survival was not significantly different between groups (HD-CT, 40 deaths; SD-CT, 49 deaths).

Conclusion.—There was a trend for better event-free survival for HD-CT (P = not significant). Further follow-up and a meta-analysis of all randomized trials will show the effect of HD-CT compared with SD-CT as adjuvant treatment in patients with high-risk primary breast cancer.

▶ Front-line chemotherapy for breast carcinoma continues to be an evolving area of management. Although these 3 studies (Abstracts 2–32 to 2–34) do not provide definitive information for a change in the standard of care, they do provide useful information for purposes of clinical decision making. Alba et al (Abstract 2–32) evaluate the relative merits of concurrent versus sequential use of an anthracycline and a taxane. As has been the case in other similar trials, no differences in efficacy were observed. The sequential regimen was associated with less febrile neutropenia. These data support the validity of the sequential rather than concurrent use of chemotherapeutic agents. It must be emphasized, however, that the regimen here does not use the second agent at relapse but rather as a part of a sequential combination regimen (3 cycles of one agent followed immediately by 3 cycles of the other agent). This is not necessarily the same as single-agent therapy followed by another single agent as salvage therapy at relapse; rather, it is likely simply another way of delivering combination chemotherapy. The appeal of such an approach is that it facilitates the addition of new agents in sequence later without the worry of overlapping acute toxicities associated with the concurrent use of drugs.

The randomized trial by Winer et al (Abstract 2–33) compared 175 mg/m^2 to 210 mg/m^2 to 250 mg/m^2 of paclitaxel in metastatic breast cancer. Response rates and survival were the same for all 3, and there was only a marginal advantage in time to progression for higher doses. Toxicity, as one would expect, escalated significantly as dose increased. The optimal dose and schedule for paclitaxel would thus appear to be the same as in ovarian carcinoma: 175 mg/m^2 over 3 hours every 3 weeks.

The trial of Zander et al (Abstract 2–34) evaluated HD-CT with stem cell support as adjuvant therapy for women with breast carcinoma and 10 or more positive nodes. High-dose cyclophosphamide, thiotepa, and mitoxantrone produced no statistically significant advantages in efficacy. This result is consistent with other reports of HD-CT in breast carcinoma and does not support the use of this approach outside clinical trials.

J. T. Thigpen, MD

Compliance With Consensus Recommendations for Systemic Therapy Is Associated With Improved Survival of Women With Node-Negative Breast Cancer

Hébert-Croteau N, Brisson J, Latreille J, et al (Institut Natl de Santé Publique Du Québec, Canada; Hôpital Charles LeMoyne; Québec, Canada; Centre Intégré de Lutte Contre Le Cancer De La Montérégie, Greenfield Park, Canada; et al)

J Clin Oncol 22:3685-3693, 2004 2–35

Introduction.—The impact of consensus recommendations for systemic therapy on disease outcome is not clearly elucidated. Time trends in systemic adjuvant therapy among women diagnosed with localized, node-negative breast cancer were evaluated to determine whether adherence to guidelines is linked with improved survival.

Methods.—Data were obtained by medical record review, linkage with administrative databases, and queries to attending physicians regarding women diagnosed with invasive node-negative breast cancer from 1988 to 1989, 1991 to 1992, and 1993 to 1994. Guidelines from the 1992 St Galien conference were regarded as standard of care. Survival was estimated by Kaplan-Meier and Cox proportional hazards analyses.

Results.—Of 1541 women evaluated, 358 died before December 1999. The median follow-up was 6.8 years. The 7-year event-free survival was 66%; overall survival was 81%. Survival was 88%, 84%, and 74% in women who were at minimal, moderate, or high risk of recurrent disease. Most women at minimal risk were treated according to consensus (98.4% of 370). By comparison, adjusted hazard ratios of death were 1.0 (95% confidence interval [CI], 0.6-1.7) and 2.3 (95% CI, 1.3-4.0) among women at moderate risk treated according to the consensus, or not, respectively. Among women at high risk, adjusted hazard ratios of death were 2.0 (95% CI, 1.4-2.8) and 2.7 (95% CI, 1.9-3.9), respectively. Both risk category ($P < .0005$) and compliance with guidelines ($P < .0005$) were independently predictive of survival (Fig 1).

Conclusion.—Treatment according to consensus guidelines is linked with improved survival of women with breast cancer. Adoption of guidelines would be a beneficial strategy for disease control.

▶ Therapeutic guidelines have not always been well received by the medical community. An argument against their use is that guidelines do not promote "tailoring" of treatment to the individual patient's health status. This study suggests that patients treated according to a relatively general guideline pro-

FIGURE 1.

A

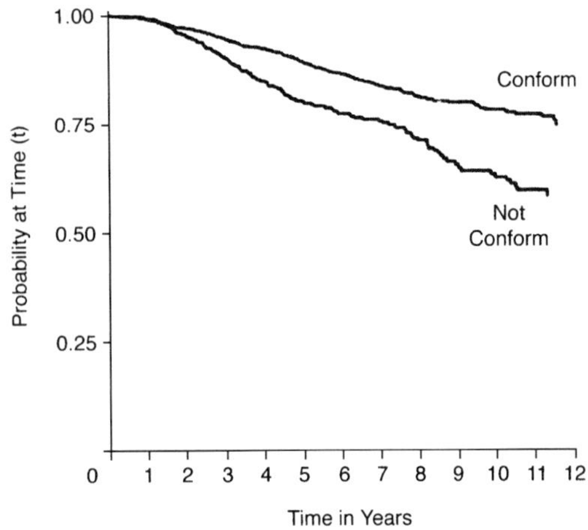

YEARS	1	3	5	7	10
Conform to Consensus					
At Risk	778	710	639	369	144
Cum. Events	9	75	145	185	218
Not Conform to Consensus					
At Risk	378	342	303	189	86
Cum. Events	3	37	76	90	115

B

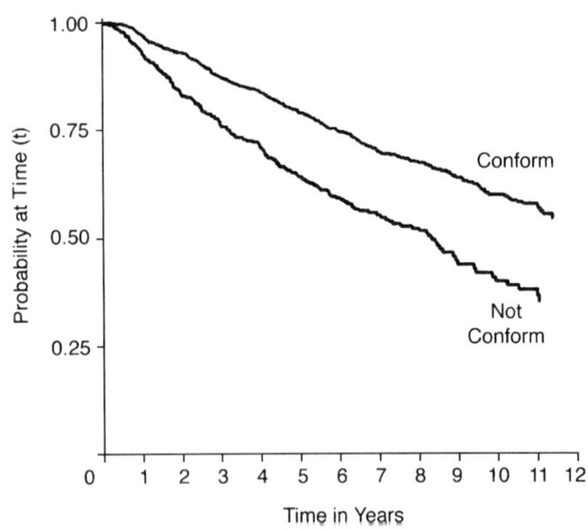

YEARS	1	3	5	7	10
Conform to Consensus					
At Risk	1102	960	808	405	146
Cum. Events	32	140	231	306	341
Not Conform to Consensus					
At Risk	346	276	217	109	40
Cum. Events	25	87	130	156	177

posed by the 1992 St Galien Consensus Conference[1] had better survival than those treated outside the guideline. In addition, the relatively simple risk stratification schema used in the St Galien Consensus Conference, which incorporated age, tumor size, receptor status, and histologic grade, was sufficient to identify patients with statistically different risks of breast cancer recurrence. The findings of this study are particularly noteworthy since the consensus process was one of expert consensus that took place over a brief time interval, indicating that relatively low-cost, rapid development of guidelines does have the ability to affect clinical care.

M. Morrow, MD

Reference

1. Glick JH, Gelber RD, Goldhirsh A, et al: Meeting highlights: Adjuvant therapy for primary breast cancer. *J Natl Cancer Inst* 84:1479-1485, 1992.

FIGURE 1.—Overall survival (**A**; $P < .00005$) and event-free survival (**B**; $P < .00005$) according to conformity of treatment with guidelines. *P* value is for comparison of women treated according to consensus vs otherwise for each outcome. *Abbreviation: Cum*, Cumulative. (Courtesy of Hébert-Croteau N, Brisson J, Latreille J, et al: Compliance with consensus recommendations for systemic therapy is associated with improved survival of women with node-negative breast cancer. *J Clin Oncol* 22:3685-3693, 2004. Reprinted with permission from the American Society of Clinical Oncology.)

3 Gynecology

Ovarian

Prognostic Significance of *p53* Mutation and p53 Overexpression in Advanced Epithelial Ovarian Cancer: A Gynecologic Oncology Group Study

Havrilesky L, Darcy KM, Hamdan H, et al (Duke Univ, Durham, NC; Roswell Park Cancer Inst, Buffalo, NY; Quest Diagnostics Nichols Inst, San Juan Capistrano, Calif; et al)

J Clin Oncol 21:3814-3825, 2003 3–1

Background.—Mutations of the *p53* gene are often found in ovarian and other cancers. This multifunctional tumor suppressor normally interacts with various proteins that contribute to transcriptional regulation, DNA repair, cell-cycle progression, apoptosis, and proteosome-mediated protein degradation. The role of normal and altered *p53* in cancer is under investigation, with much debate over links between *p53* gene mutations and patient outcomes. The prognostic significance attached to *p53* mutations and its overexpression in advanced epithelial ovarian cancers were evaluated.

Methods.—The study included 125 patients with primary tumors who participated in a Gynecologic Oncology Group randomized phase III treatment protocol. RNA or genomic DNA extracted from frozen samples of their tumors were subjected to mutational analysis of *p53*. Overexpression of *p53* in fixed tumor was evaluated using an immunohistochemical assay.

Results.—Of 109 frozen ovarian tumors, 84 (77%) had a mutation in exons 2 to 11 of *p53*. Three of these had 2 distinct mutations; the other 81 had a single mutation. Mutations were often observed (60% of the 124 cancers tested) in exons 5 to 8, the DNA-binding domain. Eleven percent of patients had mutations outside of this region. Fifty-five percent of the tumors tested had nuclear staining consistent with *p53* overexpression in more than 30% of the cancer cells, with strong staining found in 75% to 100% of the cancer cells in most cases. The presence of a missense mutation in exons 2 to 11 of the *p53* gene and the overexpression of the p53 protein were especially strongly connected. Ninety-six percent of the tumors with missense mutation(s) within these exons that overexpressed *p53* had extensive overexpression. Mutation within exons 2 to 11 of *p53* was associated with histologic subtype. Mutation within exons 5 to 8 was associated with both histologic subtype and poorer initial performance score. Overexpression of *p53* was often found in tumors with poorer initial performance status and lower histologic grade. Extensive *p53* overexpression showed no correlation with any patient or tumor characteristics evaluated. Compared to no mutation, a mutation in exons 2 to 11 of *p53* was linked to a 70% reduction in the risk of death for women who had primary advanced epithelial ovarian cancer. However, this advantage disappeared about 2.5 years after diagnosis. In addition, compared to no mutation, a mutation in exons 5 to 8 of *p53* was linked to a reduction in death risk that increased with time. No relationship was found between the overexpression of *p53* and patient outcome.

Conclusions.—Alterations in the *p53* gene are often found in women with advanced epithelial ovarian cancer. In short-term follow-up, patients who have such a mutation have a survival benefit over those who lack a mutation, but the benefit disappears with long-term follow-up. The overexpression of *p53* is not associated with any survival benefit or decrement. Further roles for *p53* in regulating therapeutic responsiveness and patient outcome have yet to be determined.

The Impact of p53 Protein Core Domain Structural Alteration on Ovarian Cancer Survival

Rose SL, Robertson AD, Goodheart MJ, et al (Univ of Iowa, Iowa City)
Clin Cancer Res 9:4139-4144, 2003 3–2

Background.—Improved diagnostic and therapeutic approaches are anticipated if molecular prognostic markers can be identified for ovarian cancer. Among the factors under investigation is the *p53* gene, which is a tumor suppressor gene whose mutations are found in up to 50% of all human cancers. About 60% of all ovarian malignancies have mutations of *p53*. Survival with a *p53* missense mutation varies greatly from patient to patient. However, a *p53*-null mutation predicts an adverse prognosis for advanced stage ovarian cancer. A structure function analysis of the p53 protein was used to assess ovarian cancer survival to determine whether all missense mutations were equivalent.

Methods.—*p53* gene sequencing was done using 267 consecutive ovarian cancers. The International Agency for Research on Cancer *p53* Mutational Database was used because it specifies the effects of *p53* mutations on *p53* core domain structure. The effect of the individual missense mutations was thus identified and classified as explained or not explained in structural or functional terms on the basis of their predicted effects on protein folding, protein-DNA contacts, or mutation in highly conserved residues. Classification of null mutations was based on their mechanism of origin.

Results.—Eighty-two missense and 43 null *p53* gene mutations were found. Of the 82 patients with the missense mutations, 63% have died of their disease; of the 43 patients with null mutations, 81% are dead of their disease. Alterations in the p53 protein explained the effects of 76% of the missense mutations, leaving 24% unexplained. Explained mutations did not show any links to stage, grade, residual disease, or nonserous tumor histology. Twenty-eight percent of the explained mutations were in highly conserved regions of the p53 core protein. No difference in survival was noted between patients with explained and those with unexplained mutations. No relationships were found between survival and structurally explained or unexplained mutations, between missense mutations at highly conserved residues or not highly conserved residues, or between missense mutations at DNA binding residues and those at non-DNA binding residues. The median survival with a mutation resulting from a point mutation was the same as that found with a mutation resulting from a frameshift mechanism. Survival was significantly compromised when a null mutation of any type was present, with a median of 1.9 years rather than the 4.0 years found for the presence of any missense mutation.

Conclusions.—Because survival was independent of missense mutation type and mechanism of null mutation, the proposition that not all missense mutations are equivalent was not supported. Structural alterations in the p53 core domain resulting from missense point mutation were not functionally equivalent to *p53*-null mutations. The mutation mechanism for a *p53*-null mutation did not correlate with the poor prognosis that accompanies *p53*-null alterations.

▶ These 2 studies by Havrilesky et al and Rose et al (Abstracts 3–1 and 3–2) examined ovarian carcinoma specimens with regard to *p53* mutations and overexpression in an effort to understand better this most common of genetic alterations in advanced ovarian carcinoma. The *p53* gene is a tumor suppressor gene. Null mutations of the *p53* gene are associated with poor outcome. Rose and colleagues (Abstract 3–2) postulated that *p53* missense mutations in critical loci that result in modifications of protein structure would have an adverse prognostic impact as compared to those missense mutations involving less critical portions of the gene. For reasons that are not clear, no correlation between such mutations and outcome could be identified in a study of 125 tumor specimens. Only null mutations were clearly associated with an adverse outcome. Havrilesky and colleagues from the Gynecologic Oncology Group (Abstract 3–1) actually identified a short-term survival benefit from missense mutations in exons 2 through 11. If the mutation was associated with overexpression of *p53*, this short-term survival benefit was not observed. The 2 trials demonstrate once again how common *p53* mutations are, but neither sheds light on the impact of specific mutations other than *p53*-null mutations on outcome. Further studies will be required to provide a better understanding of this common genetic alteration in its various forms.

J. T. Thigpen, MD

Biology of Epithelial Ovarian Cancer: Implications for Screening Women at High Genetic Risk

Hogg R, Friedlander M (Prince of Wales Hosp, Sydney, Australia)

J Clin Oncol 22:1315-1327, 2004 3–3

Background.—The 5-year survival rate for women with stage I ovarian cancer is greater than 85% but that for women with advanced ovarian cancer is only 25%. Therefore, it has been assumed that finding these cancers at an earlier stage would improve survival. However, real differences are found between the various histologic subtypes of invasive epithelial ovarian cancer, and these have been ignored in the screening programs to date. The published literature was evaluated to determine the clinicopathologic features of screening-detected ovarian cancers in women who are at high population or genetic risk for the development of ovarian cancer.

Methods.—The studies were published between 1988 and April 2003. The population screened and the primary screening modalities used formed the basis for categorizing the studies. Items sought in each study were the histologic type, stage, and grade of cancer detected on screening. Included in the review were studies of prophylactically removed ovaries from women at high risk of ovarian cancer.

Results.—Most ovarian cancers identified by CA125 screening in the general population and in women with increased genetic risk were not early stage high-grade serous tumors. The tumors found on screening were primarily high-stage cancers. Risk groups could be formed on the basis of an algorithm to determine the probability of ovarian cancer, which incorporated the individual's age and rate of change of CA125 level and the absolute CA125 value. With transvaginal US screening of the ovaries plus measurement of CA125, a more common approach than CA125 alone, most (44%) primary ovarian cancers were stage I and were borderline, germ-cell, or granulosa-cell tumors. Only 29 were invasive epithelial ovarian cancers. Serous cancers or adenocarcinomas were relatively scarce among the stage I tumors. Among a heterogeneous group of women scanned annually or every 6 months beginning at age 25 or 30 years, most of the cancers diagnosed for histologic subtype and grade were documented as grade 3 serous cancers. When high-risk women were screened, only one quarter of the cancers found were stage I at diagnosis. Many solid tumors progressed inexorably from stage I to stage IV, but stage I ovarian tumors differed biologically from advanced stage cancers. These biologic differences may explain the better prognosis rather than early diagnosis. Women found to have early stage tumors also tended to have significantly larger primary tumors than women with advanced-stage disease. In addition, advanced-stage disease tended to be poorly differentiated, and early stage disease was more likely to be well or moderately differentiated. Diploidy was more likely in stage I tumors and aneuploidy in advanced-stage tumors. The advanced-stage tumors were also more likely to be serous and undifferentiated, whereas the early stage lesions accounted for 75% of the mucinous, endometroid, and clear-cell carcinomas and only 20% of the serous cancers.

Conclusions.—Clinicopathologic differences may influence survival in women with ovarian cancer more than screening for early diagnosis. Prospective screening trials in high-risk populations are advisable. The most effective management approach is bilateral salpingo-oophorectomy. Women with a high genetic risk who are screened routinely require thorough briefing on the lack of proven benefit and low likelihood of detecting early stage serous cancers.

► This study examined the clinicopathologic features (histology, stage, and grade) of screen-detected ovarian cancers in 31 published screening studies between 1988 and 2003. Of the stage I tumors detected by screening, almost half were either borderline ovarian tumors, granulose-cell tumors, or germ-cell tumors. Of stage I invasive celomic epithelial carcinomas, most were other than serous tumors. Since most ovarian cancers that occur in the high-risk population are serous celomic epithelial carcinomas, and these are infrequently detected by screening, this further diminishes the potential for current screening methods to reduce the mortality rate in high-risk women. These observations have major implications for discussions of screening with serial CA125 and transvaginal US in that they indicate a low likelihood of benefit.

J. T. Thigpen, MD

Prediction of Optimal Versus Suboptimal Cytoreduction of Advanced-Stage Serous Ovarian Cancer With the Use of Microarrays

Berchuck A, Iversen ES, Lancaster JM, et al (Duke Univ, Durham, NC)

Am J Obstet Gynecol 190:910-925, 2004 3–4

Background.—Substantial improvements in median survival time have been obtained for advanced-stage ovarian cancer even though cure rates have not changed notably for 25 years. Surgical debulking has been suggested as contributing to the improved survival. However, it is possible that the underlying tumor biological condition predetermines outcome, with surgical debulking simply more feasible in cancers that are less virulent or more responsive to chemotherapy. The analysis of arrays of genes has led to predictions concerning clinical phenotypes in various solid tumors. Patterns of gene expression were evaluated to see if they can differentiate optimally from suboptimally debulked advanced-stage serous ovarian cancers. If distinct molecular patterns were to exist, they would support the contribution of biological differences rather than cytoreduction in determining outcome.

Methods.—RNA was obtained from 44 advanced-stage serous ovarian cancers and assessed with microarrays containing more than 22,000 genes. Nineteen of the cancers represented optimal and 25 suboptimal debulked tumors. On the basis of the relationship between genes and debulking status, the top 120 differentially expressed genes were identified. A predictive model was constructed using these 120 genes and subjected to out-of-sample cross-validation procedures.

Results.—Of the survivors who lived less than 3 years, the 5 optimally debulked patients had a median survival of 22 months, and the 16 suboptimally debulked patients had a median survival of 16 months. For long-term survivors, the 14 optimally debulked patients had a median survival of 104 months, and the 9 suboptimally debulked patients had a median survival of 91 months. Of the top 120 genes, 17 had greater than 2-fold differences in expression between optimal and suboptimal cancers. Thirty-two genes were used to construct a predictive model. The model misclassified 5 (20%) of 25 suboptimally debulked samples and 7 (37%) of 19 optimally debulked samples. Overall, the panel of 32 genes had a 72.7% predictive accuracy. Data that were based on clusters of coordinately expressed genes had a predictive accuracy of 75%.

Conclusions.—Patterns of gene expression to differentiate optimally and suboptimally debulked cancers were sought for 44 advanced serous ovarian cancers. Some support is offered for the hypothesis that improved survival related to optimal debulking is at least partly the result of underlying biological characteristics of the tumors.

▶ This study looks at differential gene expression as a means of identifying those patients with advanced ovarian carcinoma most likely to benefit from surgical cytoreduction. The data suggest that the patterns of differential expression of 32 genes predict optimal versus suboptimal surgical cytoreduction 72.7% of the time. This is said to suggest that favorable outcome from surgical cytoreduction is due, at least in part, to the underlying biology of the disease. These results could not be confirmed by a similar study[1] presented at the 2004 meeting of the American Society of Clinical Oncology. This second trial involved 70 patients with advanced ovarian carcinoma (45 optimal and 25 suboptimal). Instead of the 32 differentially expressed genes found in the Berchuck trial, this second study identified only 4 differentially expressed genes, 7 after correction for grade. These conflicting results leave the task of studies of gene expression with an uncertain role in identifying those who are most likely to benefit from surgical cytoreduction. Also in doubt is the part played by biology in determining the outcome related to the volume of disease after surgery.

J. T. Thigpen, MD

Reference

1. Levine DA, Bonome T, Olshen AB, et al: Gene expression profiling of advanced ovarian cancers to predict the outcome of primary surgical cytoreduction. *J Clin Oncol* 2004 ASCO Annual Meeting Proceedings, vol 22, no. 14S (July 15 Supplement), 2004:5000.

Systematic Review of Management Options for Women With a Hereditary Predisposition to Ovarian Cancer

Rosen B, for the Cancer Care Ontario's Practice Guidelines Initiative Gynecology Cancer Disease Site Group (Princess Margaret Hosp, Toronto; et al)

Gynecol Oncol 93:280-286, 2004 3–5

Background.—Women with 2 first-degree relatives with ovarian or breast cancer have been identified as women with *BRCA1* and *BRCA2* germ line mutations. Women with these mutations have an increased lifetime risk of ovarian cancer. About 10% of ovarian cancer cases are attributed to inheriting a *BRCA1* or *BRCA2* mutation. As a preventive measure, these women were advised to undergo prophylactic or elective oophorectomy. However, this recommendation did not specify which approach should be used and whether the procedure should also include a hysterectomy. To identify the management options for women who are genetically predisposed for the development of ovarian cancer, a search was done of the current literature.

Methods.—The literature search included MEDLINE, CANCERLIT, and the Cochrane Library databases. The articles selected offered randomized controlled trials or meta-analyses comparing elective or prophylactic oophorectomy to other approaches to prevent ovarian cancer in genetically high-risk women or were phase II trials, cohort studies, or case series focused on the outcome of such prophylactic oophorectomy in these women.

Results.—Two retrospective and 2 prospective cohort studies were identified. The aim of each was to determine whether prophylactic oophorectomy reduced the lifetime risk of developing ovarian cancer. All 4 studies found a protective effect for prophylactic oophorectomy against ovarian cancer, but only 2 documented a statistically significant reduction in risk. The complications accompanying prophylactic oophorectomy included bleeding, injury to pelvic organs, and infection. Overall complication rates for laparoscopy ranged from 0.22% to 4.0%. Early onset of menopause, with its attending risks, was the major long-term adverse effect after prophylactic oophorectomy. No surgical prophylactic approach was found to be more preferable than others. Women are faced with the choice of bilateral salpingo-oophorectomy, peritoneal lavage for cytology during prophylactic oophorectomy, and bilateral salpingo-oophorectomy at the time of hysterectomy. Various added benefits attended the use of prophylactic surgery for women with *BRCA1* and *BRCA2* germ line mutations, including a lower relative risk of breast cancer and the possible detection of early disease. In addition, women suffered significantly less cancer anxiety when they had the surgery. Alternatives to prophylactic surgery include oral contraceptives and tubal ligation. The risk reduction with oral contraceptives is reportedly as high as 60% or as low as none. The risk reduction with tubal ligation involves only carriers of *BRCA1* mutations. The odds ratio for tubal ligation in 1 study was 0.39 for ovarian cancer. Combined tubal ligation and past use of an oral contraceptive had an odds ratio of 0.28. Tubal ligation did not offer a protective effect in carriers of *BRCA2* mutations.

Conclusions.—No significant benefit in protection against the development of ovarian cancer was consistently identified for prophylactic oophorectomy. The complications that attend this procedure can be significant, including most notably early menopause. In addition, any remnant of ovarian tissue presents a risk of developing cancer.

▶ This article reviews the results of 4 cohort studies examining the potential role of prophylactic oophorectomy in preventing breast and ovarian carcinoma in women with confirmed *BRCA1* or *BRCA2* mutations. Each study found a reduction in the risk of breast and ovarian carcinoma associated with prophylactic oophorectomy; two of the studies established statistically significant reductions. Discussion of this option with patients with confirmed mutations should convey these observations of benefit and should also discuss the long-term adverse effects associated with the early onset of menopause.

J. T. Thigpen, MD

Mucinous Epithelial Ovarian Cancer: A Separate Entity Requiring Specific Treatment

Hess V, A'Hern R, Nasiri N, et al (Royal Marsden Hosp, London)

J Clin Oncol 22:1040-1044, 2004 3–6

Background.—From 7% to 14% of all primary epithelial ovarian cancers are mucinous epithelial ovarian cancer (mEOC). The first-line treatment for these cancers is the same as for other, more common histopathologic groups and involves surgery followed by platinum-based chemotherapy. Few cases of mEOC have been included in the randomized clinical trials for advanced disease, so little is known about the effectiveness of this treatment that is specifically for advanced cases of mEOC. The efficacy of this therapy was determined.

Methods.—The study included 81 patients, comprising 27 cases and 54 control patients, all of whom received platinum-based chemotherapy. The patients with advanced mEOC (cases) were classified as stage III or IV. The control subjects had other histologic subtypes of EOC. The response rates and progression-free survival rates (PFS) of the patients with advanced mEOC were compared with those of the patients with other histologic subtypes.

Results.—About one third of each group received single-agent platinum therapy. Fifty-two percent of the patients in the study group and 81% of the control patients had fewer than the planned 6 cycles. The difference may indicate the relative chemoresistance of mEOC and the differing progression rates in the 2 patient groups. Sixty-three percent of those with mEOC had disease progression while receiving platinum-based chemotherapy. The overall response rate for the mEOC group was 26.3%; that for control patients was 64.9%. The mEOC group had 1 patient who had a complete response and the control group had 6. In comparison to the control group, the odds ratio for response for the mEOC group was 0.19. Stage was the only factor with any importance for predicting response. The median PFS was 5.7 and 14.1 months for the mEOC and control groups, respectively. The hazard ratio (HR) for risk of progression for mEOC patients compared to controls was 2.94. The median overall survival (OS) was 12.0 months for the mEOC group and 36.7 months for the control group. A significantly higher risk of death was found for the mEOC group compared to control patients. Disease stage was found to be statistically significant for OS on both univariate and multivariate analysis.

Conclusions.—Patients with mEOC respond less well to platinum-based chemotherapy than patients with other EOC subtypes. Those with advanced mEOC have worse PFS and OS than patients with other EOC subtypes. Thus, platinum-based chemotherapy does not achieve the effect against mEOC that it does with other EOC subtypes. mEOC is diagnosed at an early stage more often than other EOC subtypes and offers a better overall prognosis. However, with advanced disease, survival is poorer than with the other subtypes. Cases of advanced mEOC should perhaps be excluded from future trials of first-line chemotherapy or be analyzed as a separate group. Some of the regimens used for gastrointestinal cancers may be more effective than platinum-based chemotherapy for these ovarian cancers.

▶ This study of invasive mEOC identifies this entity with a much poorer response and survival with platinum-based chemotherapy than that observed with serous and endometrioid tumors. The authors hypothesize that regimens similar to those currently in use in colon carcinomas might offer a better therapeutic alternative, although they are able to cite only 1 study of alternative chemotherapy (a phase II trial from Japan reporting a 52% response rate to irinotecan plus mitomycin).[1] The challenge for randomized trials of such combinations as the 5-fluorouracil/leucovorin plus oxaliplatin (FOLFOX regimen) is that mucinous carcinomas are relatively uncommon among advanced tumors in most countries. For now, the best one can do is to note that outcome is substantially worse for this histologic subtype and to speculate about the potential benefit of such alternative regimens.

J. T. Thigpen, MD

Reference

1. Shimizu Y, Umezawa S, Hasumi K: A phase II study of combined CPT-11 and mitomycin-C in platinum refractory clear cell and mucinous ovarian carcinoma. *Ann Acad Med Singapore* 27:650-656, 1998.

Preoperative Detection of Peripherally Circulating Cancer Cells and Its Prognostic Significance in Ovarian Cancer

Judson PL, Geller MA, Bliss RL, et al (Univ of Minnesota, Minneapolis)
Gynecol Oncol 91:389-394, 2003 3–7

Background.—In several solid tumors, the finding of occult metastasis in bone marrow or peripheral blood strongly predicts reduced disease-free and

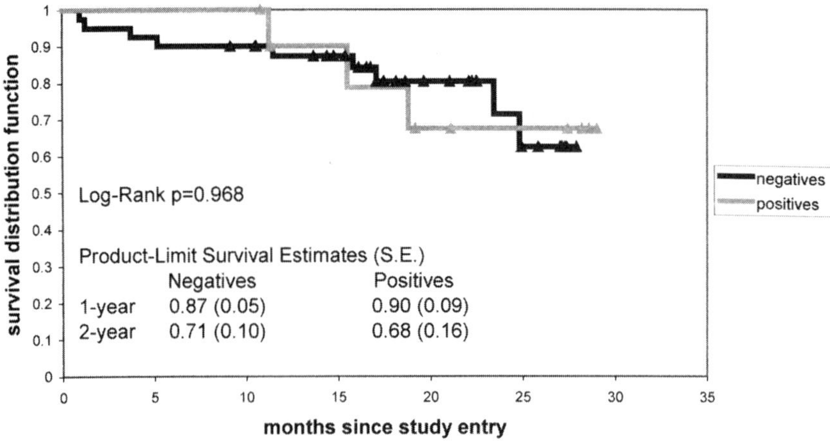

FIGURE 1.—Overall survival in newly diagnosed ovarian cancer by circulating ovarian cancer cells. (Reprinted by permission of the publisher from Judson PL, Geller MA, Bliss RL, et al: Preoperative detection of peripherally circulating cancer cells and its prognostic significance in ovarian cancer. *Gynecol Oncol* 91:389-394, 2003. Copyright 2003 by Elsevier Science Inc.)

overall survival. The incidence of circulating ovarian or primary peritoneal cancer cells in the peripheral blood at diagnosis or recurrence was determined, and the prognostic significance of these occult metastases established.

Methods.—Ninety-one women believed to have new or recurrent epithelial ovarian or primary peritoneal carcinoma were studied. Peripheral blood was obtained, and a tumor-enriched immunocytochemical assay applied.

Findings.—Sixty-four women had epithelial ovarian or primary peritoneal cancer, of whom 12 (18.7%) had evidence of circulating cancer cells in

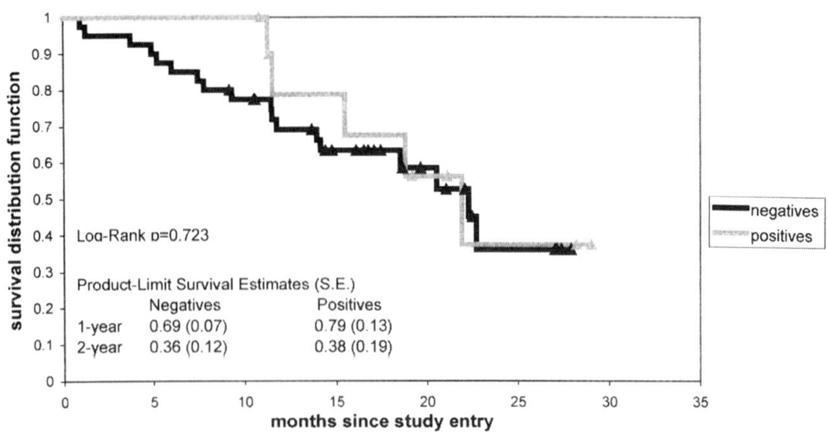

FIGURE 2.—Disease-free survival in newly diagnosed ovarian cancer by circulating ovarian cancer cells. (Reprinted by permission of the publisher from Judson PL, Geller MA, Bliss RL, et al: Preoperative detection of peripherally circulating cancer cells and its prognostic significance in ovarian cancer. *Gynecol Oncol* 91:389-394, 2003. Copyright 2003 by Elsevier Science Inc.)

peripheral blood. Compared with women without circulating cancer cells, those with such cells had statistically more grade 3 tumors. At a mean 18.7 months, survival curves did not differ between women with and without circulating cancer cells (Figs 1 and 2).

Conclusions.—Circulating cancer cells can be found in the peripheral blood of some patients with ovarian and primary peritoneal cancer. The clinical utility of assessing patients' peripheral blood for circulating cancer cells has not been established.

▶ It has been known for several decades that patients who have malignant disease often have circulating neoplastic cells in the blood. This has been reported even in patients who are thought to have localized disease, raising the question of whether or not those cells are actually viable, ie, will they "take" when they land in a specific organ. The answer to that is not clear, because many malignancies do not appear to metastasize despite the presence of these cells in the blood.

These investigators from the University of Minnesota looked carefully at 91 women undergoing treatment for what was thought to be primary peritoneal or epithelial ovarian tumor. Almost 20%, 12 of 64 women, had morphologic and immunocytochemical evidence of circulating cancer cells in their blood. With a mean follow-up of 18.7 months, the interesting thing is that survival and disease-free survival were not significantly different in the two groups of patients.

It is clear that it cannot be good to have circulating cells, but the question from this study is whether it is really bad. I guess it depends on the mutations that those cells possess.

E. Glatstein, MD

Long-term Follow-up of Women With Ovarian Cancer After Positive Second-Look Laparotomy

Dowdy SC, Constantinou CL, Hartmann LC, et al (Mayo Clinic, Rochester, Minn)

Gynecol Oncol 91:563-568, 2003 3–8

Background.—Second-look laparotomy (SLL) has had various applications, with its principal use now being the periodic evaluation of ovarian carcinoma. SLL itself has had little or no effect on survival rate, but it has been incorporated into several therapeutic schema. The information obtained in SLL has the theoretical advantage that it can be used to determine which patients are candidates for added therapy. Prognostic variables and adjuvant treatment in patients with a positive finding at SLL were assessed. In addition, the characteristics of a group of women who lack evidence of disease after prolonged follow-up were identified.

Methods.—The study included 150 patients who had persistent disease at SLL from 1977 to 1989. A retrospective chart review of these cases retrieved clinical data for assessment.

Results.—Of the 150 patients, 145 (96.7%) of the women have died, with the median survival being 18 months after SLL. The median follow-up for the 5 patients still living was 15.4 years. One of these patients has stable disease, and the other 4 are disease free. Univariate analysis identified tumor grade as a significant predictor of survival. Fifty percent of the patients with grade 1 lesions but only 8% of those with Broder's grade 4 lesions were alive at 5 years. The hazard of death for patients with the higher-grade lesions was 6.32 times that for patients with the lower-grade lesions. The tumor volume before and after SLL (pre/post SLL tumor volume) was predictive of survival. Patients with microscopic tumor at SLL had a survival rate of 31%; those with 1 cm or less of disease cytoreduced to microscopic disease had a survival rate of 24%. The survival of those with 1 cm or less of disease who had cytoreduction to microscopic disease was significantly better than that for women who did not have cytoreduction to microscopic size. The results for patients who did not have cytoreduction were no better than those for patients whose disease at SLL was greater than 1 cm. No significant impact on survival rate was noted. Treatment with intraperitoneal P32 was especially predictive of survival, with other salvage therapy also improving survival prognostication. Patients with low residual tumor burdens and low-grade disease received both P32 and whole abdominal radiation therapy, but only grade and residual tumor size were predictive of survival. All of the patients who are alive were young, had low-grade tumors, had initial disease measuring 1 cm or less at SLL, and had cytoreduction to microscopic disease. P32 was given to 1 patient, and 3 received whole abdominal radiation therapy.

Conclusions.—Therapy with P32 did not improve survival in patients with a positive SLL. Similarly, no advantage was noted in survival in using whole abdominal radiation therapy, and this approach has significant morbidity, such as small bowel obstruction. Improved survival was related to low-grade disease and low tumor burden after cytoreduction.

The Relationship Between Serum Vascular Endothelial Growth Factor, Persistent Disease, and Survival at Second-Look Laparotomy in Ovarian Cancer

Secord AA, Sayer R, Snyder SA, et al (Duke Univ, Durham, NC; Northwestern Univ, Chicago)

Gynecol Oncol 94:74-79, 2004 3–9

Background.—The utility of second-look laparotomy (SLL) in patients with epithelial ovarian cancer is limited, as recurrent disease will still develop in more than half of patients whose laparotomy results are negative. Markers of vascular angiogenesis and hemostasis might be more useful for monitoring disease status. Thus, the utility of vascular endothelial growth factor (VEGF) and D-dimer levels for predicting outcomes in patients with ovarian cancer was investigated.

Methods.—The medical records of 62 women with epithelial ovarian cancer (median age, 56 years) who completed first-line chemotherapy and underwent SLL between May 1983 and April 1993 were reviewed. All were in clinical remission at the time of SLL. Blood samples had been obtained within 2 months (median, 14 days) of SLL, and serum levels of VEGF, D-dimer, and CA125 were measured. Patients were followed up for a median of 15 years to determine disease-free and overall survival rate.

Results.—SLL findings were positive in 40 (64.6%) patients. During follow-up, disease recurrence or progression developed in 80% of patients with positive SLL findings compared with that of 20% of patients with negative findings on SLL. The median VEGF levels in the patients with negative SLL findings were not significantly different from those in patients with positive SLL findings (264 vs 390 pg/mL, respectively). Also not significantly different were median D-dimer levels (250 vs 395 ng/mL) or CA125 levels (10.8 vs 13.4 U/mL). The median survival time was 35 months. D-dimer levels were not predictive of disease-free or overall survival. High CA125 levels were predictive of worse disease-free and worse overall survival. After stratification according to median CA125 level (10.4 U/mL), disease-free survival was significantly longer in patients with low CA125 level (median, 14 months) than in patients with high CA125 levels (median, 9.6 months). Similarly, overall survival was almost 1.5 times longer for patients with low CA125 levels than for those with high CA125 levels. High VEGF levels were predictive of worse overall survival but were not predictive of disease-free survival. After stratification according to median VEGF level (341 pg/mL), survival was significantly longer for patients with low VEGF levels (median, 14 months) than for patients with high VEGF levels (median, 9.7 months). In multivariate regression models, after adjustment for CA125 level, VEGF level was a significant and independent predictor of overall survival.

Conclusion.—The serum VEGF level after first-line chemotherapy in patients with epithelial ovarian cancer may be a marker of persistent disease and is an independent predictor of overall survival in these patients.

▶ SLL had previously been a standard part of the management of advanced ovarian carcinoma. The rationale for the procedure was the establishment of actual disease status in those patients who achieve a clinical complete response with initial chemotherapy for purposes of further therapeutic decision making and the removal of isolated gross residual disease in selected patients (secondary surgical cytoreduction). Dowdy and colleagues (Abstract 3–8) examined long-term outcome in patients with positive SLLs between 1977 and 1989 to determine whether the SLL led to a treatment decision that afforded the patient benefit. Among 145 patients, salvage therapy did not influence subsequent survival. Secondary surgical cytoreduction, in particular, did not appear to influence outcome except in those patients with small-volume residual (gross disease < 1-cm diameter), which could be cytoreduced to microscopic residual only. Factors which did predict outcome included tumor grade and pre- and post-SLL tumor size. In a second study of patients who had undergone a SLL, Secord and colleagues (Abstract 3–9) identified an additional factor that appears to predict for outcome. The median serum levels of VEGF were correlated with the finding of a positive SLL with higher levels associated with positive second-look and shorter survival. These observations suggest that the SLL does not provide either benefit or information useful in determining appropriate further management of these patients. However, they do support the potential future role of biological factors, such as VEGF, in determining prognosis.

J. T. Thigpen, MD

Clinically Occult Recurrent Ovarian Cancer: Patient Selection for Secondary Cytoreductive Surgery Using Combined PET/CT

Bristow RE, del Carmen MG, Pannu HK, et al (Johns Hopkins Univ, Baltimore, Md)

Gynecol Oncol 90:519-528, 2003 3–10

Background.—Careful biochemical and radiographic monitoring is routinely performed for patients with ovarian cancer in complete clinical remission. However, the value of early detection of recurrent disease is unclear. The utility of combined positron emission tomography (PET) and CT for identifying ovarian cancer tumors of 1 cm or greater in patients with clinically occult recurrent disease by conventional CT imaging was assessed.

Methods.—The study included 22 patients (median age, 55 years) with epithelial ovarian cancer, increasing serum CA125 levels, and negative or equivocal conventional CT imaging 6 months or more after primary treatment. Of the 22 patients, 91% had International Federation of Gynecology and Obstetrics (FIGO) stage IIIC/IV disease. All underwent combined PET/CT imaging followed by surgical re-examination.

Findings.—Serum CA125 levels increased a median of 24 U/mL. Conventional CT was negative in 15 patients and was equivocal in 7. Eighteen patients were subsequently found to have recurrent ovarian cancer 1 cm or greater at the time of surgery. The median maximal tumor diameter was 2.3 cm. Overall, the patient-based accuracy of PET/CT was 81.8% for detecting recurrent disease of 1 cm or greater. The sensitivity of this combination was 83.3%, and the positive predictive value, 93.8%. Complete cytoreduction to no gross residual tumor was achieved in 72.2% of patients with recurrent disease of 1 cm or greater (Fig 1).

Conclusions.—The combination of PET and CT has a high sensitivity and positive predictive value in detecting potentially respectable, macroscopic recurrent ovarian cancer in patients with biochemical evidence of disease recurrence and negative or equivocal conventional CT findings. The early detection of macroscopic recurrent cancer may facilitate complete surgical cytoreduction in carefully selected patients.

▶ This article from a group of strong investigators from Johns Hopkins assesses the PET/CT scanning combination in the detection of occult recurrent ovarian carcinoma. They evaluated 22 patients who had increasing CA125 levels but no clear radiologic evidence with CT only of recurrent intra-abdominal neoplasm. They then underwent the PET/CT imaging technique, and in 18 of the 22 patients, a lesion of at least 1 cm was detected.

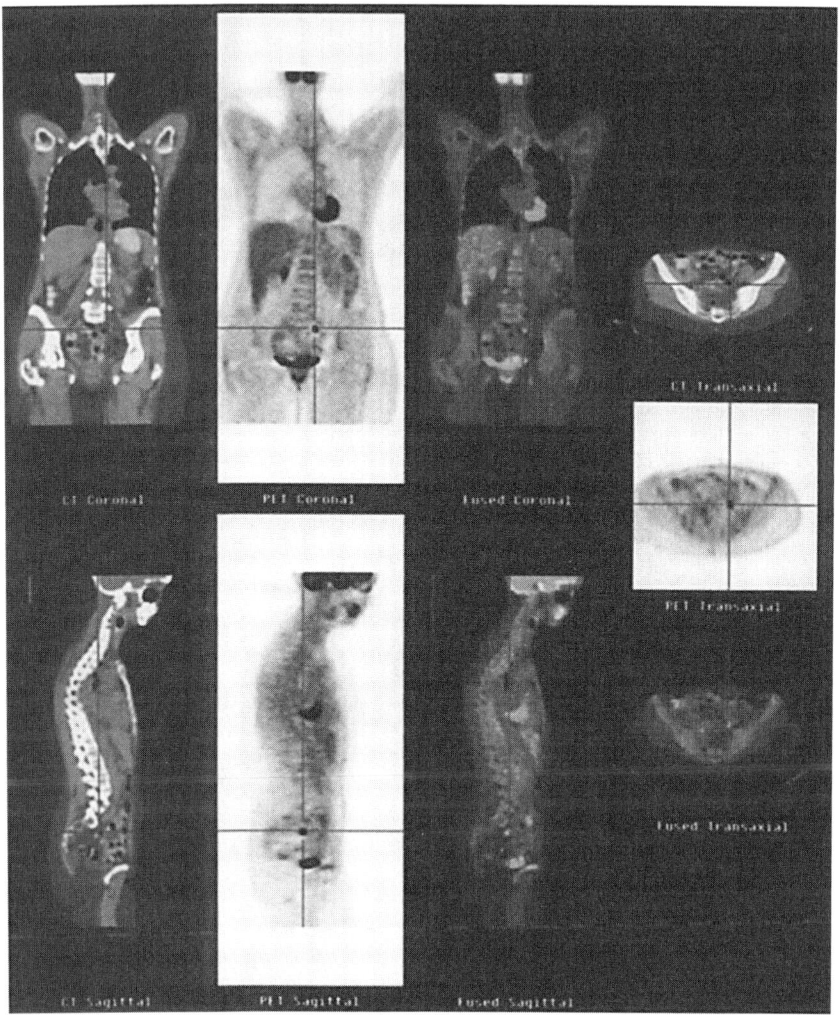

FIGURE 1.—Combined PET/CT images showing sagittal, coronal, and transaxial views of CT, PET, and fused PET/CT. At surgery, a 2.5-cm tumor nodule of recurrent Stage IIIC serous ovarian cancer was resected from the sigmoid colon mesentery. *Abbreviation: PET*, Positron emission tomography. (Reprinted by permission of the publisher from Bristow RE, del Carmen MG, Pannu HK, et al: Clinically occult recurrent ovarian cancer: Patient selection for secondary cytoreductive surgery using combined PET/CT. *Gynecol Oncol* 90:519-528, 2003. Copyright 2003, by Elsevier Science Inc.)

This is probably the first time I have been able to see any reasonable evidence that PET/CT as a combination study might have some advantages over both separate investigations. The illustrations shown are reasonably convincing of the potential merits of this study. Whether this is really a significant improvement over 2 separate studies is still not clear to me, but if you want to actually biopsy the area in question it is probably helpful. On the other hand, one hesitates to estimate what it will cost the patient and our insurance system.

E. Glatstein, MD

Paclitaxel 175 or 225 mg per Meters Squared With Carboplatin in Advanced Ovarian Cancer: A Randomized Trial

Bolis G, Scarfone G, Polverino G, et al (Università di Milano, Italy; Istituto Nazionale Tumori, Italy; Ospedale S Raffaele, Milano, Italy; et al)

J Clin Oncol 22:686-690, 2004 3–11

Background.—The optimal chemotherapy for treating advanced ovarian cancer has involved the use of cisplatinum and paclitaxel. The combination of carboplatin plus paclitaxel has recently been shown to have equal efficacy and less toxicity than the cisplatinum plus paclitaxel regimen. The use of escalating doses of paclitaxel combined with fixed doses of carboplatin has been proposed. The effect of various doses of paclitaxel plus fixed doses of carboplatin for ovarian cancer therapy was investigated in a large, randomized clinical trial where carboplatin was given before paclitaxel.

Methods.—The study included 502 women with histologically confirmed epithelial ovarian cancer stages IIB to IV who were randomly selected to receive 2 different regimens of carboplatin plus paclitaxel. One group received carboplatin according to the following formula: target area under the free carboplatin plasma concentration versus time curve (AUC) = 6 × (glomerular filtration rate + 25) mg/m^2 (AUC6) plus 175 mg/m^2 of paclitaxel for 6 cycles every 21 days. The second group received carboplatin AUC6 plus 225 mg/m^2 of paclitaxel for 6 cycles every 21 days.

Results.—The response to chemotherapy did not differ between treatment groups. One hundred thirty-two patients in the 175-mg/m^2 group and 147 patients in the 225-mg/m^2 group had a complete response. Similar proportions of these women in each group experienced progression of their disease. The progression-free survival rates in the 175-mg/m^2 and 225-mg/m^2 groups after 4 years were 41.5% and 39.2%, respectively. Four-year survival rates were 46.2% in the 175-mg/m^2 group and 47.3% in the 225-mg/m^2 group. Similar rates of response were found for women in both groups who had residual tumor. Thrombocytopenia grade 3 to 4 developed in 40 of the women receiving 175-mg/m^2 doses and 49 of those receiving 225-mg/m^2 doses, which was not a significant difference between the 2 groups.

Conclusions.—No significant difference in response or survival rate was found in women given varying doses of paclitaxel and fixed doses of carboplatin. The group receiving the higher dose experienced significantly greater neurotoxicity than the group receiving the lower dose.

► This randomized trial examined the value of higher-dose paclitaxel in combination with carboplatin for the treatment of advanced ovarian carcinoma. No benefit was observed for paclitaxel 225 mg/m^2 over 3 hours plus carboplatin AUC 6 as compared to paclitaxel 175 mg/m^2 over 3 hours plus carboplatin AUC

6. Significantly greater neurotoxicity was observed with the higher dose. The authors conclude that the higher dose offers no advantage and a less favorable toxicity profile. This is not a surprising outcome in light of prior published results. A Gynecologic Oncology Group trial compared 175 mg/m^2 to 250 mg/m^2 of paclitaxel as single agent therapy for platinum-resistant recurrent or persistent disease and found no advantage for the higher dose.[1] A meta-analysis presented at the 1996 meeting of the American Society of Clinical Oncology by Rowinsky and colleagues noted no advantage for doses higher than 175 mg/m^2.[2] Furthermore, previous reports of an interaction between paclitaxel and carboplatin that reduces the amount of myelosuppression seen with carboplatin raises serious questions about the potentially adverse effect of higher doses of paclitaxel on the antitumor efficacy of the carboplatin. The bottom line is that, based on the best evidence available, there is no need to use doses of paclitaxel higher than 175 mg/m^2 every 3 weeks in the treatment of ovarian carcinoma.

J. T. Thigpen, MD

References

1. Omura GA, Brady MF, Look KY, et al: Phase III trial of paclitaxel at two dose levels, the higher dose accompanied by filgrastim at two dose levels in platinum-pretreated epithelial ovarian cancer: An intergroup study. *J Clin Oncol* 21:2843-2848, 2003.
2. Rowinsky EK, Mackey MK, Goodman SN: Meta-analysis of paclitaxel (P) dose-response and dose intensity (DI) in recurrent or refractory ovarian cancer. Presented at 1996 ASCO Annual Meeting, Abstract No. 770.

Topotecan Compared With No Therapy After Response to Surgery and Carboplatin/Paclitaxel in Patients With Ovarian Cancer: Multicenter Italian Trials in Ovarian Cancer (MITO-1) Randomized Study

De Placido S, Scambia G, Di Vagno G, et al (Università Federico II di Napoli, Italy; Ospedale Cardarelli, Italy; Istituto Nazionale Tumori di Napoli, Italy; et al)
J Clin Oncol 22:2635-2642, 2004 3–12

Background.—Worldwide, surgery followed by chemotherapy with paclitaxel plus carboplatin is first-line treatment for patients with epithelial ovarian cancer. This approach results in a clinical response in up to 80% of patients, yet the 5-year survival rate is only 20% to 40%. A major cause of chemotherapy failure is drug resistance. Topotecan is not cross resistant with paclitaxel or carboplatin and has induced responses in up to 30% of patients refractory or resistant to initial paclitaxel and carboplatin treatment. Whether topotecan might be effective as consolidation therapy after first-line paclitaxel and carboplatin chemotherapy for epithelial ovarian cancer was investigated.

Methods.—The subjects in this phase III study were 273 women (median age, 56 years) with epithelial ovarian cancer. At diagnosis, most patients had advanced disease (stage III, 65%; stage IV, 10%), and all had an Eastern Cooperative Oncology Group performance status of 2 or less. All patients underwent primary surgery; after surgery, 46% had no residual disease, 20% had been optimally debulked, and 34% had disease 1 cm or more. In addition, 20% of patients had interval debulking surgery after 3 cycles of standard chemotherapy. All patients underwent 6 cycles of standard paclitaxel plus carboplatin chemotherapy, and had complete (87.2%) or partial (12.8%) responses. After first-line chemotherapy, patients were randomly assigned in a 1:1 ratio either to observation (control group) or to additional chemotherapy with topotecan (1.5 mg/m^2 on days 1-5 every 3 weeks for 4 cycles). Progression-free survival in the topotecan group was compared with that of the control group.

Results.—During a median follow-up of 28 months, 153 (56.0%) patients had disease progression, and 73 (26.7%) died. Progression-free survival did not differ significantly between the observation and topotecan groups (28.4 vs 18.2 months, respectively). After data adjustment for residual disease, interval debulking, and response to first-line chemotherapy, the risk of disease progression was 18% higher in the topotecan group (hazard ratio 1.18). The most frequent adverse events associated with topotecan were neutropenia (58%, grades 3 or 4) and thrombocytopenia (24%, grades 3 or 4).

Conclusion.—Consolidation chemotherapy with topotecan after first-line standard paclitaxel plus cisplatin chemotherapy does not improve progression-free survival rates in patients with advanced ovarian cancer.

Randomized Phase II Trial of Two High-Dose Chemotherapy Regimens With Stem Cell Transplantation for the Treatment of Advanced Ovarian Cancer in First Remission or Chemosensitive Relapse: A Southwest Oncology Group Study

Stiff PJ, Shpall EJ, Liu PY, et al (Loyola Univ, Maywood, IL; Univ of Colorado, Denver; Southwest Oncology Group Statistical Ctr, Seattle; et al)

Gynecol Oncol 94:98-106, 2004 3–13

Background.—High-dose chemotherapy and stem cell transplantation have each shown some benefits for patients with recurrent or persistent advanced ovarian cancer. A phase II study was undertaken to examine the efficacy and safety of 2 high-dose chemotherapy regimens combined with stem cell transplantation in patients with recurrent or persistent stage III/IV ovarian cancer.

Methods.—The study included 58 women younger than 65 years (median age, 49 years) with recurrent stage III/IV ovarian cancer despite initial standard chemotherapy, or who relapsed more than 6 months after having a complete response to standard chemotherapy. About half the patients were low risk (ie, maximal tumor diameter $\leq$ 0.5 cm, platinum-sensitive tumor). Patients were assigned randomly to receive 1 of the following 2 high-dose chemotherapy regimens: CMC (n = 32), carboplatin (300 mg/m^2 per day on days 1-5), mitoxantrone (25 mg/m^2 on days 1, 3, and 5), and cyclophosphamide (40 mg/kg on days 1, 3, and 5), or CTC (n = 26), cisplatin (55 mg/m^2 per day on days 3-5), thiotepa (600 mg/m^2 on day 2), and cyclophosphamide (1875 mg/m^2 per day on days 3-5). On days 9-11, all patients underwent hematopoietic stem cell transfusion, and began taking filgrastim; filgrastim was continued until the absolute neutrophil count was more than 2000/mm^3 on 3 consecutive days. Patients were followed up to determine progression-free and overall survival.

Results.—Two patients in each group died of transplant-related complications. Among the survivors, patients in the CMC group had longer progression-free survival time (median, 13 vs 8 months) and overall survival (29 vs 22 months) than those in the CTC group. In multivariate analyses, normal CA125 levels at stem cell transplantation and a complete response to primary therapy were significant independent predictors of improved progression-free survival. Normal CA125 levels at transplantation and platinum sensitivity were significant independent predictors of improved overall survival. Hematologic toxicity was similar in both groups, but the CTC group was more likely to have grade III/IV nausea or vomiting (29% vs 7%), grade III/IV diarrhea (42% vs 19%), and stomatitis (41% vs 15%). In addition, grade IV nephrotoxicity developed in 2 of the survivors in the CTC group.

Conclusion.—The CMC regimen was associated with better progression-free and overall survival time than the CTC regimen for these patients with relapsed or persistent advanced ovarian cancer after primary therapy. Still, median progression-free survival in the CMC group was only about a year, and median overall survival in both groups was about 2.5 years.

► Current front-line therapy for advanced ovarian carcinoma succeeds in establishing a clinical complete remission in roughly 75% of these patients. Unfortunately, 75% of these clinical complete remissions will relapse. Over the last 2 decades, multiple studies have attempted to identify effective consolidation or maintenance therapy to prevent these relapses. De Placido and colleagues (Abstract 3–12) present the results of 1 of these efforts, a randomized trial assigning patients with either a clinical complete response (87%) or partial response (13%) to either 4 cycles of topotecan or no further therapy. The study showed no significant advantage for the consolidation with topotecan. These results are corroborated by a second study of consolidation topotecan conducted by the AGO (German cooperative group) and presented at the 2003 American Society of Clinical Oncology meeting.[1] This second trial also found no advantage for consolidation with topotecan. An alternative approach to consolidation is the use of high-dose chemotherapy with stem-cell support. Stiff and colleagues (Abstract 3–13) in the Southwest Oncology Group present the results of a randomized phase II trial of 2 high-dose chemotherapy regimens given as either consolidation therapy or as treatment for chemosensitive relapse. This study produced relatively short progression-free survivals and overall survivals comparable to what one would expect with standard platinum-based therapy used for treatment of a platinum-sensitive relapse. The role of this approach to consolidation was dealt a further blow at the 2004 meeting of the American Society of Clinical Oncology, at which the results of a

European randomized phase III study of high-dose chemotherapy with stem-cell support as consolidation therapy for those with a clinical complete remission showed no advantage over continuation of standard platinum-based therapy.[2] To date, the only positive phase III trial of consolidation or maintenance therapy is the Southwest Oncology Group/Gynecologic Oncology Group (SWOG/GOG) study of 12 versus 3 additional cycles of paclitaxel in those with a clinical complete response to front-line paclitaxel/carboplatin.[3] This study found a superior progression-free survival and reduced relapse rate associated with the more prolonged 12 cycles of maintenance paclitaxel.

J. T. Thigpen, MD

References

1. Meier W, for the AGO Ovarian Cancer Study Group: Topotecan vs treosulfan in recurrent ovarian cancer (OC) after initial therapy with platinum and paclitaxel. A prospective randomized phase III study. Abstract no. 1810, *Proc Am Clin Oncol* p 450, 2003.
2. Cure H, Battista C, Guastalla JP, et al: Phase III randomized trial of high-dose chemotherapy (HDC) and peripheral blood stem cell (PBSC) support as consolidation in patients (pts) with advanced ovarian cancer (AOC): 5-year follow-up of a GINECO/FNCLCC/SFGM-TC study. *J Clin Oncol*, 2004 ASCO Annual Meeting Proceedings (Post-Meeting Edition), vol 22, No. 14S (July 15 Supplement), 2004:5006.
3. Markman M, Liu PY, Wilczynski S, et al: Phase III randomized trial of 12 versus 3 months of maintenance paclitaxel in patients with advanced ovarian cancer after complete response to platinum and paclitaxel-based chemotherapy: A Southwest Oncology Group and Gynecologic Oncology Group trial. *J Clin Oncol* 21:2460-2465, 2003.

The Role of Topotecan for Extending the Platinum-Free Interval in Recurrent Ovarian Cancer: An In Vitro Model

Horowitz NS, Hua J, Gibb RK (Washington Univ, St Louis)
Gynecol Oncol 94:67-73, 2004 3–14

Background.—Some researchers believe lengthening the platinum-free interval in women with recurrent ovarian cancer improves their response to subsequent platinum-based therapies. This possibility, however, has not been rigorously studied. An in vitro model was used to examine the molecular genetic alterations associated with intrinsic and acquired resistance to platinum in recurrent ovarian cancer, with the goal of understanding the effects of treatment-free interval and retreatment with platinum or a novel second-line agent, topotecan.

Methods.—Human ovarian cancer cell line A2780 was rendered resistant to cisplatin by exposure to increasing concentrations of the drug. A2780 cells and cisplatin-resistant A2780 (A2780-CR) cells were separately seeded in culture plates, then exposed to increasing concentrations of cisplatin plus paclitaxel or of topotecan. After 7 days, cells were cultured in drug-free media for 3 weeks, then replated and exposed to clinically relevant concentrations of cisplatin or topotecan. The dose lethal to 50% or more of cells (LD_{50})

was determined in a cytotoxic tetrazolium dye (MTT) assay. Cells surviving this step were again cultured in drug-free medium for another 4 weeks, and a second MTT assay was performed to assess the LD_{50}. Messenger RNA (mRNA) was extracted by means of a reagent, and its expression was evaluated by reverse transcription-polymerase chain reaction and Northern blot hybridization. Resistance was evaluated by measuring expression of the multidrug-resistant gene (*MDR-1*), multidrug-resistant protein (MRP), and topoisomerase-I.

Results.—The LD_{50} to cisplatin in the A2780 cells exposed to topotecan was the same as that in the A2780-CR cells exposed to topotecan, indicating the A2780-CR cells had no intrinsic resistance to topotecan. With cisplatin treatment, the first MTT assay (drug-free interval of 3 weeks) showed A2780-CR cells exposed to higher concentrations of cisplatin became more resistant to this drug, whereas A2780-CR cells exposed to lower cisplatin concentrations became more sensitive to the drug ($P < .01$). The second MTT assay showed the LD_{50} for cisplatin decreased significantly in all samples after a 4-week drug-free period, regardless of the initial cisplatin concentration. In contrast, the first MTT assay showed only 1 of 3 A2780-CR cell lines had a lower LD_{50} after topotecan. But in the second MTT assay, all 3 strains were extremely sensitive to topotecan. Still, regardless of initial treatment, LD_{50} values in the second MTT assay were significantly lower than those in the first assay. mRNA expression of MRP and topoisomerase-I did not differ in either cell line according to type or concentration of chemotherapeutic drug. However, mRNA for *MDR-1* was not amplified in A2780 cells, but was significantly overexpressed in A2780-CR cells initially treated with low doses of cisplatin and paclitaxel.

Conclusion.—The acquired resistance to cisplatin in the A2780 ovarian cancer cell line is an unstable phenotype that is gained or lost depending on the chemotherapeutic agent and the drug-free interval, and some cells do become more sensitive to treatment after a drug-free interval. However, reversal of resistance cannot be explained simply by the loss of *MDR-1* expression. These findings offer hope that agents with mechanisms of action different from those of cisplatin can extend the platinum-free interval and improve survival rate for patients with recurrent ovarian cancer.

▶ For some time, the concept of "prolonging the platinum-free interval" by the use of alternative drugs to prolong artificially the time free from platinum agents to restore or enhance the sensitivity of ovarian cancer to the platinum compounds has been used to encourage the use of these alternative drugs earlier in the treatment history of a patient with recurrent ovarian cancer. While the concept has enjoyed some acceptance in the oncology community, there has been little evidence to support the validity of the approach. Horowitz and colleagues provide for the first time some evidence to support the potential for therapy with topotecan to allow the restoration of platinum sensitivity. While this does not establish prolonging the platinum-free interval as the approach of choice to the management of recurrent ovarian carcinoma, it should encourage further studies designed to test this hypothesis.

J. T. Thigpen, MD

Topotecan Dosing Guidelines in Ovarian Cancer: Reduction and Management of Hematologic Toxicity

Armstrong DK (Johns Hopkins Univ, Baltimore, Md)

Oncologist 9:33-42, 2004 3–15

Background.—The use of topotecan is effective in many patients with recurrent ovarian cancer, but grade III/IV myelosuppression limits tolerability. The hematologic toxicity associated with topotecan as second-line therapy, and techniques for managing myelosuppression were reviewed.

Hematologic Toxicity With Topotecan.—The recommended dose of topotecan for treating recurrent ovarian cancer is 1.5 mg/m^2 infused IV for 30 minutes during days 1-5 of a 21-day course. Despite a high incidence of severe leukopenia, neutropenia, and thrombocytopenia with topotecan, myelosuppression with this drug is predictable, manageable, and not cumulative. Certain factors increase a patient's risk of developing hematologic toxicity, including older age, impaired renal function, prior radiation therapy, prior platinum therapy, and a longer duration of primary chemotherapy. Thus, guidelines recommend reducing topotecan starting doses to 1.0 or 1.25 mg/m^2 for patients at high risk of myelosuppression.

Management of Myelosuppression.—In addition to dosage reductions, other techniques can help manage hematologic toxicity. Hematopoietic growth factors reduce the incidence of neutropenic fever, and transfusion therapy improves anemia and thrombocytopenia. In addition, alternative dosing schedules, such as a 3-day course or once-weekly dosing, may be effective but less myelotoxic than the currently approved regimen and are being investigated. However, until data from phase III trials are available, alternative-dosing schedules should be considered investigational.

▶ This review examines alternative doses and schedules of topotecan and provides a reasonably good summary of the data on these. The article correctly concludes that schedules alternative to the 5-day schedule in the package insert remain experimental at the present time and should be studied further in settings that allow thorough examination of their efficacy relative to the 5-day schedule. This is especially true in light of phase II data that suggest lower response rates with the shorter schedules and the weekly schedule.

J. T. Thigpen, MD

Survival Outcomes in Patients With Recurrent Ovarian Cancer Who Were Treated With Chemoresistance Assay–Guided Chemotherapy

Loizzi V, Chan JK, Osann K, et al (Univ of California, Orange)

Am J Obstet Gynecol 189:1301-1307, 2003 3–16

Background.—Ovarian cancer is the most lethal gynecologic malignancy in the United States, causing approximately 14,500 deaths each year. Patients with ovarian cancer who have relapse are often characterized as having platinum-resistant (PR) disease or platinum-sensitive (PS) disease, depending on the interval to progression after initial platinum-based chemotherapy. Patients with PS disease tend to have a more favorable prognosis with a better response to second-line chemotherapy than do patients with PR diseases. However, the best strategy for the selection of second-line chemotherapy after relapse has not been defined. The outcome of patients with recurrent ovarian carcinoma after extreme drug resistance assay-directed therapy was determined.

Methods.—The study was conducted in 50 women who were treated with chemotherapy on the basis of extreme drug-resistance assay and 50 well-balanced control subjects who received empirical treatment. Data were collected from hospital charts, clinic follow-up records, and tumor registry databases. Most patients were treated with single-agent chemotherapy because there is no evidence of a benefit for the use of combination chemotherapy in the treatment of recurrent ovarian carcinoma. Complete response to second-line chemotherapy was defined as the disappearance of all measurable disease for at least 4 weeks. Partial response was defined as a decrease of more than 50% in all measurable lesions for at least 4 weeks with no increase in any tumors or appearance of new lesions during this period. Progressive disease was defined as an increase of more than 50% in any measurable lesions or the appearance of 1 or more new lesions.

Results.—In the PS group, patients with extreme drug resistance-directed therapy had an overall response rate of 65%, whereas the response rate in those patients who were treated empirically was 35%. In the PR group, there was no improved outcome in the patients who underwent assay-guided therapy. Multivariate analysis showed that PS disease, extreme drug resistance-guided therapy, and early stage of disease were independent predictors for improved survival.

Conclusions.—This retrospective analysis showed that an improved outcome in patients with recurrent ovarian carcinoma who have PS disease and who underwent extreme drug resistance-directed chemotherapy. There is a need for randomized, prospective, controlled trials.

▶ This retrospective study examined therapy for recurrent ovarian carcinoma guided by a chemoresistance assay as compared with historical controls treated empirically. The data suggest that assay-guided therapy produces a much higher frequency of response to treatment and superior progression-free and overall survival. As with all retrospective studies, there is potential for unrecognized bias that can explain the observations. What is needed is a well-designed randomized clinical trial examining the value of these in vitro assays. Until such a trial is completed, it is difficult to recommend the routine use of these assays to direct therapy even in the salvage setting.

J. T. Thigpen, MD

Cardiac Safety Profile of Prolonged (≥6 Cycles) Pegylated Liposomal Doxorubicin Administration in Patients With Gynecologic Malignancies

Uyar D, Kulp B, Peterson G, et al (Cleveland Clinic Found, Ohio)
Gynecol Oncol 94:147-151, 2004 3–17

Introduction.—Pegylated liposomal doxorubicin (PLD) is an active cytotoxic agent used to treat recurrent or resistant ovarian carcinoma and metastatic endometrial cancer. It has a relatively favorable toxicity profile. PLD is less cardiotoxic than doxorubicin, but the safety of its prolonged administration is not known. The experience with delivery of PLD over an extended period was retrospectively examined in women with gynecologic malignancies.

Methods.—The medical records of 22 patients with gynecologic malignancies treated between 1997 and 2003 with prolonged (≥6 cycles) use of PLD were reviewed. PLD was administered in doses ranging from 20 to 40 mg/m^2 (infused over 1-2 hours); treatment was repeated every 4 to 6 weeks. During therapy, patients underwent routine assessments for toxicity, including performance of multigated acquisition scans for determination of left ventricular heart ejection fraction.

Results.—Of 22 patients who met inclusion criteria, 18 had ovarian cancer, 3 had primary peritoneal cancer, and 1 had endometrial cancer. Patients received a median of 4 (range, 1-8) chemotherapy regimens before starting PLD. No patients were previously treated with doxorubicin. The median number of PLD cycles and cumulative dose of PLD were 8 (range, 6-26) and 483 mg/m^2 (256-1699 mg/m^2), respectively. Fourteen patients (64%) underwent 1 or more multigated acquisition scans. There was no clinical evidence of heart failure in any participants. There was no need for dose reduction because of cardiac dysfunction in any patient; none had a reduction in left ventricular ejection fraction to less than 50% or a 10% or greater reduction compared with baseline value.

Conclusion.—Prolonged PLD therapy is possible in carefully selected patients with advanced gynecologic malignancies. Cardiac dysfunction does not seem to be a toxicity in this setting. The development of evidence-based guidelines for monitoring cardiac function would be helpful in this patient population.

► Uyar et al evaluated the potential cardiotoxicity of PLD in a series of 22 patients with extensive prior treatment with agents other than an anthracycline. No cumulative cardiac toxicity was observed after a median of 8 cycles and a range of 6 to 26 cycles at doses ranging from 20 mg/m^2 to 40 mg/m^2 per course. While this does not establish definitively that there is not some higher cumulative dose beyond which cardiac toxicity becomes a problem, it provides evidence that, over the usual range of courses of therapy, cardiotoxicity does not appear to be a concern.

J. T. Thigpen, MD

Phase 2 Trial of Single Agent Docetaxel in Platinum and Paclitaxel-Refractory Ovarian Cancer, Fallopian Tube Cancer, and Primary Carcinoma of the Peritoneum

Markman M, Zanotti K, Webster K, et al (Cleveland Clinic Foundation, Ohio)

Gynecol Oncol 91:573-576, 2003 3–18

Background.—Paclitaxel and docetaxel are each active in platinum- and paclitaxel-resistant ovarian cancer, and cross-resistance between these 2 taxanes appears to be limited. Thus, the efficacy of docetaxel in patients with platinum- and paclitaxel-resistant ovarian cancer was investigated in a phase II trial.

Methods.—The study included 30 women, 40 to 80 years old, with advanced ovarian cancer (n = 20) or primary carcinoma of the peritoneum (n = 10). In all cases, the patients had not responded to primary chemotherapy with platinum and paclitaxel, or the disease progressed within 3 months of treatment. The patients received an initial dose of docetaxel, 75 mg/m^2 infused IV for 1 hour. In 3 patients who had received extensive prior therapy and had evidence of excessive bone marrow suppression, the initial dose was only 60 mg/m^2. Treatment was repeated every 3 weeks, and doses were reduced by 10 mg/m^2 when serious neutropenia occurred.

Results.—The patients received between 1 and 7 courses of docetaxel (median, 3 courses). Three (10%) patients achieved both an objective response (based on CA-125 levels) and symptomatic improvement. Responses in these 3 patients lasted 3 to 6 months. Dose reductions caused by treatment-related adverse events were required in 7 patients. The most common adverse events were grade IV neutropenia (n = 9, 30%), neutropenic fever (n = 2, 7%), and grades II/III/IV fatigue (n = 5, 17%).

Conclusion.—Single-agent docetaxel was of benefit for 10% of the women, although it was not effective in all patients with platinum- and paclitaxel-resistant ovarian cancer. The initial dose of docetaxel used in this study (75 mg/m^2) is lower than that in 2 other phase II trials (100 mg/m^2), and the incidence of grade IV neutropenia and febrile neutropenia was considerably lower in the current trial. Thus, for appropriate selected patients, IV docetaxel at doses of 60 to 100 mg/m^2 should be considered for patients with ovarian cancer refractory to conventional first-line chemotherapy.

► This phase II trial of docetaxel in patients with platinum and paclitaxel-refractory ovarian carcinoma demonstrates that docetaxel is active in patients who are no longer responsive to the other commonly used taxanes. Similar results have been achieved with an alteration in the schedule of paclitaxel. Weekly paclitaxel has been shown to have activity for patients with either breast or ovarian carcinoma who have failed to respond to paclitaxel given every 3 weeks.

J. T. Thigpen, MD

Treatment of High-Risk Gestational Trophoblastic Neoplasia With Etoposide, Methotrexate, Actinomycin D, Cyclophosphamide, and Vincristine Chemotherapy

Escobar PF, Lurain JR, Singh DK, et al (Northwestern Univ, Chicago)
Gynecol Oncol 91:552-557, 2003 3–19

Background.—Patients with high-risk metastatic trophoblastic tumors have recently been treated with etoposide, high-dose methotrexate, actinomycin D, cyclophosphamide, and vincristine (EMA-CO). The efficacy and toxicity of this regimen are reported in a group of 45 patients with high-risk gestational trophoblastic neoplasia.

Study Design.—The study group consisted of 45 patients, aged 15 to 50 years, with high-risk gestational trophoblastic neoplasia who were treated with EMA-CO. Of these patients, 25 were treated with EMA-CO primarily and 20 were treated after failure to respond to single-agent chemotherapy. Patients with partial responses or who had resistance to therapy develop were treated with regimens that included cisplatin. Adjuvant surgery and radiotherapy were used for some patients. Survival, clinical response, and toxicity were retrospectively analyzed.

Findings.—The overall survival rate was 91%, with 92% for primary treatment and 90% for secondary treatment. A complete response to EMA-CO occurred in 71%; 20% had resistance develop but achieved remission with cisplatin-based therapy, whereas 9% died of widespread metastatic disease. Prognostic factors included duration from pregnancy to treatment, metastatic site, and World Health Organization score. EMA-CO therapy was not associated with life-threatening toxicity, caused grade 3 to 4 hematologic toxicity in only 1.6% of cycles, and caused neutropenia necessitating a 1-week treatment delay in only 13.5% of cycles.

Conclusions.—EMA-CO chemotherapy, with adjuvant radiotherapy and surgery when necessary, results in overall cure rates of more than 80% in patients with high-risk gestational trophoblastic neoplasia. Approximately 20% of patients will relapse or have treatment failure, and these patients often respond to cisplatin-based chemotherapy and surgery. EMA-CO based therapy is effective and well tolerated for patients with high-risk gestational trophoblastic neoplasia.

▶ This study evaluates the efficacy of a combination of etoposide, methotrexate, actinomycin D, cyclophosphamide, and vincristine in 45 women with high-risk metastatic gestational trophoblastic disease. The authors report a high complete response rate of 71% and a survival rate of 91% at a median follow-up of 36 months. These data indicate that this regimen is highly active, and many regard it as the current regimen of choice in high-risk metastatic patients (high-risk features include duration of disease >6 months, high human chorionic gonadotropin level of >100,000 mIU/mL, metastases to brain or liver, and a World Health Organization score of >7). There are, however, several caveats to this. First, there are too few of these patients to permit large trials; hence, conclusions about relative merit of regimens are drawn from relatively small phase II trials. Second, while it is clear that the addition of etoposide seems to increase the efficacy, the role of cisplatin has not been adequately explored; it is not a part of the EMA-CO regimen. Third, the relative merits of each drug and the particular dose and schedule as a part of the combination have never been examined; hence, it may be possible to simplify the regimen significantly. With these caveats, EMA-CO should be regarded as a very active regimen in these patients and, at least for now, a reasonable choice of therapy.

J. T. Thigpen, MD

Carcinosarcoma of the Ovary: 19 Years of Prospective Data From a Single Center

Brown E, Stewart M, Rye T, et al (Univ of Edinburgh, Scotland; Little France, Edinburgh, Scotland; Inst of Health Sciences, Oxford, England)

Cancer 100:2148-2153, 2004 3–20

Background.—Malignant mixed mesodermal tumors (MMMTs), which are also called carcinosarcomas, are found throughout the female genital tract, most often the uterus, but are rare in comparison with other gynecologic tumors. The combination theory of pathogenesis credits a common epithelial stem cell for both malignant elements, and the collision theory postulates that 2 distinct malignant cell populations of different origins are responsible. Ovarian carcinosarcomas are similar to other ovarian carcinomas in presentation and pattern of spread, but patients with carcinosarcoma develop recurrences quickly and have a poor prognosis, with long-term survival unlikely. The clinical characteristics, management, and outcome of 65 patients with MMMT were compared with those of 746 patients with serous adenocarcinoma (SAC).

Methods.—The patients received a diagnosis of MMMT or SAC between 1984 and 2002. Variables were documented at baseline prospectively. Chemotherapy responses, progression-free survival (PFS), and cause-specific survival were determined and compared between patients with MMMT and those with SAC.

Results.—A significant difference was found in the mean age at diagnosis of patients with MMMT (66.6 years) and SAC (62.0 years). The distribution of disease by stage was similar between the 2 groups. Radiologically measurable disease remained in 14 patients with stage III/IV MMMT (27%) and 302 patients with stage III/IV SAC (49%). The overall objective response rate was 25% for MMMT and 60% for SAC. The rate of complete response was 8% for MMMT and 21% for SAC; the rates for partial response were 17% and 39%, respectively. Fifty-eight percent of MMMT patients had progressive disease; only 24% of SAC patients had progressive disease. No change occurred in 2 MMMT patients or 42 SAC patients. CA 125 assay found 41% of the MMMT patients and 63% of the SAC patients responded to platinum-based chemotherapy. The median survival was 8.2 months for the MMMT group and 20.7 months for the SAC group; this was a significant difference. Patients with MMMT also had a significantly shorter median

PFS of 6.4 months, compared with a PFS of 12.1 months for the SAC group. When optimal debulking was achieved during the initial surgery, patients with MMMT had a median survival of 14.8 months; when this was not accomplished, the median survival was only 3.1 months. Achieving optimal debulking was thus a highly significant factor determining outcome.

Conclusions.—The carcinosarcomas differ significantly from SACs with regard to age at onset, response to platinum-based chemotherapy, clinical course, and survival. MMMTs are much more aggressive and carry a worse survival than SACs. The factor found to be significantly predictive of outcome is optimal debulking of the tumor at the initial surgery.

Survival of Women Diagnosed With Malignant, Mixed Mullerian Tumors of the Ovary (OMMMT)

Barnholts-Sloan JS, Morris R, Malone JM Jr, et al (Wayne State Univ, Detroit)

Gynecol Oncol 93:506-512, 2004 3–21

Background.—Age at diagnosis, stage of disease, race, tumor grade, and histologic type all influence the prognosis and survival of patients with ovarian cancer. One of the most highly malignant forms of ovarian cancer, although occurring rarely, is malignant, mixed mullerian tumor of the ovary (OMMMT), which is also called ovarian carcinosarcoma. This tumor has a highly aggressive course, and affected patients have a median survival between 17 and 27 months. Management has been similar to that for epithelial ovarian cancers (EOCs), including initial surgical cytoreduction followed by chemotherapy in the adjuvant and relapsed settings. The optimal chemotherapy regimen and its impact on survival are as yet undetermined. Data from the population-based Surveillance, Epidemiology, and End Results Program were used to evaluate the survival of women with OMMMT in comparison with that of women with advanced-stage EOC.

Methods.—The data were drawn from 14,025 women who received a diagnosis of primary invasive ovarian cancer between 1988 and 1997. OMMMT was present in 382 of these women, and 13,643 had EOC. Prognostic variables were identified by histologic subtype. Risk of death from OMMMT or EOC was assessed.

Results.—The women with OMMMT were about 3% of the entire sample. No difference between those with OMMMT and EOC were found for distribution by race or stage of disease at diagnosis. Women with OMMMT were older at diagnosis (≥70 years) than those with EOC. The proportion of women with OMMMT who had primary surgery was significantly greater (96%) than that for women with EOC (83%). Women with OMMMT had a significantly poorer survival, with a 69% increased risk of death from any cause compared with women with EOC. The median survival was 18 months and 40 months, respectively, for OMMMT and EOC. The types of surgery performed were similar, although fewer women with OMMMT had “no surgery/biopsy only” approaches. Eighty-one percent of advanced-stage EOC and 85% of advanced-stage OMMMT cases had tumor debulking. Patients with high-grade OMMMT had a median survival of 18 months, whereas those with high-grade EOC had a median survival of 30 months. Compared with women with early stage, high-grade EOC, women with early stage OMMMT had a 30% increased risk of death. Those with advanced-stage OMMMT had a 60% increased risk of death compared with those with advanced-stage high-grade EOC. Very poor median survival (13 months) was also noted for OMMMT.

Conclusions.—Postmenopausal women are the group most likely to have OMMMT. Most patients with EOC or OMMMT had advanced-stage disease at diagnosis. The risk of death from any cause was significantly increased for women with OMMMT whether they were compared with women with EOC of any grade or stage, or with women with high-grade EOC only. The median survival for advanced-stage OMMMT was very poor, only 13 months.

Cisplatin as Initial Chemotherapy in Ovarian Carcinosarcomas: A Gynecologic Oncology Group Study

Thigpen JT, Blessing JA, DeGeest K, et al (Univ of Mississippi, Jackson; Roswell Park Cancer Inst, Buffalo, NY; Rush Med College, Chicago; et al)

Gynecol Oncol 93:336-339, 2004 3–22

Background.—Carcinosarcoma of the ovary is rare. An analysis of the largest series of carcinosarcomas of the ovary treated with cisplatin is described.

Study Design.—The study group consisted of 136 patients with carcinosarcoma of the ovary who received IV cisplatin, 50 mg/m^2, every 3 weeks until unacceptable toxicity, disease progression, death, or loss to follow-up. End points of the study included objective response, progression-free survival, and overall survival.

Findings.—Of the 44 patients with carcinosarcoma evaluable for response, 2% had a complete response and 18% had a partial response. An additional 23% had stable disease, whereas 57% had disease increase. The median progression-free survival in 130 evaluable patients was 5.2 months and median survival was 11.7 months. Adverse effects included leukopenia, neutropenia, thrombocytopenia, anemia, nausea and vomiting, azotemia, neurotoxicity, fever, and tinnitus.

Conclusions.—Cisplatin has activity against carcinosarcoma of the ovary. Because this disease is rare, further studies of cytotoxic agents will be difficult, but because the activity of cisplatin was similar to that of the more common uterine carcinosarcomas, similar therapies may be useful.

► This group of 3 articles (Abstracts 3–20 to 3–22) concerns ovarian carcinosarcoma, a relatively rare cancer of the ovary that constitutes less than 2% of ovarian malignancies. Brown et al (Abstract 3–20) report a review of 65 patients with ovarian carcinosarcoma seen at the Edinburgh Cancer Center between 1984 and 2002. These patients, when compared with serous carcinoma of the ovary, have shorter progression-free and overall survival times. Optimal debulking conferred a significantly better survival. Barnholtz-Sloan et al (Abstract 3–21) reported on 382 patients with ovarian carcinosarcoma and found similarly poor survival compared with celomic epithelial ovarian carcinoma. Because of the rarity of these tumors, there have been virtually no concerted prospective phase II or III studies of the use of systemic therapy. Thigpen et al (Abstract 3–22) report one of the first such series to show clear activity for a particular agent. Single-agent cisplatin at a dose of 50 mg/m^2 every 3 weeks produced 1 complete and 8 partial responses among 44 patients (20% response rate) with disseminated or recurrent disease. This response rate is identical to that observed in a Gynecologic Oncology Group study of the same drug in the same dose and schedule in patients with carcinosarcomas of the uterus. This suggests that the more extensive prospective literature available on carcinosarcomas of uterine origin can probably be applied to those lesions arising in the ovary.

J. T. Thigpen, MD

Uterine

A Phase III Trial of Surgery With or Without Adjunctive External Pelvic Radiation Therapy in Intermediate Risk Endometrial Adenocarcinoma: A Gynecologic Oncology Group Study

Keys HM, Roberts JA, Brunetto VL, et al (Albany Medical College, NY; Stanford Univ, Calif; Roswell Park Cancer Inst, Buffalo, NY; et al)
Gynecol Oncol 92:744-751, 2004 3–23

Background.—Adenocarcinoma of the endometrium is diagnosed in more than 36,000 women each year, most of whom have received postoperative radiation to minimize relapses. Evidence is increasing that women with noninvasive endometrial adenocarcinoma have a very low risk of recurrent disease and do not need radiation therapy (RT). The usefulness of RT given postoperatively to women with stages IB, IC, and II endometrial cancer was assessed.

Methods.—After surgery, 448 patients with a diagnosis of intermediate-risk endometrial adenocarcinoma were randomly assigned to receive either no additional therapy (NAT) or whole pelvic RT. In a refinement of the classification, a high-intermediate-risk (HIR) subgroup of patients included (1) patients with moderate to poorly differentiated tumor, lymphovascular invasion, and outer third myometrial invasion; (2) patients aged 50 years or older with at least 2 of the above risk factors; or (3) patients aged 70 years or older with any risk factor listed above. Toxic reactions, recurrences, and overall survival were documented.

Results.—Three hundred ninety-two women were divided into the 2 treatment groups. The median follow-up was 68 months, with 15 patients alive after recurrence a median of 80 months after treatment. Twenty-four were lost to follow-up after a median of 50 months. Women who received RT had a 58% lower risk of recurrence of disease than those receiving NAT. Most recurrences developed within 18 months of the initial treatment. The

RT group had a 24-month estimated cumulative incidence of recurrence of 3%; the cumulative incidence of recurrence for the NAT group was 12%. In the NAT group, there were 13 recurrences in the vaginal vault, but only 2 in the RT group. The estimated cumulative incidence of isolated local (vaginal or other pelvic) recurrence was 1.6% for the RT group and 7.4% for the NAT group at 24 months. The risk of death was an estimated 14% less with RT than with NAT, although this was not statistically significant. At 48 months, the overall survival was 92% for the RT group and 86% for the NAT group. Nineteen of 36 deaths in the NAT group and 15 of the 30 in the RT group resulted from causes other than endometrial cancer or treatment. One third of the women were in the HIR subgroup, but almost two thirds of the recurrences and two thirds of the cancer-related deaths occurred in this subgroup. Among the women in the HIR subgroup, the overall death rate was somewhat lower with RT than with NAT. Women receiving RT had more frequent and more severe toxic reactions than those receiving NAT. Two deaths in the RT group were attributed to radiation-related intestinal injury.

Conclusions.—In a comparison of whole pelvic RT and NAT for patients at high-intermediate risk for endometrial adenocarcinoma recurrence, adjuvant RT produced better outcomes in terms of risk of recurrence. Patients at lower risk of recurrence may experience adverse effects that are greater than the benefit obtained.

Cost-Effectiveness Analysis of the Treatment for Intermediate Risk Endometrial Cancer: Postoperative Brachytherapy vs. Observation

Fanning J, Hoffman ML, Andrews SJ, et al (Med College of Ohio, Akron; Summa Health System, Akron, Ohio)

Gynecol Oncol 93:632-636, 2004 3–24

Background.—About 55% of the estimated 40,100 new cases of endometrial cancer identified in a year are low-risk tumors that require no adjuvant treatment after surgery. Another 33% are intermediate-risk cancers for which various treatment approaches have been recommended. The use of surgical staging and postoperative vaginal cuff brachytherapy without teletherapy produced a 5-year progression-free survival rate of 97% in these women at intermediate risk. More recent results have suggested that full surgical staging with lymphadenectomy but no postoperative radiation therapy is sufficient. Those who develop vaginal recurrence are treated with teletherapy and brachytherapy, achieving a salvage rate of 57% to 63%. A cost-effectiveness analysis was performed to compare the survival, morbidity, and cost of treating patients with intermediate-risk endometrial cancer who have postoperative vaginal cuff brachytherapy, with the survival, morbidity, and cost for those who undergo observation and treatment for vaginal recurrence as needed.

Methods.—The definition of intermediate-risk endometrial cancer included stage IC, IG3, and II tumors confined to the uterus with more than 50% myometrial invasion, poor differentiation, or cervical metastasis. The treatment included hysterectomy, oophorectomy, and lymphadenectomy. In strategy 1, patients had postoperative vaginal cuff brachytherapy; in strategy 2, observation was conducted. Strategy 2 patients who had vaginal recurrence underwent a diagnostic workup, teletherapy, and brachytherapy. Brachytherapy was delivered by low-dose rate (strategy 2A) or high-dose rate (strategy 2B). The 6 principles of cost-effectiveness analysis were observed, including explicit description of costs, explicit description of benefits, detailed description of costs, adjustment for different time periods, sensitivity analysis, and cost ratio analysis. The analysis used actual payer costs rather than charges.

Results.—Observation was accompanied by a decline in survival of 3% if no postoperative brachytherapy was done. Projected radiation complication rates for the 2 strategies were comparable. By not treating patients with postoperative low-dose rate brachytherapy and treating only those who develop vaginal recurrence, the cost was diminished by 31%. These decreased costs are possible because only 8% of patients develop vaginal cuff recurrence, even though teletherapy has significantly more complications than brachytherapy. The cost per life saved was $38,764, which was less than the usually used benchmark of $50,000 per life saved.

Conclusions.—The reduction in cost achieved by following an observation strategy was 31%. The radiation complication rate was similar in the 2 approaches, and the decline in survival was only 3%. The cost per life saved was less than the usual benchmark, maintaining the acceptability of postoperative high-dose rate brachytherapy as an intervention for intermediate-risk patients with endometrial cancer.

▶ This phase III trial from the Gynecologic Oncology Group (GOG) (Abstract 3–23) randomized endometrial carcinoma patients with an approximate 15% recurrence rate after surgery alone, to surgery followed by either pelvic radiation or no further therapy. Among the 392 eligible patients with stages IB, IC, or II disease, pelvic radiation led to a reduced recurrence rate at 2 years (3% vs 12%). The estimated survival rate at 4 years was 86% with no adjuvant therapy and 92% with radiation. The best results were seen in those patients with risk factors that predict for a higher risk of recurrence (high grade, lymphovascular space invasion, outer third myometrial invasion). These results provide the first solid evidence for a role of external beam radiation in intermediate-risk endometrial carcinoma (stages IA grade 3, IB, IC, and II). Two editorials accompanying the article present thoroughly the pros and cons of the debate that has ensued over these results.

Shortly after the publication of the GOG trial, a study by Fanning and colleagues (Abstract 3–24) examined the cost of immediate versus delayed brachytherapy in this intermediate-risk group of endometrial carcinoma patients. This study found that withholding brachytherapy and using it only in those who actually develop vaginal metastases resulted in a 31% decrease in cost with a similar radiation complication rate, but a 3% decrease in survival. These issues should be discussed with patients in considering what treatment options should be used in an individual case.

J. T. Thigpen, MD

Improved Outcome at 10 Years for Serous-Papillary/Clear Cell or High-risk Endometrial Cancer Patients Treated by Adjuvant High-dose Whole Abdomino-pelvic Irradiation

Martinez AA, Weiner S, Podratz K, et al (William Beaumont Hosp, Royal Oak, Mich; Mayo Clinic, Rochester, Minn)

Gynecol Oncol 90:537-546, 2003 3–25

Background.—The risk of endometrial cancer recurrence and death from disease is increased in women with high-grade histologic findings and/or aggressive cell types, deep myometrial invasion, cervical involvement, and/or extreme disease. Ten-year outcomes of treatment with adjuvant high-dose whole abdominal irradiation (the WAPI technique) with a pelvic/vaginal boost in patients with stage I to III endometrial carcinoma at high risk for intra-abdominopelvic recurrence are reported.

Methods.—One hundred thirty-two patients were enrolled in the prospective, nonrandomized trial and treated with adjuvant WAPI between November 1981 and October 2001 (Fig 1). Thirty-two percent of the women had stage I or II disease, and 68%, stage III. Deep myometrial invasion was present in 52% of the patients, positive peritoneal cytology in 38%, high-grade lesions in 67%, positive pelvic/paraaortic lymph nodes in 19%, and serous-papillary or clear cell histology in 45%. Patients were observed for a mean of 6.4 years.

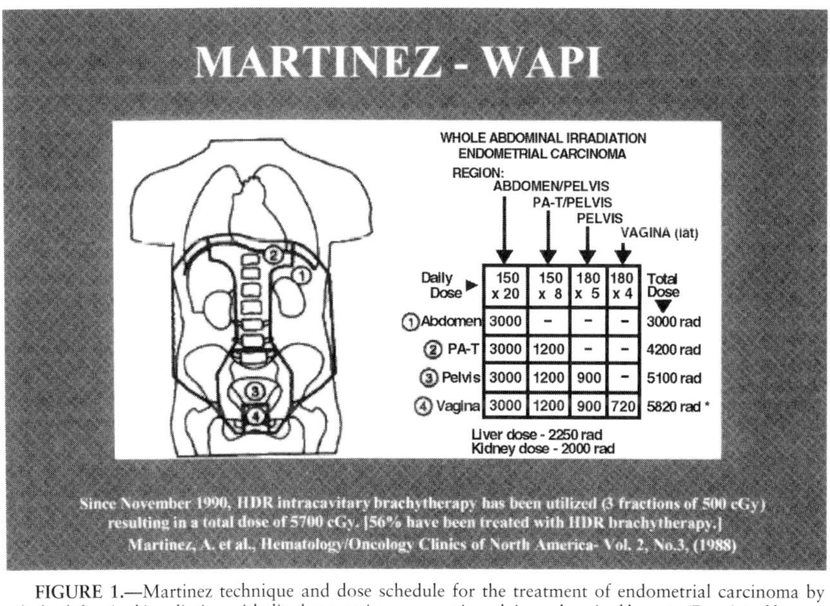

FIGURE 1.—Martinez technique and dose schedule for the treatment of endometrial carcinoma by whole abdominal irradiation with diaphragmatic, para-aortic, pelvic, and vaginal boosts. (Reprinted by permission of the publisher from Martinez AA, Weiner S, Podratz K, et al: Improved outcome at 10 years for serous-papillary/clear cell or high-risk endometrial cancer patients treated by adjuvant high-dose whole abdomino-pelvic irradiation. *Gynecol Oncol* 90:537-546, 2003. Copyright 2003 by Elsevier Science.)

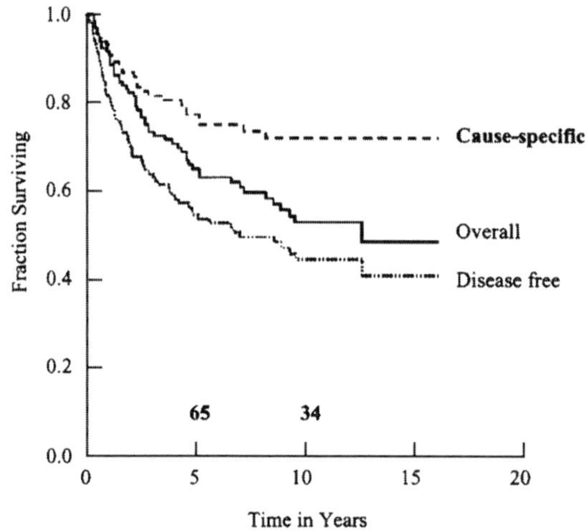

FIGURE 2.—Actuarial analysis of overall survival, cause-specific survival, and disease-free survival for 132 patients. Number of patients remaining in cause-specific survival calculation are indicated on the X-axis. (Reprinted by permission of the publisher from Martinez AA, Weiner S, Podratz K, et al: Improved outcome at 10 years for serous-papillary/clear cell or high-risk endometrial cancer patients treated by adjuvant high-dose whole abdomino-pelvic irradiation. *Gynecol Oncol* 90:537-546, 2003. Copyright 2003 by Elsevier Science.)

Findings.—Overall, cause-specific survival (CSS) was 77% at 5 years and 72% at 10 years. Disease-free survival (DFS) was 55% and 45%, respectively (Figs 2 and 3). When patients were stratified by histologic findings, the 5- and 10-year CSS was 75% and 70%, respectively, among those with adenocarcinoma, and 80% and 74% among those with serous-papillary/clear cell (Fig 6). The DFS for adenocarcinoma was 59% at 5 years and 49% at 20 years; for serous-papillary/clear cell, these rates were 49% and 38%, respec-

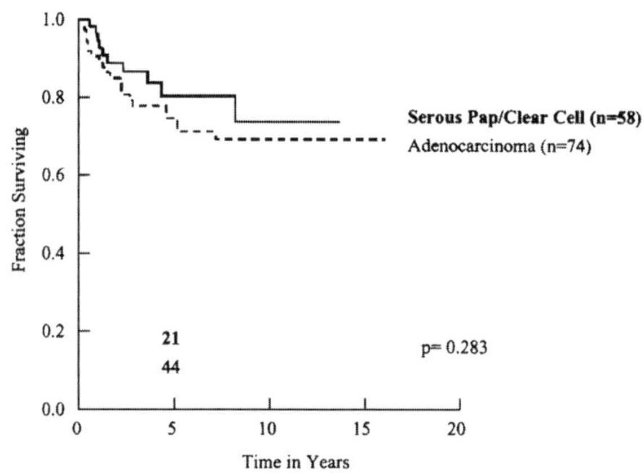

FIGURE 3.—Actuarial analysis of cause-specific survival of 132 patients stratified by histology. Number of patients remaining in calculation at 5 years is indicated on the X-axis. (Reprinted by permission of the publisher from Martinez AA, Weiner S, Podratz K, et al: Improved outcome at 10 years for serous-papillary/clear cell or high-risk endometrial cancer patients treated by adjuvant high-dose whole abdomino-pelvic irradiation. *Gynecol Oncol* 90:537-546, 2003. Copyright 2003 by Elsevier Science.)

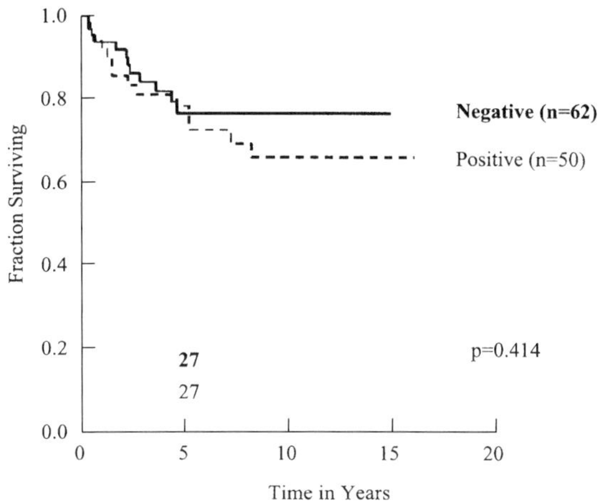

FIGURE 6.—Actuarial analysis of cause-specific survival of 112 patients stratified by peritoneal cytology. Number of patients remaining in calculation are indicated on the X-axis. (Reprinted by permission of the publisher from Martinez AA, Weiner S, Podratz K, et al: Improved outcome at 10 years for serous-papillary/clear cell or high-risk endometrial cancer patients treated by adjuvant high-dose whole abdomino-pelvic irradiation. *Gynecol Oncol* 90:537-546, 2003. Copyright 2003 by Elsevier Science.)

tively. Among patients with surgical stage I to II disease, the CSS was 83% for adenocarcinoma and 89% for serous-papillary disease at 5 years. Among patients with stage III disease, these rates were 73% and 62%. Relapses occurred in 35% of the patients. In 59% of the patients, the first site of failure was the abdomen or pelvis (Table 6). When the patients were stratified by histologic variant, disease recurred in 34% of patients with adenocarcinoma and in 41% with serous-papillary disease. A multivariate regression analysis indicated that advancing age was the only significant prognostic factor for CSS and DFS. Fourteen percent of the patients experienced chronic grade 3 to 4 toxicity (Table 8). In 2%, grade 3 renal toxicity developed.

Conclusions.—High-dose adjuvant WAPI appears to be a very effective treatment for women with stage I to III endometrial carcinoma and risk fac-

TABLE 6.—Patterns of Failure by First Site

	Adenocarcinoma		Serous-Papillary/CC		All Patients	
Site	No. Patients	% Failure	No. Patients	% Failure	No. Patients	% Failure
Abdomen/pelvis	10	40	11	52	21	46
Extra abd LNs	3	12	4	19	7	15
Vagina	4	16	2	10	6	13
Lung	7	28	3	14	10	22
Other	1	4	1	5	2	4
Total	25	54	21	46	46	100

Abbreviations: CC, Clear cell carcinoma; *extra abd LNs:* extraabdomino-pelvic lymph nodes.

(Reprinted by permission of the publisher from Martinez AA, Weiner S, Podratz K, et al: Improved outcome at 10 years for serous-papillary/clear cell or high-risk endometrial cancer patients treated by adjuvant high-dose whole abdomino-pelvic irradiation. *Gynecol Oncol* 90:537-546, 2003. Copyright 2003 by Elsevier Science.)

TABLE 8.—Analysis of Chronic Toxicity Using the RTOG Criteria

Toxicity	None (%)	Grade 1 (%)	Grade 2 (%)	Grade 3 (%)	Grade 4 (%)
Bowel	64 (50)	38 (30)	8 (6)	17 (13)	1 (1)
Liver	68 (53)	46 (36)	13 (10)	1 (1)	0 (0)
Lung	77 (60)	44 (34)	6 (5)	1 (1)	0 (0)
Kidney	120 (94)	4 (3)	1 (1)	3 (2)	0 (0)
Bladder	111 (87)	13 (10)	2 (1.5)	2 (1.5)	0 (0)

(Reprinted by permission of the publisher from Martinez AA, Weiner S, Podratz K, et al: Improved outcome at 10 years for serous-papillary/clear cell or high-risk endometrial cancer patients treated by adjuvant high-dose whole abdomino-pelvic irradiation. *Gynecol Oncol* 90:537-546, 2003. Copyright 2003 by Elsevier Science.)

tors for intra-abdominopelvic recurrence (Table 9). The 10-year outcomes of this treatment were excellent in the current series. The low rate of long-term complications and the high CSS make high-dose WAPI the treatment of choice for such patients.

▶ This is a very provocative article from solid investigators focusing on the outcome of patients with endometrial carcinoma stages I-III, with high risk features for intra-abdominal or pelvic recurrence. This will include patients who have serous-papillary or clear cell histologic types. The patients consist of 132 patients receiving whole abdominal pelvic irradiation with actuarial data out to 10 years. Forty-three of these patients were FIGO stage I and II but 8 were stage III. Half the patients had deep myometrial invasion, over one third of patients had positive peritoneal cytology, and two thirds of the patients had high-grade lesions. Almost 20% had positive nodes. The data are impressive because chemotherapy was not given until time of relapse. The authors spent a lot of time discussing technique, because whole abdominal pelvic radiotherapy is heavily operator dependent, as this article illustrates in great detail.

E. Glatstein, MD

TABLE 9.—Comparison of Time-Dose-Fractionation Values for Selected Whole Abdomino-Pelvic Irradiation Techniques

Site	High-Dose WAPI	GOG-WART	% Dose Reduction*
Abdomen	42	38-42	0-10
Liver	32-59	38-42	0-40
Diaphragm	42-59	0	100
PA-Nodes	59	38-62	0-40
Pelvis	73	57-62	18-28
Vagina	98	57-62	58-72

Note: Time-dose fractionation calculations were performed by Colin Orton, PhD

*% dose reduction between high-dose WAPI and low-dose GOG-WART techniques.

Abbreviation: PA-Nodes, Para-aortic nodes.

(Reprinted by permission of the publisher from Martinez AA, Weiner S, Podratz K, et al: Improved outcome at 10 years for serous-papillary/clear cell or high-risk endometrial cancer patients treated by adjuvant high-dose whole abdomino-pelvic irradiation. *Gynecol Oncol* 90:537-546, 2003. Copyright 2003 by Elsevier Science.)

Phase III Trial of Doxorubicin Plus Cisplatin With or Without Paclitaxel Plus Filgrastim in Advanced Endometrial Carcinoma: A Gynecologic Oncology Group Study

Fleming GF, Brunetto VL, Cella D, et al (Univ of Chicago; Northwestern Univ, Evanston, Ill; Roswell Park Cancer Inst, Buffalo, NY; et al)

J Clin Oncol 22:2159-2166, 2004 3–26

Background.—Patients with metastatic endometrial carcinoma are currently treated with doxorubicin plus cisplatin (AP). This prospective, randomized clinical trial compared AP to TAP (addition of paclitaxel plus filgrastim for hematopoietic support) for the treatment of 263 chemotherapy naive patients with stage III, stage IV, or recurrent endometrial carcinoma.

Study Design.—The study group consisted of 263 women with endometrial cancer who were randomly assigned to receive either AP or TAP. The average follow-up was 32 months. Peripheral neuropathy was monitored. The primary end point was overall survival (OS), with progression-free survival (PFS) and response rate (RR) as secondary end points. Data were analyzed by intention to treat.

Findings.—The RR, PFS, and OS were all significantly improved in the TAP treatment group compared with the AP treatment group. Treatment was well tolerated hematologically. Neurologic toxicity was worse for patients in the TAP group, with 12% having grade 3 and 27% grade 2 peripheral neuropathy.

Conclusion.—TAP chemotherapy was superior to AP chemotherapy for RR, PFS, and OS in patients with advanced or recurrent endometrial carcinoma. TAP requires growth factor support to control hematologic toxicity, but when filgrastim was used, hematologic toxicity and cardiac toxicity were not limiting. However, neurotoxicity was common among patients receiving TAP and should be closely monitored.

▶ Fleming et al in the Gynecologic Oncology Group (GOG) present the results of the third in a series of randomized phase III trials of chemotherapy in advanced or recurrent endometrial carcinoma. The initial trial in this series compared doxorubicin alone with doxorubicin plus cisplatin (GOG Protocol 107) and reported a superior response rate and PFS without a difference in survival with the doublet. The second in the series randomized patients to either doxorubicin/cisplatin or doxorubicin/paclitaxel (GOG Protocol 163) and found no significant differences except for an apparent toxicity advantage for doxorubicin/cisplatin. This third trial in the series compared doxorubicin/cisplatin to the 3-drug combination of paclitaxel/doxorubicin/cisplatin with G-CSF support (GOG Protocol 177). The triplet significantly enhances RR, PFS, and OS with some increase in toxicity, particularly neurotoxicity. This study establishes the 3-drug combination as the treatment of choice in patients with advanced or recurrent endometrial carcinoma. An ongoing GOG study (GOG Protocol 209) seeks to simplify the triplet by comparing the 3-drug regimen to a doublet of paclitaxel plus carboplatin. At the present time, however, there is no randomized phase III evidence to support the use of the doublet in place of the 3-drug regimen outside of clinical trial.

J. T. Thigpen, MD

Uterine Papillary Serous Carcinoma (UPSC): A Single Institution Review of 129 Cases

Slomovitz BM, Burke TW, Eifel PJ, et al (Univ of Texas, Houston)
Gynecol Oncol 91:463-469, 2003 3–27

Background.—About 5% of all endometrial cancers are uterine papillary serous carcinoma (UPSC), which is an aggressive histologic subtype that accounts for a disproportionately high number of recurrences and deaths. The clinical and pathologic characteristics of patients with UPSC were identified, with correlations then sought with overall survival (OS).

Methods.—Between 1989 and 2002, 129 patients with stages I through IV UPSC were surgically staged at M. D. Anderson Cancer Center. A review of their medical records and pathology reports identified the clinical and pathologic findings characteristic of such patients. OS data were noted, along with factors predictive of outcome.

Results.—Patients ranged in age from 44 to 93 years (median age, 68 years), and most were postmenopausal. Abnormal bleeding was the presenting symptom in 66.7% of all cases, with abdominal symptoms found in 36% of patients with stage IV disease. Disease stage was not correlated with race, median weight, diabetes, parity, or smoking. Twenty-two percent of the patients had a personal or family history of breast cancer. Stage I disease was found in 40.3% of patients, stage II in 3.9%, stage III in 31.8%, and stage IVB in 24.0%. OS and progression-free survival correlated with disease stage. A considerable difference was found between the OS rate for patients with stage IA disease (82%) and those with stage IC disease (34%). Deep myometrial invasion was seen in stages II through IV disease, and lymphatic and vascular space invasion was linked to extrauterine spread and the presence of high-stage disease. Analysis of the effect of pathologic prognostic features on OS identified deep myometrial invasion and nodal involvement as predictive of a worse prognosis. The tumors of most stage IV patients had pure UPSC histology, as did most with no myometrial invasion. Twenty-five percent of patients had no uterine invasion, and 38% of these patients had extrauterine disease. Abdominal disease, most often affecting the omentum, was found in 69% of those with extrauterine disease. Lymph node metastases were identified in 19% of patients with noninvasive uterine disease. Fifteen of 32 patients with no myometrial invasion had tumors involving endometrial polyps. The median survival for stage III patients who received chemotherapy was 69.7 months, compared with 29.4 months for those who did not receive chemotherapy. Chemotherapy did not increase OS among stage I, II, or IV patients. Radiotherapy did not increase either OS or progression-free survival. Seventy-four percent of the stage IA patients were treated with observation alone. At 5 years, the survival rate for stage IA patients was 80.4%. Twenty-one percent had a documented recurrence, 3 of which were in patients who did not receive radiation therapy.

Conclusions.—The clinical and pathologic characteristics of UPSC are distinct from those of other endometrial cancers, requiring separate analysis. Some patients who have minimal uterine disease and no serious pathologic risk factors develop distant metastasis, recurrence, and mortality. Disease limited to the uterus carries a worse prognosis than for similar endometrioid tumors. Patients with advanced-stage disease require systemic therapy, and chemotherapy for stage III patients improves survival significantly. Tumors with pure UPSC histology and those with mixed histology and a serous component require differential consideration from other types of endometrial cancer in clinical trials.

Her-2/*neu* Overexpression and Amplification in Uterine Papillary Serous Carcinoma

Slomovitz BM, Broaddus RR, Burke TW, et al (Univ of Texas, Houston)
J Clin Oncol 22:3126-3132, 2004 3–28

Background.—More than 50% of the recurrences and deaths resulting from endometrial cancer are attributable to uterine papillary serous carcinoma (UPSC). The overall survival (OS) of women with UPSC is 46% at 5 years. Other characteristics of UPSC include early metastasis and resistance to therapy. Some investigations have suggested that the human Her-2/*neu* gene product may be overexpressed in many endometrial cancers, particularly UPSC. Her-2/*neu* expression was assessed with immunohistochemistry (IHC) in a large series of UPSCs. The effect of gene amplification on Her-2/*neu* expression and any possible prognostic value were also evaluated.

Methods.—IHC methods documented Her-2/*neu* expression in tumor tissues from 68 patients with UPSC. The definition of overexpression used was complete membrane staining in more than 10% of the cells. Fluorescence in situ hybridization (FISH) was used to evaluate gene amplification in all tumors with Her-2/*neu* overexpression. Medical records were used to obtain clinical and pathologic correlates.

Results.—IHC identified Her-2/*neu* overexpression in 12 patients (18%). The tumors in 2 patients (17%) had specific gene amplification, and those in 8 patients (75%) had aneuploidy of chromosome 17. Both tumors with Her-2/*neu* amplification were also aneuploid. Half of the 12 patients with Her-2/*neu* overexpression had a personal history of breast cancer, whereas only 13% of Her-2/*neu*–negative cases had such a history. No clinical or pathologic characteristics distinguished the 2 patients with gene amplification of Her-2/*neu* from the other patients, and neither had a personal or family history of breast cancer. Thirty-seven patients died during the 1- to 162-month follow-up (median, 28.6 months). In 27 cases, the death was related to endometrial cancer. Patients with Her-2/*neu*–positive tumors had a median OS of 18 months, and those with Her-2/*neu*–negative tumors had a median OS of 48 months. A significant relationship was noted between Her-2/*neu* overexpression, lymph vascular space invasion, lymph node status, and high disease stage and a shorter OS. Among 42 patients with stage III or IV disease, the median survival was 17 months with Her-2/*neu*–positive tumors and 39 months with Her-2/*neu*–negative tumors. Advanced-stage disease and Her-2/*neu* overexpression were the only factors identified on multivariate proportional hazards modeling to predict a shorter OS.

Conclusions.—The incidence of Her-2/*neu* overexpression in this large population of women with UPSC was 18%. Only rarely was gene amplification seen. Her-2/*neu* overexpression was identified as a prognostic marker for UPSC. A worse prognosis attended positive IHC expression.

▶ These 2 articles (Abstracts 3–27 and 3–28) from the Department of Gynecologic Oncology at M. D. Anderson Cancer Center examine a subset of endometrial cancer patients whose tumors exhibit papillary serous histology. The first article (Abstract 3–27) reviews 129 cases surgically staged at M. D. Anderson Cancer Center over a 14-year period ending in 2002. Important associated prognostic factors were similar to those for other types of endometrial carcinoma: International Federation of Gynecology and Obstetrics (FIGO) stage, nodal status, lymphatic and vascular space invasion, and depth of myometrial invasion. Complete surgical staging was deemed to be critical in this histologic type because the traditional risk factors did not predict the presence or absence of metastatic disease. For example, the 25% of patients without uterine invasion had a 38% incidence of extrauterine disease, far greater than is seen with the more common histologic types. This series supports the relatively poor prognosis of UPSCs compared with other, more common histologic types of endometrial carcinomas.

The second article (Abstract 3–28) examined the frequency and nature of Her-2/*neu* overexpression. In a series of 68 UPSCs, 12 (18%) demonstrated overexpression by IHC, but only 2 of these showed gene amplification by FISH. Her-2/*neu* overexpression was associated with a poorer outcome. The study did not address the use of trastuzumab treatment.

Taken together, these 2 articles support the reported poor prognosis of UPSC and provide a basis for studies of monoclonal antibody therapy directed against Her-2/*neu*.

J. T. Thigpen, MD

Surveillance, Epidemiology, and End Results Analysis of 2677 Cases of Uterine Sarcoma 1989-1999

Brooks SE, Zhan M, Cote T, et al (Univ of Maryland, Baltimore, Md; Food and Drug Administration, Rockville, Md)

Gynecol Oncol 93:204-208, 2004 3–29

Background.—Uterine sarcomas account for 4% to 9% of all invasive uterine cancers. Black women have been noted to have an excess incidence of leiomyosarcoma and mixed mesodermal sarcoma compared with white women, but details concerning survival, distribution of stages, and treatment are lacking. Data from the Surveillance, Epidemiology, and End Results program were evaluated to determine demographic, histologic, treatment, and survival parameters for women of various races with uterine sarcoma.

Methods.—Included in the family of uterine sarcoma were leiomyosarcoma, carcinosarcoma, high-grade endometrial stromal sarcoma, adenosarcoma, and sarcoma not otherwise specified. The cases were identified in women aged 35 years or older. Race-specific age-adjusted incidence, histologic distribution, extent of disease when diagnosed, and race-specific survival were documented.

Results.—Eight percent of the primary uterine malignancies for the years surveyed were uterine sarcomas. These were found in 2098 white women, 420 black women, and 159 women of other races. White women were significantly older at diagnosis (64.2 years) than black women (62.7 years) or those of other races (58.5 years). The age-adjusted incidence rates were $7.0/10^5$ for black women, $3.6/10^5$ for white women, and $2.7/10^5$ for women of other races. Carcinosarcoma was more common with increasing age, with age-adjusted incidence rates of $0.7/10^5$, $2.1/10^5$, and $0.5/10^5$ for white, black, and other women aged 35 to 64 years, but $4.9/10^5$, $11.1/10^5$, and $2.4/10^5$, respectively, at age 65 years or older. The incidences differed between racial groups for leiomyosarcoma and carcinosarcoma only. At diagnosis, most women had stage I disease, which was found in 54% of whites and 45% of blacks. Stage II disease was present at diagnosis for 7% of whites and 11% of blacks. The distribution of stage III and IV disease did not differ by racial group. Stage I disease was found in 80% of women with adenosarcoma, 55% of women with leiomyosarcoma, and 51% of women with carcinosarcoma. Fifty percent of white women and 53% of black women had surgery, and 21% of white women and 18% of black women had radiation therapy plus surgery. At 5 years, the relative survival was better for white women (53%) than for black women (42%); the rate for women of other races was 49%. Black women with stage I disease had a survival of 63%, whereas white women had a survival of 73%, a significant difference. Survival statistics did not differ by racial group for stage II to IV disease. Linking survival to type of treatment, no racial differences in survival were found.

Conclusions.—A higher incidence of uterine sarcomas was found in black women compared with white women, but the survival rates of black and white patients who were given comparable treatments were similar. Carcinosarcoma and leiomyosarcoma were identified as the most common types of uterine sarcoma. More than 50% of women with these sarcomas have stage I disease, with black women less likely to have stage I disease than white women. The poorer survival of black women may be attributable to lower referral rates for or use of radiation therapy or other adjuvant treatments. Women whose disease extends beyond the uterus should receive adjuvant therapy.

Phase II Trial of Gemcitabine as Second-Line Chemotherapy of Uterine Leiomyosarcoma: A Gynecologic Onclogy Group (GOG) Study

Look KY, Sandler A, Blessing JA, et al (Indiana Univ, Indianapolis; Vanderbilt Univ, Nashville, Tenn; Roswell Park Cancer Inst, Buffalo, NY; et al)

Gynecol Oncol 92:644-647, 2004 3–30

Background.—It is estimated that uterine leiomyosarcoma (LMS) represents 1% of all uterine malignancies. Uterine LMS is generally treated with total abdominal hysterectomy and bilateral salpingo-oophorectomy. Most patients with clinical stage I and II disease can develop recurrences. Systemic cytotoxic therapy may be an option for patients with recurrent uterine LMS, with doxorubicin and ifosfamide being the most commonly used agents. Gemcitabine is a cytosine arabinoside analogue that inhibits DNA synthesis and limits the ability of DNA repair enzymes to remove altered DNA. A phase II trial of gemcitabine was initiated by the Gynecologic Oncology Group to determine the drug's response rate and toxicity profile in patients with persistent or recurrent unresectable uterine LMS.

Methods.—The 48 patients ranged in age from 31 to 82 years (median, 52.5 years). All received gemcitabine, 1000 mg/m^2, administered IV over 30 minutes on days 1, 8, and 15, with cycles repeated every 28 days. A toxicity assessment was done in 44 patients, and toxicity and response evaluations were done in 42 patients.

Results.—Patients received a median of 2 cycles of treatment; the range was 1 to 13 cycles. Treatment was well tolerated with no deaths related to therapy. Of the 33 patients experiencing leukopenia, the median white blood cell count nadir was 2400. Of the 19 who had thrombocytopenia, the median platelet nadir was 68,000. Only neutropenia, nausea and vomiting, and dermatologic responses reached grade 4 toxicity. Measurable disease was found in pelvic locations in 9 cases and extrapelvic locations in 35 cases. One patient had a complete response, and 8 patients had a partial response. The overall response rate was 20.5%. Responses lasted a median of 4.9 months, and 15.9% of patients had stable disease. The response rate for those having previous irradiation was 18%, and that for patients not having irradiation was 21%. Six responses were outside the pelvis and 3 within the pelvis.

Conclusions.—Patients with persistent or recurrent uterine LMS may benefit from the use of gemcitabine. The overall response rate was 20.5%, with 1 complete and 8 partial responses to therapy. The treatment and the treatment schedule were both well tolerated.

► The article by Brooks et al (Abstract 3–29) examines Surveillance, Epidemiology, and End Results (SEER) data for the years 1989-1999 on uterine sarcomas. Significant observations include an increased age-adjusted incidence twice as high in blacks as whites, and a survival advantage for women with stages II to IV disease who received radiation in addition to surgery. These observations held for both of the 2 most common histologic types, carcinosarcomas and leiomyosarcomas. The second article by Look et al (Abstract 3–30) reports significant activity for gemcitabine in the second most common histologic type, leiomyosarcomas (1 complete response and 8 partial responses among 44 patients), as a part of the ongoing Gynecologic Oncology Group investigation of the activity of a series of single agents in each of the 2 major histologies (carcinosarcomas and leiomyosarcomas) in patients with disseminated or recurrent disease. The results of this series of phase II trials have identified doxorubicin and gemcitabine as having significant activity in leiomyosarcomas, and ifosfamide, cisplatin, and paclitaxel as having significant activity in carcinosarcomas.

J. T. Thigpen, MD

Cervix

Cervical Cancer Screening Among Women Without a Cervix

Sirovich BE, Welch HG (VA Outcomes Group, White River Junction, Vt; Dartmouth College, Hanover, NH)
JAMA 291:2990-2993, 2004 3–31

Background.—The Papanicolaou (Pap) smear screening for cervical cancer has become a widely accepted cancer screening test. In the United States, all women have historically been considered to be eligible for Pap smear screening, including millions of women who have undergone complete hysterectomy and who are not at risk of cervical cancer. In 1996, the US Preventive Services Task Force recommended that routine Pap smear screening is unnecessary in these women. Whether Pap smear screening among women who have undergone hysterectomy has decreased since publication of that recommendation was determined.

Methods.—Data from the Behavioral Risk Factor Surveillance System (1992-2002) were used. This system is an annual, population-based telephone survey of adults in the United States conducted by the Centers for Disease Control and Prevention. Data about timing, type, and indication for hysterectomies were obtained from the Nationwide Inpatient Sample and other sources.

Results.—Hysterectomies have been performed in 22 million women aged 18 years and older in the United States, representing 21% of the population. The proportion of these women who reported a current Pap smear did not change in the 10 years of the study. In 1992, 68.5% of women who had undergone hysterectomy reported having had a Pap smear in the past 3 years; in 2002, 69.1% had had a Pap smear during the same period. After adjustment for Pap smears that might have been performed before a recent hysterectomy and hysterectomies that spared the cervix or were performed for cervical neoplasia, it was estimated that almost 10 million women, or half of all women who have undergone hysterectomy, are being screened unnecessarily.

Conclusions.—Pap smear screening is being performed in many women in the United States who are not at risk of cervical cancer. The recommendations published by the US Preventive Services Task Force regarding cervical cancer screening in women without a cervix either have not been read or have been ignored.

► Pap screening has been one of the most successful models for cancer screening since first introduced more than 60 years ago. Indeed, the routine use of Pap smears is widely accepted by women in this country as part of their regular examinations. For women who have undergone hysterectomy with resection of the cervix, it is intuitively obvious that a Pap smear would not be important. Nonetheless, despite this information, it is curious to know that these women continue to be screened on a regular basis by their primary care providers. This is not insignificant, as it accounts for almost 10 million women in the United States. If we are to have an impact on our health care dollars, we must be careful to avoid inappropriate screening for asymptomatic individuals.

P. J. Loehrer, Sr, MD

Occult Supraclavicular Lymph Node Metastasis Identified by FDG-PET in Patients With Carcinoma of the Uterine Cervix

Tran BN, Grigsby PW, Dehdashti F, et al (Washington Univ, St Louis, Mo)

Gynecol Oncol 90:572-576, 2003 3–32

Background.—Fewer than 5% of patients with invasive carcinoma of the uterine cervix will have left supraclavicular lymph node metastasis. However, this frequency is much greater in patients who undergo cervical cancer surgical staging and are found to have positive para-aortic lymph nodes. The frequency of prognostic significance of occult supraclavicular lymph node metastases detected by fluorodeoxyglucose positron emission tomography (FDG-PET) in patients with cervical carcinoma was determined.

Methods.—The study included 186 patients diagnosed as having cervical cancer between 1998 and 2002 who underwent whole-body FDG-PET before treatment. In 14 patients, abnormal FDG uptake was noted in left supraclavicular lymph nodes without palpable disease. These patients underwent US-guided fine-needle aspiration of the left supraclavicular lymph nodes. Seven patients received definitive irradiation and concurrent chemotherapy, and 6 were treated with palliative intent. One patient refused treatment.

Findings.—Overall, a frequency of 8% of FDG-positive left supraclavicular lymph nodes was seen. In all 14 patients, metastasis was verified pathologically. Abnormal FDG uptake in left supraclavicular lymph nodes had a positive predictive value of 100%. In 19% of all patients, FDG uptake was abnormal in para-aortic lymph nodes. Positive FDG uptake in the left supraclavicular lymph nodes occurred with a 40% frequency in patients with para-aortic lymph node uptake and 15% in patients with stage IIIb disease (Fig 1). The median overall survival was 7.5 months. At the most recent follow-up, only 3 patients were alive with disease. The remaining 11 had died. Metastatic disease developed in all patients, most often in the bone and lung.

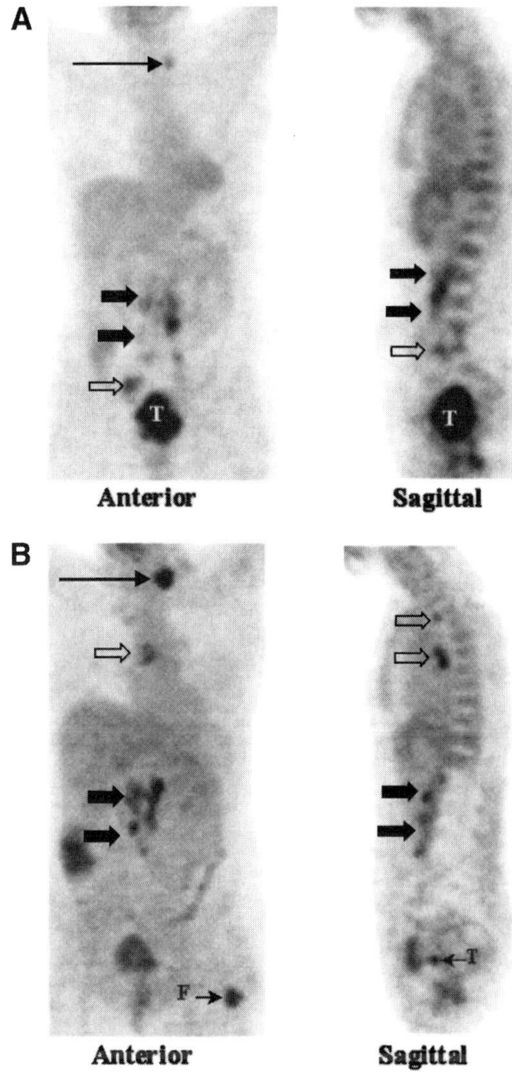

FIGURE 1.—Fifty-two year-old woman with newly diagnosed stage IIIb cervical carcinoma. (**A**) Anterior and sagittal images from pretherapy FDG-PET study show a large, lobulated focus of markedly increased FDG uptake in the cervical tumor. There are multiple metastases involving pelvic (*open arrow*), para-aortic (*solid arrows*), and left supraclavicular lymph nodes (*long arrow*). This patient underwent chemotherapy and radiotherapy to the pelvic and to a para-aortic port up to the L1 level. (**B**) Three months after completion of therapy, the patient was noted to have a palpable mass in the left supraclavicular region. Anterior and sagittal images from posttherapy FDG-PET study show further increased FDG uptake in the left supraclavicular region (*long arrow*). There are multiple metastases involving the mediastinum (*open arrows*) and para-aortic lymph nodes (*solid arrows*) in the upper abdomen as well as worsening of the previously noted metastases to the para-aortic lymph nodes in this region. There is a new metastatic focus in the left proximal femur (*F*). There is only a small focus of residual disease at the site of the primary tumor (*T*). Decreased activity in the lumbosacral marrow is due to radiation therapy. *Abbreviation: FDG-PET*, Fluorodeoxyglucose positron emission tomography. (Reprinted by permission of the publisher from Tran BN, Grigsby PW, Dehdashti F, et al: Occult supraclavicular lymph node metastasis identified by FDG-PET in patients with carcinoma of the uterine cervix. *Gynecol Oncol* 90:572-576, 2003. Copyright 2003 by Elsevier Science Inc.)

Conclusions.—Abnormal FDG uptake in left supraclavicular lymph nodes had a positive predictive value of 100%. Despite aggressive treatment, the prognosis for these patients is dismal.

► These investigators from Washington University in St Louis report on 186 patients with newly diagnosed carcinoma of the cervix who underwent whole body PET scanning with FDG. Fourteen of them showed an abnormal FDG uptake in the left supraclavicular lymph nodes. Apparently none of them had palpable disease, but all of them appeared to have para-aortic node positivity, which would seem to be logical.

E. Glatstein, MD

Staging of Advanced Cervical Carcinoma Using MRI—Predictors of Outcome After Radical Radiotherapy

Taylor MB, Carrington BM, Davidson SE, et al (Christie Hosp NHS Trust, Withington, Manchester, England)
Clin Radiol 58:532-541, 2003 3–33

Background.—Magnetic resonance imaging (MRI) is increasingly used to stage cervical carcinoma. The prognostic significance of MRI findings in the staging of cervical carcinoma was investigated.

Methods.—The MR images of 99 patients with cervical carcinoma were examined. Tumor involvement of the pelvic structures was noted, and lymph node sites, short axis diameters, and signal characteristics were documented. Staging by MRI was compared with clinical staging.

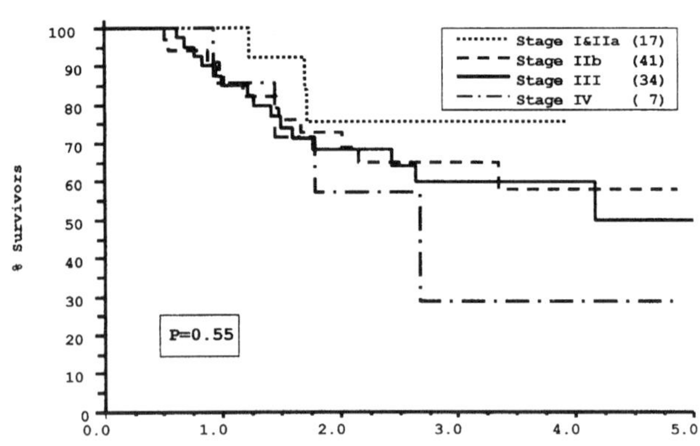

Stage I&IIa	17	14	8	5	0	0
Stage II	41	35	21	13	7	1
Stage III	34	29	19	10	5	0
Stage IV	7	6	3	1	1	1

FIGURE 1.—Disease-specific survival by clinical stage. (Reprinted by permission of the publisher from Taylor MB, Carrington BM, Davidson SE, et al: Staging of advanced cervical carcinoma using MRI—Predictors of outcome after radical radiotherapy. *Clin Radiol* 58: 532-541, 2003. Copyright 2003 by Elsevier Science Inc.)

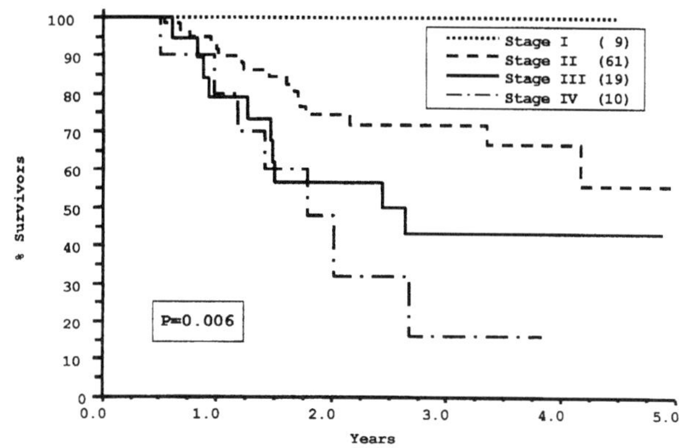

Stage I	9	7	6	5	1	0
Stage II	61	54	33	18	8	1
Stage III	19	15	9	5	4	1
Stage IV	10	8	3	1	0	0

FIGURE 2.—Disease-specific survival by MRI stage. (Reprinted by permission of the publisher from Taylor MB, Carrington BM, Davidson SE, et al: Staging of advanced cervical carcinoma using MRI—Predictors of outcome after radical radiotherapy. *Clin Radiol* 58: 532-541, 2003. Copyright 2003 by Elsevier Science Inc.)

Findings.—Staging by MRI correlated with disease-specific survival (DSS) and disease-free survival (DFS) (Figs 1 and 2). Clinical staging did not show these correlations. Pelvic nodes 10 mm or greater and juxtaregional or distant nodes 8 mm or greater in the short axis were most strongly related to survival. Poor DSS and DFS were significantly associated with tumor involvement of pelvic bowel loops, pelvic sidewall, and bladder mucosa. Tumor dimensions and bladder muscle involvement alone did not correlate with poor survival (Fig 7).

Conclusions.—Staging with MRI better predicts survival than does clinical staging in patients undergoing radiotherapy for cervical carcinoma. Valuable prognostic information can be obtained with MRI assessment of lymph node enlargement and tumor involvement of pelvic structures.

▶ This is a group of solid investigators from the Christie Hospital in Manchester, UK. They evaluated patients with carcinoma of the cervix, comparing clinical staging to staging by MRI technology. It was demonstrated in the group of 99 patients who underwent radiation alone that MR was better at predicting outcome than clinical staging. This is not shocking, because MR has the capability of addressing the issue of nodes, for which the clinical staging does a relatively poor job. The staging per se, is demonstrated in Table 1, and it emphasizes just how little attention is paid to nodes. It is also unfortunate that in Table 4 they have node IIA patients, and all their stage I patients went to surgery thereby negating some of the intention of the study. The other issue is criteria used for abnormality. In the end, there is really only one criterion that they have and that is size. Exactly what size has to do with involvement is unclear, at least until nodes become very large. There are many benign reasons

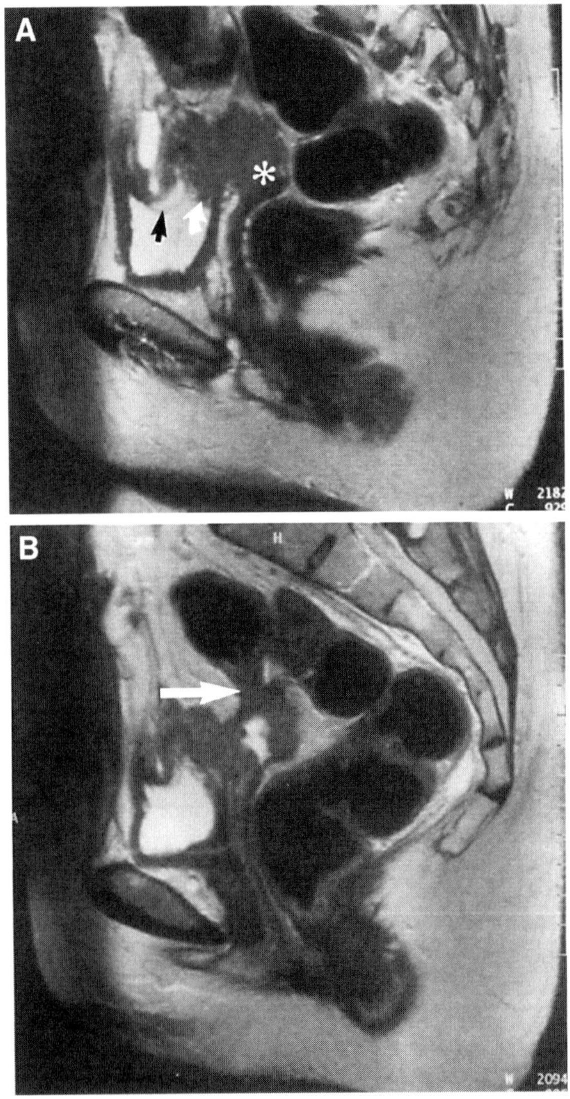

FIGURE 7.—(**A**) Parasagittal T2-weighted MRI in a patient with previous subtotal hysterectomy showing a cervical tumor destroying the low-signal-intensity bladder muscle wall and directly involving the bladder mucosa (*white arrow*). Bladder mucosal edema is seen superiorly (*black arrow*). The tumor also extends to the upper vagina (asterisk). (**B**) Parasagittal T2-weighted image in the same patient shows the tumor also extending superiorly from the cervix to directly involve a loop of sigmoid colon (*arrow*). (Reprinted by permission of the publisher from Taylor MB, Carrington BM, Davidson SE, et al: Staging of advanced cervical carcinoma using MRI—Predictors of outcome after radical radiotherapy. *Clin Radiol* 58: 532-541, 2003.

why someone can have a lymph node that is a centimeter more in size. This is not only in the long dimension but even in the short dimension.

In any event, the illustrations in this article are interesting and provocative for those of us who try to evaluate patients using radiologic techniques.

E. Glatstein, MD

Surgical–Pathological Predictors of Disease-Free Survival and Risk Groupings for IB2 Cervical Cancer: Do the Traditional Models Still Apply?

Kamelle SA, Rutledge TL, Tillmanns TD, et al (Oklahoma Health Sciences Ctr; Washington Univ, St Louis)

Gynecol Oncol 94:249-255, 2004 3–34

Background.—Tumor size in cervical cancer is predictive of disease recurrence, leading to the use of size as an accepted criterion by which to differentiate stages. The Gynecologic Oncology Group (GOG) established risk factors for stage I cervical cancers, but the sample on which these factors were based was predominantly B1 tumors, with few 3 cm or larger and even fewer 4 cm or larger. Such standards do not apply to bulky stage IB cancers. The independent surgical or pathologic factors predictive of recurrence of bulky stage IB cervical cancers were identified, then evaluated for fit in traditional early-stage cervical cancer risk models.

Methods.—The tumor registries of 2 institutions were the source for data on 86 patients who had stage IB2 cervical cancer diagnosed between 1990 and 2000. Patients ranged in age from 19 to 67 years (median, 42 years), and most were white and used tobacco. Three classification groups were identified: high-risk (HR), who had positive nodes, parametria, or margins; intermediate-risk (IR), some of whom had positive lymph vascular space involvement (LVSI) with cervical stromal invasion (CSI) and some of whom had no LVSI with or without CSI; and low-risk (LR), who had none of the HR or IR characteristics. Measures included disease-free survival (DFS). Follow-up extended for a median of 25 months.

Results.—Seventy-two percent of the tumors were squamous, 17% were adenosquamous, and 11% were adenocarcinomas. High-risk factors for recurrence were identified in 55% of the patients, 92% had tumors with middle or outer third CSI, and 60% had LVSI. Overall DFS was 75% at 2 years. No significant difference was found between the DFS for patients with tumors less than 5 cm (86%) and the DFS for patients with tumors 5 cm or greater (72%). Patients whose tumors measured 6 cm or greater showed a trend toward a shorter DFS compared with patients whose tumors were less than 6 cm. Neoadjuvant chemotherapy or radiation did not improve DFS. DFS was only 55% when patients had positive lymph nodes but was 81% when the lymph nodes were negative. Significantly shorter DFS accompanied tumor in the parametria (53%) and finding at least two thirds CSI (68%) compared with less than two thirds CSI (93%). LVSI-positive patients had a DFS at 25 months of 62% and LVSI-negative patients had a DVS of 93%. LVSI was found to be the only significant independent predictor of recurrence. None of the low-risk group had recurrences, but 9 and 11 recurrences, respectively, were reported for the intermediate- and high-risk groups. DFS for the 3 groups were 100%, 83%, and 62%. For the 29 patients without LVSI, DFS was 97%, with only 1 recurrence.

Conclusions.—The risk linked to tumor size and CSI for bulky cervical cancers proved to be less important than the risk accompanying LVSI. Patients with IR stage I may benefit from classification according to LVSI only. Radical hysterectomy was sufficient treatment for the 34% of patients who were in the IR group but had no LVSI.

▶ This study of 86 patients with stage IB2 disease suggests that this patient population can be divided into 3 groups: LR (6%), IR (60%), and HR (34%). The data suggest that LR patients and those IR patients with no involvement of lymphovascular spaces do well with surgery alone and do not require the use of concurrent chemoradiation. All other IR patients and those patients at high risk do less well and perhaps should be considered for concurrent chemoradiation at the very least after surgery if surgery is to be done. Given the recent recommendation that patients with stage IB2 disease should receive concurrent chemoradiation, these observations suggest that at least some subsets of stage IB2 patients can be treated more conservatively. Larger trials evaluating a number of prognostic markers are needed to sort out those stage IB2 patients most likely to benefit from concurrent chemoradiation from those who do well with surgery alone. It is unlikely that the presence or absence of LVIS alone will suffice to distinguish subsets requiring a less aggressive approach.

J. T. Thigpen, MD

Association of Hemoglobin Level With Survival in Cervical Carcinoma Patients Treated With Concurrent Cisplatin and Radiotherapy: A Gynecologic Oncology Group Study

Winter WE III, Maxwell GL, Tian C, et al (Walter Reed Army Med Ctr, Washington, DC; Roswell Park Cancer Inst, Buffalo, NY; Toronto-Sunnybrook Regional Cancer Ctr)

Gynecol Oncol 94:495-501, 2004 3–35

Background.—The incidence of cervical cancer has decreased since the implementation of screening programs, but approximately 25% of patients will be diagnosed with locally advanced disease. Several randomized trials have shown that treatment regimens combining radiotherapy with cisplatin-containing chemotherapy improve rates of survival and progression-free interval in women with stage IIB through IVA cervix cancer. Disease recurrence in patients with locally advanced cervical cancer has been associated with anemia before and during radiotherapy alone, and retrospective studies have suggested that poor survival associated with anemia may be improved with the correction of hematologic indices. Whether there is an association of hemoglobin level before or during concurrent cisplatin and radiotherapy with disease outcome in women with locally advanced cervical cancer and whether the association is particularly significant at a specific point in the course of treatment was determined.

Methods.—This retrospective review included 494 patients treated in 2 consecutive prospective Gynecologic Oncology Group (GOG) trials. Demographic data, pathologic information, treatment-related factors, and hemoglobin values were collected at baseline and during each week of therapy. Cox proportional hazards modeling was performed to evaluate the effects of hemoglobin level on progression-free survival. Among the combined patients, 278 (56%) received a diagnosis of stage II disease and 216 (44%) received a diagnosis of stage II/IV disease.

Results.—After controlling for age, race, performance status, disease stage, tumor size, cell type, and duration of radiotherapy, mean hemoglobin values during treatment were predictive of disease progression. The pretreatment level was not significant when hemoglobin levels during treatment were predictive of disease progression. The pretreatment level was not a significant factor when hemoglobin levels during treatment were included in the multivariate analysis. Division of the 6-week treatment course into 2-week periods (early, middle, and late) showed that hemoglobin values during the late period were most predictive of disease progression.

Conclusions.—Hemoglobin levels during combined radiotherapy and cisplatin therapy were found to be independent predictors of treatment outcome in patients with advanced cervical carcinoma. The pretreatment level was not a significant predictive factor for outcome when hemoglobin levels during treatment were included in the multivariate regression model. Hemoglobin levels in the final stage of treatment were the most predictive of disease recurrence and patient survival.

▶ Winter et al, on behalf of the GOG, reviewed 494 patients on 2 GOG randomized phase III trials of concurrent chemoradiation to examine the impact of anemia on therapeutic results. After controlling for all known major prognostic factors other than anemia, the investigators found that low hemoglobin levels during the final 2 weeks of chemoradiation were associated with a greater likelihood of disease progression. This observation of the adverse impact of low hemoglobin levels on treatment effects supports other retrospective studies that have shown a similar adverse impact in patients with carcinoma of the cervix. By extension, these observations would support the recommendation that hemoglobin levels be maintained above 12 g/dL during chemoradiation to optimize therapeutic outcome.

J. T. Thigpen, MD

Pelvic Irradiation With Concurrent Chemotherapy Versus Pelvic and Para-aortic Irradiation for High-Risk Cervical Cancer: An Update of Radiation Therapy Oncology Group Trial (RTOG) 90-01

Eifel PJ, Winter K, Morris M, et al (Univ of Texas, Houston; Radiation Therapy Oncology Group, Philadelphia; Washington University, St Louis; et al)
J Clin Oncol 22:872-880, 2004 3–36

Background.—The results of several recent trials of concurrent administration of cisplatin and fluorouracil in addition to radiotherapy for locoregionally advanced carcinoma of the cervix have led to issuance of a clinical alert from the National Institutes of Health and stimulated a significant change in the standard of care for many patients with carcinoma of the cervix. Mature results were reported from a randomized trial that compared extended-field radiotherapy (EFRT) with pelvic radiotherapy with concomitant fluorouracil and cisplatin (CTRT) in women with locoregionally advanced carcinomas of the uterine cervix.

Methods.—A total of 403 women with cervical cancer were randomly assigned to receive either EFRT or CTRT. All of the patients had stage IIB to IVA disease, stage IB to IIA disease with a tumor diameter of 5 cm or larger, or positive pelvic lymph nodes. The patients were stratified by stage and by the method used in evaluation of lymph nodes.

Results.—The median follow-up time for the 228 surviving patients was 6.6 years. The overall survival rate for patients treated with CTRT was significantly greater than that for patients with EFRT (67% vs 41%). The overall reduction in risk of disease recurrence for patients who received CTRT was 51%. Among patients with stage IB to IIB disease, those who received CTRT had better overall and disease-free survival than those treated with EFRT. Among patients with stage III to IVA disease, those randomly assigned to CTRT had better disease-free survival and showed a trend toward better overall survival. The rate of serious complications was similar for the 2 groups.

Conclusion.—The survival rate of women with locally advanced cervical cancer is significantly improved by the addition of fluorouracil and cisplatin to radiotherapy without an increase in the rate of late treatment side effects.

▶ This report is the updated analysis of one of the 5 randomized studies that established concurrent chemoradiation as the treatment of choice for patients with stages IB-IVA carcinoma of the cervix. At a median follow-up of 6.6 years in this report, both relapse-free and overall survival remain significantly better with concurrent chemoradiation than with radiation alone; and serious late complications were similar between the 2 treatment arms of the study. This confirms the benefits of platinum-based concurrent chemoradiation for carcinoma of the cervix.

J. T. Thigpen, MD

Phase III Study of Cisplatin With or Without Paclitaxel in Stage IVB, Recurrent, or Persistent Squamous Cell Carcinoma of the Cervix: A Gynecologic Oncology Group Study

Moore DH, Blessing JA, McQuellon RP, et al (Indiana Univ, Indianapolis; Roswell Park Cancer Inst, Buffalo, NY; Mem Sloan-Kettering Cancer Ctr, New York; et al)

J Clin Oncol 22:3113-3119, 2004 3–37

Background.—Fewer than 20% of patients who have advanced, persistent, or recurrent squamous cell cervical cancer survive 1 year. Cisplatin has been considered the most active drug in treating cervical cancer and achieves initial response rates up to 50%, but more recently the rates have been between 20% to 30%. The response rate rose from 19% for cisplatin alone to 33% with cisplatin plus ifosfamide. The progression-free survival (PFS) was also higher with the combined therapy, but adverse side effects were more numerous as well. Paclitaxel has also been combined with cisplatin (C+P) and achieved a 46% response rate for solid tumors such as cancers of the ovary, breast, and endometrium. In a randomized phase III trial, cisplatin was compared with C+P for response rate, PFS, and survival in patients who have advanced squamous cell carcinoma of the cervix. Treatment-related toxicity, health-related quality of life (QOL), and pain during chemotherapy were also assessed for the 2 regimens.

Methods.—Two hundred sixty-four patients participated. All had measurable disease, performance status (PS) between 0 and 2, and adequate hematologic hepatic and renal function. Treatment was administered every 3 weeks for 6 cycles. Cisplatin 50 mg/m^2 treatment was randomly assigned to 134 patients and C+P (cisplatin 50 mg/m^2, paclitaxel 135 mg/m^2) to 130 patients. Before each cycle, the tumors were measured and QOL was assessed.

Results.—Radiation therapy was given to 92% of the cisplatin group and 91% of the C+P group. Nineteen percent of those receiving cisplatin (6% complete and 13% partial) and 36% of those receiving C+P (15% complete and 21% partial) had objective responses to the regimen. No significant differences were found between the 2 groups regarding objective responses. Cisplatin had a median PFS of 2.8 months; C+P had a median PFS of 4.9 months. The median survival was similar for the 2 groups, 8.8 months for the cisplatin group and 9.7 months for the C+P group. Myelosuppression was the most common adverse side effect in both groups and included grade 3 to 4 anemia and neutropenia. Patients receiving combination therapy were more likely to have myelosuppression than those taking cisplatin only. Nausea and vomiting developed in both groups at equal rates. Only 60% of the sample completed QOL information, with the rate declining as treatment progressed. A disproportionate number of patients receiving cisplatin chose to drop out of the QOL aspect of the investigation. Patients who completed the fourth QOL evaluation were those who had achieved a better clinical response and had stable or slightly improving QOL over time. More than 30% of patients who did not complete the QOL assessment had not responded to treatment and their QOL had progressively worsened. Worse

QOL was not linked to treatment. Higher response rate was not related to a worsened QOL.

Conclusions.—Objective response rate, PFS, and sustained QOL were better with the C+P combination than with cisplatin alone. Overall survival was not improved. A comparison of health-related QOL would be advisable in future trials among patients with stage IB, recurrent, or persistent squamous cell carcinoma of the cervix.

▶ Moore et al in the Gynecologic Oncology Group present the results of a randomized phase III trial comparing cisplatin alone to C+P in the treatment of advanced or recurrent squamous cell carcinoma of the cervix. In this trial, the doublet produced a superior response rate and a superior PFS with no difference in overall survival. QOL was not significantly different between the 2 regimens. This establishes combination chemotherapy as the treatment of choice in patients with recurrent or advanced squamous cell carcinoma of the cervix; but it should be noted that the differences in response rate and PFS were modest, although statistically significant. This doublet will be tested in comparison to other active doublets (eg, topotecan/cisplatin) in these patients in a recently activated Gynecologic Oncology Group study, but the ultimate goal is better therapy through the identification of new and more active agents, including biologic agents.

J. T. Thigpen, MD

Evaluation of Vinorelbine in Persistent or Recurrent Squamous Cell Carcinoma of the Cervix: A Gynecologic Oncology Group Study

Muggia FM, Blessing JA, Method M, et al (New York Univ; Roswell Park Cancer Inst, Buffalo, NY; Uniformed Services Univ of the Health Sciences, Bethesda, Md; et al)

Gynecol Oncol 92:639-643, 2004 3–38

Background.—When carcinoma of the uterine cervix is initially found at locally advanced stages, recurrences are more likely, with a similar increase in morbidity and mortality after surgery, radiation, or the combination. Adding cisplatin-based chemotherapy has improved outcomes and suggested the use of other drugs. The semisynthetic vinca alkaloid vinorelbine is under investigation for use in advanced or recurrent squamous cell carcinoma of the cervix. Patients who failed standard chemotherapy were given vinorelbine in a days 1 and 8 every-21-days regimen and the results were assessed.

Methods.—Initially, 25 patients were included, receiving vinorelbine 30 mg/m^2 on days 1 and 8 every 21 days. A second stage accrual of patients was planned if the activity with the first 25 patients was sufficient.

Results.—A total of 44 patients were enrolled in 2 stages. Patients completed a median of 2.0 cycles (range, 1-10 cycles). Fourteen cases required the dose to be reduced to 20 mg/m^2, and doses were delayed in 12 patients and omitted in 10. The overall response rate was 13.7%, with 1 complete response and 5 partials. At the completion of treatment, 22.7% of the patients had stable disease; at reassessment, 59.1% had increasing disease. The most common toxic reaction was neutropenia grades 3 and 4, which occurred in 41% of patients. All but 17 patients had anemia. Twenty-seven percent of patients had neurotoxicity. Twelve patients reported pain, and a few grade 3 or 4 events may have been related to disease or infection. Five instances of alopecia developed. The nausea, vomiting, and other gastrointestinal effects reported rarely exceeded grade 3 in severity.

Conclusions.—The 13.7% response rate with vinorelbine indicates moderate activity as a single agent in previously treated squamous cell cervical cancer. Only 41% of patients had neutropenia that was drug-related and more than moderate in severity. Rarely was the neuropathy that affected 27% of patients severe. Further evaluation of the use of vinorelbine in a days 1 and 8 schedule for squamous cell carcinoma of the cervix is needed.

► This phase II trial of vinorelbine in squamous cell carcinoma of the cervix found modest activity (1 complete and 5 partial responses among 44 patients, for a 13.7% response rate). This result has led to the inclusion of a doublet of vinorelbine plus cisplatin as 1 of 4 arms of an ongoing Gynecologic Oncology Group phase III trial in advanced or recurrent carcinoma of the cervix.

J. T. Thigpen, MD

4 Genitourinary

Prostate

Prevalence of Prostate Cancer Among Men With a Prostate-Specific Antigen Level ≤4.0 ng Per Milliliter

Thompson IM, Pauler DK, Goodman PJ, et al (Univ of Texas, San Antonio; Fred Hutchinson Cancer Research Center, Seattle; Univ of Colorado, Denver; et al)
N Engl J Med 350:2239-2246, 2004 4–1

Introduction.—The optimal upper limit of the normal range for prostate-specific antigen (PSA) has not been determined. The prevalence of prostate cancer was examined in the Prostate Cancer Prevention Trial among men who had a PSA level of 4.0 ng/mL or less.

Methods.—Of 18,882 men enrolled in this phase III, double-blind, placebo-controlled trial, 9459 were randomly assigned to receive a placebo and underwent annual measurement of PSA and digital examination and prostate biopsy after being in the trial for 7 years. It was this cohort that was followed for prevalence of prostate cancer among participants with PSA levels below 4.0 ng/mL. Of the 9459 who received placebo rather than active treatment (which was 5 mg finasteride daily), 2950 never had a PSA level above 4.0 ng/mL or an abnormal digital rectal examination.

Results.—The age range of the 2950 men evaluated was 62 to 91 years. Prostate cancer was diagnosed in 449 (15.2%). Of thcsc, 67 (14.9%) had a Gleason score of 7 or more. The incidence of prostate cancer was 6.6% in men with a PSA level of up to 0.5 ng/mL, 10.1% among those with values of 1.1 to 2.0 ng/mL, 23.9% in those with values of 2.1 to 3.0 ng/mL, and 26.9% in those with values of 3.1 to 4.0 ng/mL. The incidence of high-grade cancers rose from 12.5% of cancers associated with a PSA level of 0.5 ng/mL or less to 25.0% of cancers linked with a PSA level of 3.1 to 4.0 ng/mL.

Conclusion.—Biopsy-identified prostate cancer, including high-grade cancers, is not rare among men with PSA levels of 4.0 ng/mL or lower, levels that are generally regarded as being in the normal range.

► Prostate cancer represents the second leading cause of cancer-related death in this country. As with most cancers, earlier diagnosis should lead to greater likelihood for cure. Prostate cancer is an anathema. At the core of the controversy is that many patients with prostate cancer live and die with it but not from it.

This article by Thompson et al demonstrates that up to 15% of men with a PSA within normal limits have prostate cancer on biopsy. If you are a believer in PSA-based screening, this study opens the door to biopsy in more men. If you are a "PSA agnostic," you will question the specificity of PSA and the routine use of this in early detection. The authors state "the large difference between a man's risk of death from prostate cancer (3%-4%) and his lifetime risk of the diagnosis of prostate cancer (16.7%) suggests that many prostate cancers detected in routine practice may be clinically unimportant." In essence, we need better markers than PSA to detect earlier "clinically important" prostate cancer.

P. J. Loehrer, Sr, MD

Natural History of Early, Localized Prostate Cancer

Johansson J-E, Andrén O, Andersson S-O, et al (Örebro Univ Hosp, Sweden; Karolinska Inst, Stockholm; Univ Hosp, Uppsala, Sweden; et al)

JAMA 291:2713-2719, 2004 4–2

Introduction.—Without understanding the natural history of prostate cancer diagnosed at an early, localized stage, patient counseling and clinical management are challenging. Little is known concerning disease progression and mortality beyond 10 to 15 years of watchful waiting. The long-term natural history of untreated, early stage prostate cancer was evaluated in a population-based, cohort investigation with a mean observation period of 21 years.

Methods.—A consecutive sample of 223 patients with early stage (T0-T2 NX MO classification), initially untreated prostate cancer was monitored. Patients with tumor progression underwent hormonal treatment with either orchiectomy or estrogens if they were symptomatic. The primary outcome measure was progression-free, cause-specific, and overall survival.

Results.—After complete follow-up, 39 (17%) patients had generalized disease. The course for most cancers was indolent during the initial 10 to 15 years. Further follow-up from 15 years (49 patients were still alive) to 20 years showed a marked reduction in cumulative progression-free survival (45.0%-36.0%), survival without metastases (76.9%-51.2%), and prostate cancer–specific survival (78.7%-54.4%). The incidence of prostate cancer mortality rose from 15 of 1000 person-years (95% confidence interval [CI], 10-21) during the initial 15 years to 44 of 1000 person-years (95% CI, 22-88) beyond 15 years of follow-up (P= .01).

Conclusion.—Most prostate cancers diagnosed at an early stage have an indolent course. Local tumor progression and aggressive metastatic disease can develop during the long term. These findings support early radical treatment, particularly among patients with an estimated life expectancy of more than 15 years.

► The natural history of prostate cancer has a variable course. In elderly patients with comorbid illnesses, prostate cancer is often the least concerning problem. With increasing asymptomatic patients with prostate cancer, evaluating the natural history becomes more precious. Data such as found in this study are particularly helpful to delineate high- and low-risk patients for whom treatment can be avoided or instituted early.

P. J. Loehrer, Sr, MD

Did the Rate of Incidental Prostate Cancer Change in the Era of PSA Testing? A Retrospective Study of 1127 Patients

Zigeuner RE, Lipsky K, Riedler I, et al (Karl Franzens Univ Graz, Austria)
Urology 62:451-455, 2003 4–3

Background.—Before the introduction of prostate-specific antigen (PSA) testing, incidental prostate carcinoma was detected in up to 16% of patients with a preoperative negative digital rectal examination (DRE) undergoing transurethral resection of the prostate (TURP) or open surgery for obstructive symptoms from presumed benign prostatic enlargement (BPE). To determine the effect of routine PSA testing on the rate of incidental prostate cancer in this patient population, a retrospective study was done.

Methods.—After January 1993, data from 2422 operations for BPE, including 2283 TURP and 139 retropubic adenoma enucleations, were analyzed. Patients in whom cancer was suspected were excluded from the analysis. Preoperative DRE findings and PSA levels were assessed, and pathologic reports were reviewed. The diagnosis of incidental prostate carcinoma was based on histologic evidence of cancer and negative DRE findings in addition to a PSA level within age-specific reference ranges preoperatively.

Findings.—Overall, the diagnosis of prostate cancer was established by surgery in 13%. Of the 2422 patients, 1127 (46.5%) had both negative DRE findings and an age-specific PSA level. In this group, 6.4% of patients were found to have incidental prostate cancer (Table 1).

Conclusions.—The likelihood of finding incidental prostate cancer by surgery was 6.4%. The rate of incidental prostate cancer has been reduced by more than half in the PSA era. The low rate of incidental carcinoma today does not warrant routine histologic assessment of the prostate if PSA testing

TABLE 1.—Detection Rate of Prostate Cancer by TURP or Open Surgery Dependent on Preoperative PSA and DRE

	Patients (%)	Cancer (%)
PSA negative, DRE negative	1127 (46.5)	72 (6.4)
PSA negative, DRE positive	140 (5.8)	21 (15)
PSA elevated, DRE negative	893 (36.9)	106 (11.9)
PSA elevated, DRE positive	262 (10.8)	115 (43.9)
Total	2422 (100)	314 (13)

Abbreviations: TURP, Transurethral resection of the prostate; *PSA*, prostate-specific antigen; *DRE*, digital rectal examination.

(Reprinted from Zigeuner RE, Lipsky K, Riedler I, et al: Did the rate of incidental prostate cancer change in the era of PSA testing? A retrospective study of 1127 patients. *Urology* 62:451-455, 2003.

and DRE are negative when alternative modalities without tissue sampling are offered for treating BPE.

▶ This group of Austrian investigators has assessed the impact of the PSA test on the detection of coincidental prostate cancer in patients undergoing surgery for presumed BPE. They have over 2400 specimens, the vast majority of which represented TURPs, but 139 retropubic enucleations were also included. The diagnosis of the coincidental carcinoma of the prostate required both histologic evidence of neoplasm and negative rectal examination for cancer, as well as a PSA that was thought to be within age-specific reference range. Of these patients, over 1100 had both negative digital rectal findings and what was thought to be a normal PSA level for the age of the patient. Of the total group, 314 of 2422 patients were diagnosed as having pathologic evidence of carcinoma. That is a percentage of 13%, and for those who were negative in PSA and in the DRE, there are only 72 of the 1127 or 6.4%. Thus, a truly coincidental lesion seems to be relatively uncommon in the era of PSA evaluation. It is unfortunate that the authors did not break this information down by age factors, but the point is that PSA is a pretty reliable assessment, even when the DRE is negative.

E. Glatstein, MD

Prostate Cancer Detection Is Also Relevant in Low Prostate Specific Antigen Ranges

Lujan M, Paez A, Miravalles E, et al (Hosp Universitario de Getafe, Madrid)

Eur Urol 45:155-159, 2004 4–4

Background.—Serum prostate-specific antigen (PSA) and some of its available modalities are considered to be the optimal marker for prostate cancer screening. However, prostate biopsy is usually recommended when PSA levels are above specific cutoff points (usually 3-4 ng/mL) because of the limited detection rate that this marker is assumed to provide. There is limited evidence that cancer detection is also significant in PSA ranges below these limits. Thus far, no convincing evidence has been presented to support mass screening for prostate cancer to reduce cancer-specific mortality. The use of the free to total (f/t) PSA ratio has been shown to be a valid tool for enhancing the specificity of PSA and thus reducing the number of biopsies needed when low PSA ranges are considered. Detection rates and clinical features of the cancers detected with low PSA levels were examined in the context of a prostate cancer screening program.

Methods.—After going through a prostate cancer screening program, 1097 men attended a new prescreening round. Sextant prostate biopsy was recommended when PSA was 3 ng/mL or greater. It was also recommended that biopsy be performed when PSA was in the range of 1.0 to 2.99 ng/mL when the f/t PSA ratio was 20% or less. The detection rate was calculated, and clinical features of the cancers detected were examined.

TABLE 2.—Biopsies Performed and Cancer Detection

Total PSA Range (ng/ml)	f/t PSA Ratio	Screened Men	Biopsies Performed and Acceptance Rate	Cancers	Biopsies Per Cancer	Detection Rate
<1.0	—	497	—	—	—	—
1.0-2.99	>20%	190	—	—	—	—
	≤20%	249	159 (63.9%)	15	10.6	0.094
3.0-3.99	—	72	56 (77.8%)	12	4.7	0.214
4.0-9.99	—	86	62 (72.1%)	7	8.9	0.113
≥10.0	—	3	2 (66.7%)	0	—	0
Total	—	1097	279 (68%)	34	8.2	0.035

Note: Indication for biopsy is shown in the column headings. Detection rates have been adjusted taking into account acceptance for biopsy.

Abbreviations: PSA, Prostate-specific antigen; *f/t PSA*, free-to-total PSA ratio.

(Reprinted by permission of the publisher from Lujan M, Paez A, Miravalles E, et al: Prostate cancer detection is also relevant in low prostate specific antigen ranges. *Eur Urol* 45:155-159, 2004. Copyright 2004 by Elsevier.)

Results.—The mean age of the patients was 61.1 years. A total of 497 patients (45.3%) had a total PSA of less than 1.0 ng/mL, 439 (40%) had a total PSA between 1.0 and 2.99 ng/mL, and 161 (14.7%) had a PSA of 3.0 ng/mL or greater. Among the group of patients with a total PSA between 1.0 and 2.99 ng/mL and a f/t PSA ratio of 20% or less, a total of 249 biopsies were

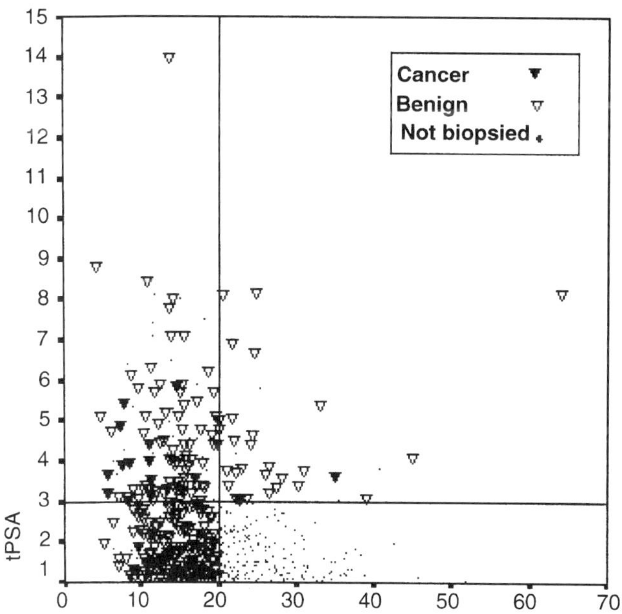

FIGURE 1.—Scatterplot showing the screening procedure and biopsy performance and outcomes in regard to total prostate-specific antigen (*tPSA*) and free to total (*f/t*) PSA ratio. (Reprinted by permission of the publisher from Lujan M, Paez A, Miravalles E, et al. Prostate cancer detection is also relevant in low prostate specific antigen ranges. *Eur Urol* 45:155-159, 2004. Copyright 2004 by Elsevier.)

TABLE 3.—Estimation of Clinical Relevance of the Cancers Detected According to Epstein et al*

	PSA Range (ng/ml)		
	1-2.99	3-3.99	≥4
Number of cancers	15	12	7
f/t PSA ratio >0.15	7 (46.7%)	4 (33.3%)	1 (14.3%)
Nonpalpable cancer	13 (86.7%)	9 (75%)	6 (85.7%)
Gleason score at biopsy <7	12 (80%)	7 (58.3%)	6 (85.7%)
<3 involved cores	10 (66.7%)	10 (83.3%)	6 (85.7%)
Probably insignificant cancer [*]	4 (26.7%)	1 (8.3%)	0 (0%)
Radical prostatectomy	5 (33.3%)	7 (58.3%)	4 (57.1%)
Extracapsular pathological stage	2 (13.3%)	1 (8.3%)	0 (0%)

Note: All cancers detected were clinically organ-confined.

*(Epstein JI, Chan DW, Sokoll LJ, et al: Nonpalpable stage T1c prostate cancer: Prediction of insignificant disease using free/total prostate specific antigen levels and needle biopsy findings. *J Urol* 160:2407-2411, 1998.)

Abbreviations: PSA, Prostate-specific antigen; *f/t PSA*, free-to-total PSA ratio.

(Reprinted by permission of the publisher from Lujan M, Paez A, Miravalles E, et al: Prostate cancer detection is also relevant in low prostate specific antigen ranges. *Eur Urol* 45:155-159, 2004. Copyright 2004 by Elsevier.)

indicated, and 159 were performed (acceptance rate, 63.9%), with 15 cancers detected (detection rate, 9.4%) (Table 2). Biopsy was recommended in 72 men with a PSA between 3.0 and 3.99 ng/mL and was performed in 56 (77.8%), with 12 tumors detected (detection rate, 21.4%) (Fig 1). All the cancers were clinically localized, and most were clinically significant (Table 3). Two cancers were found to be poorly differentiated and to have pathologically extracapsular disease.

Conclusions.—Cancer detection in lower PSA ranges is lower but nevertheless relevant. The detection of potentially aggressive cancers within these ranges is still a matter of concern. However, long-term randomized studies are needed to determine potential benefit of prostate cancer screening within PSA ranges below the traditional cutoff points of 3.0 to 4.0 ng/mL.

▶ This group of Spanish investigators looked at cancer screening and defined a group of patients whose PSA was not thought to be elevated but had an abnormal f/t PSA ratio. They were able to detect 15 cancers in patients with a PSA of less than 3 ng/mL, all of which were localized, and only 4 of which were thought to be clinically insignificant. This latter category bears some attention. If the Gleason score is low and the PSA is low and the gland does not have any palpable disease, it is easy to understand how that could be considered insignificant. A high Gleason score and a low PSA are a combination that probably needs intervention. The real issue is the projection down the road in time. Many cancers, if not all of them, progress over time, even in the prostate. What is insignificant at diagnosis may not be so insignificant down the road. Indeed, one of the real problems with the "watch and wait" approach for prostate cancer is frequently there are no criteria for intervention. What happens if the PSA continues to climb? What happens if one begins to detect a discrete nodule on physical exam, or the nodule grows? There is a point at which potential curability for an individual patient can be compromised by inaction. Our ability to predict for any one patient is less than what we would like it to be.

In any event, this is a provocative article in terms of what are our standards for diagnosis and for prediction of outcome.

E. Glatstein, MD

6-Month Androgen Suppression Plus Radiation Therapy vs Radiation Therapy Alone for Patients With Clinically Localized Prostate Cancer: A Randomized Controlled Trial

D'Amico AV, Manola J, Loffredo M, et al (Brigham and Women's Hosp, Boston; Dana Farber Cancer Inst, Boston)

JAMA 292:821-827, 2004 4–5

Introduction.—There is a survival benefit among patients with high-grade clinically localized prostate cancer who undergo 70 Gy radiation therapy combined with 3 years of androgen suppression therapy (AST). Long-term treatment with AST is associated with several adverse events. The survival benefit of 3-dimensional conformational radiation therapy (3D-CRT) alone versus combination with 6 months of AST was prospectively evaluated in 206 patients with clinically localized prostate cancer.

Methods.—Patients were randomly assigned to receive 70 Gy 3D-CRT alone or in combination with 6 months of AST. All patients had a prostate-specific antigen (PSA) level of at least 10 ng/mL, a Gleason score of at least 7, or radiographic evidence of extraprostate disease. The primary outcome

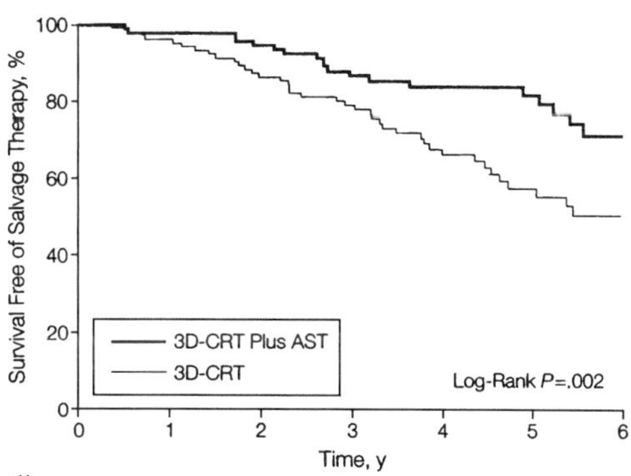

Events During Interval/ No. at Risk							
3D-CRT Plus AST	0/102	2/90	3/85	7/70	2/51	1/36	4/21
3D-CRT	0/104	4/98	10/87	7/69	10/45	5/28	4/13

FIGURE 4.—Survival without progression for 3D-CRT vs 3D-CRT plus AST. Progression was defined on the date of the institution of salvage AST. (Courtesy of D'Amico AV, Manola J, Loffredo M, et al: 6-Month androgen suppression plus radiation therapy vs radiation therapy alone for patients with clinically localized prostate cancer: A randomized controlled trial. JAMA 292:821-827, 2004. Copyright 2004 American Medical Association.)

TABLE 3.—Event Size and Hazard Ratio for Main Outcome Measures

Outcome Measure	No. of Events 3D-CRT (n = 103)	3D-CRT Plus AST (n = 98)	Hazard Ratio (95% CI)	P Value	Adjusted Hazard Ratio (95% CI)*	P Value
PSA failure	46	21	2.86 (1.69-4.86)	<.001	2.66 (1.56-4.55)	<.001
Survival free of salvage AST	43	21	2.30 (1.36-3.89)	.002	2.17 (1.28-3.69)	.004
Prostate cancer-specific mortality	6	0	NA	.02†	NA	.02†
Overall mortality	23	12	2.07 (1.02-4.20)	.04	2.04 (1.01-4.20)	.05

*Adjusted for clinical tumor category.
†Log-rank *P* value comparing cumulative incidence.
Abbreviation: NA, Not applicable because of no cancer-specific deaths in 3D-CRT plus AST.
(Courtesy of D'Amico AV, Manola J, Loffredo M, et al: 6-month androgen suppression plus radiation therapy vs radiation therapy alone for patients with clinically localized prostate cancer: A randomized controlled trial. *JAMA* 292:821-827, 2004. Copyright 2004 American Medical Association.)

measures were time to PSA failure (PSA >1.0 ng/mL and increasing >0.2 ng/mL on 2 consecutive visits) and overall survival.

Results.—After a median follow-up of 4.52 years, patients assigned to the 3D-CRT plus AST group had significantly higher survival rates (*P* = .04), lower prostate cancer–specific mortality rates (*P* = .02), and higher survival rates free of salvage AST (*P* = .002) compared with patients in the 3D-CRT group. Kaplan-Meier estimates of 5-year survival rates were 88% (95% confidence interval [CI], 80%-95%) in the combination therapy group versus 78% (95% CI, 68%-88%) in the 3D-CRT group. The rates of survival free of salvage AST at 5 years were 82% (95% CI, 73%-90%) in the combination therapy group and 57% (95% CI, 46%-69%) in the 3D-CRT group (Fig 4). The unadjusted and adjusted hazard ratios for survival without salvage AST were 2.30 (95% CI, 1.36-3.89; *P* = .002) and 2.17 (95% CI, 1.28-3.69; *P* = .004) for patients in the 3D-CRT group compared with the combination therapy group (Table 3).

Conclusion.—The addition of 6 months of AST to 70 Gy 3D-CRT provides an overall survival benefit in patients with clinically localized prostate cancer.

▶ Prospective trials demonstrating improvement in survival have been hard to come by in prostate cancer. Locally advanced prostate cancer is defined as tumor with local extension (determined clinically by the physician or radiographically). Surgery for locally advanced prostate cancer is felt to have a minimal impact on overall survival, leaving radiation therapy as the standard of care. The addition of hormonal therapy to radiation therapy has been previously explored. This study demonstrates that 5 months of androgen suppressive therapy with radiation therapy improves cancer-specific and overall survival. As with any good study, more questions arise. One such question is can similar benefits be achieved with hormonal therapy alone? The Canadians are currently evaluating this approach in which patients with locally advanced disease are treated with hormonal therapy with or without radiation therapy. Finding the optimal therapy while minimizing morbidity is the ultimate goal.

P. J. Loehrer, Sr, MD

Docetaxel and Estramustine Compared With Mitoxantrone and Prednisone for Advanced Refractory Prostate Cancer

Petrylak DP, Tangen CM, Hussain MHA, et al (Columbia Univ, New York; Southwest Oncology Group Statistical Ctr, Seattle; Univ of Michigan, Ann Arbor)

N Engl J Med 351:1513-1520, 2004 4–6

Background.—In men with progressive androgen-independent prostate cancer, mitoxantrone-based chemotherapy palliates pain but does not extend survival. Docetaxel plus estramustine with mitoxantrone plus prednisone was compared in this patient population.

Methods.—Seven hundred seventy men were assigned randomly to 1 of 2 treatments given in 21-day cycles. Three hundred thirty-eight received 280 mg of estramustine 3 times a day on days 1 through 5, 60 mg of docetaxel per square meter of body-surface area on day 2, and 60 mg of dexamethasone in 3 divided doses before docetaxel (group 1). Three hundred thirty-six patients received 12 mg of mitoxantrone per square meter on day 1 plus 5 mg of prednisone twice a day (group 2).

Findings.—Intention-to-treat analysis demonstrated an overall survival of 17.5 months in group 1 compared with 15.6 months in group 2. The corresponding hazard ratio for death was 0.80. The median time to progression in groups 1 and 2 were 6.3 and 3.2 months, respectively. Decreases in prostate-specific antigen (PSA) of at least 50% were documented in 50% of group 1 and 27% of group 2. Objective tumor responses were observed in 17% and 11%, respectively, of patients with bidimensionally measurable disease. Grade 3 or 4 neutropenic fevers, nausea and vomiting, and cardiovascular events were more common in group 1 than in group 2. Pain relief in the 2 groups was comparable.

Conclusions.—First-line treatment with estramustine and docetaxel, compared with mitoxantrone and prednisone, moderately increases survival in men with metastatic androgen-independent prostate cancer. However, this benefit must be weighed against the increased rate of adverse events.

▶ Several treatments are available. In none of these therapies, however, has prolongation of survival been demonstrated. One of the most commonly used regimens is that of mitoxantrone and prednisone that proved to have a beneficial impact on quality of life but not survival in patients with advanced hormone refractory prostate cancer.[1] This was 1 of 2 trials presented at this year's American Society of Clinical Oncology Plenary Session that demonstrated superiority of docetaxel-based chemotherapy over mitoxantrone and prednisone. A modest but significant improvement in median survival (17.5 months vs 15.6 months; *P* = .02) was noted, but more importantly, the progression-free survival and quality of life was also favorably impacted with the docetaxel regimen. It remains questionable whether estramustine is an essential part of this regimen as a benefit was not appreciated in a similarly designed trial of docetaxel plus prednisone versus mitoxantrone/prednisone.[2] For those involved in the treatment of patients with hormone refractory prostate cancer, this is an encouraging step forward.

P. J. Loehrer, Sr, MD

References

1. Pannosk IF, Osoba B, Stockler MR, et al: Chemotherapy with mitoxantrone and prednisone or prednisone alone for symptomatic hormone-resistant prostate cancer: A Canadian Randomized Trial with palliative endpoints. *Gen Clin Oncol* 14:1756-1764, 1996.
2. Eisenberger MA, DeWit R, Berry W, et al: A multicenter phase III comparison of docetaxel (D) + prednisone (P) and mitoxantrone (MTZ) + P in patients with hormone-refractory prostate cancer (HRPC). *Proc Am Soc Clin Oncol* 23:2, 2004 (abstract 4).

Testis

Outcome and Staging Evaluation in Malignant Germ Cell Tumors of the Ovary in Children and Adolescents: An Intergroup Study

Billmire D, Vinocur C, Rescorla F, et al (JW Riley Hosp for Children, Indianapolis)

J Pediatr Surg 39:424-429, 2004 4–7

Background.—Pediatric malignant germ cell tumors (GCTs) are treated with surgery and platinum-based chemotherapy. The surgical staging guidelines have been adopted from adult ovarian epithelial cancer. The role of surgical staging in pediatric malignant GCTs of the ovary was studied.

Study Design.—The study group consisted of 131 girls, aged 1.4 to 20 years, with GCT of the ovary. Those with stage I and II ovarian tumors were treated with tumor resection followed by 4 rounds of cisplatin, etoposide, and bleomycin (PEB) chemotherapy. Those with stage III and IV tumors were treated with surgical resection and randomly assigned to 4 rounds of either PEB or high-dose cisplatin, etoposide, and bleomycin (HD PEB). Second-look surgery with attempted resection could be performed after completion of chemotherapy. Surgical staging compliance was compared with outcome. Survival data were calculated by the Kaplan-Meier method.

Findings.—The 6-year survival rate was 95.1% for stage I, 93.8% for stage II, 98.3% for stage III, and 93.3% for stage IV. Surgical guidelines were followed completely in only 3 patients. Protocol noncompliance included failure to biopsy bilateral nodes, no omentectomy, no peritoneal cytology, and no contralateral ovarian biopsy. More aggressive surgery than recommended included total hysterectomy and bilateral salpingo-oophorectomy in 6 patients and retroperitoneal node dissection in 10 patients.

Conclusions.—Pediatric ovarian malignant GCTs appear to have excellent rates of survival with conservative surgery plus platinum-based chemotherapy. Survival does not appear to be affected by deviations from surgical guidelines. Revised surgical guidelines include collection of ascites or washings, excision or biopsy of nodules on peritoneal surfaces, palpation and sampling of lymph nodes, inspection of omentum and removal of abnormalities, inspection of contralateral ovary and biopsy of abnormalities, and complete resection of tumor-containing ovary with fallopian-sparing surgery if possible. Further treatment studies should focus on reducing the morbidity associated with treatment.

Randomized Comparison of Combination Chemotherapy With Etoposide, Bleomycin, and Either High-Dose or Standard-Dose Cisplatin in Children and Adolescents With High-Risk Malignant Germ Cell Tumors: A Pediatric Intergroup Study—Pediatric Oncology Group 9049 and Children's Cancer Group 8882

Cushing B, Giller R, Cullen JW, et al (Wayne State Univ, Detroit Univ of Colorado, Denver; Stanford Univ, Calif; et al)

J Clin Oncol 22:2691-2700, 2004 4–8

Background.—The Pediatric Oncology Group and the Children's Cancer Group designed this randomized trial to test the efficacy of cisplatin dose intensification for patients with high-risk malignant germ cell tumors (MGCT). Toxicity was assessed.

Study Design.—The study group consisted of 299 pediatric patients with stage II to IV MGCT of gonadal origin or stage I to IV of extra-agonal origin. All gonadal MGCTs were excised if possible. Patients were stratified according to stage, site, and metastases. They were randomly assigned to either standard cisplatin-based therapy (PEB) or high-dose cisplatin-based therapy (HDPEB) for 4 cycles. Patients with a partial response (PR) had attempted resection. If there was residual malignant disease, they received 2 more cycles of their chemotherapy regimen. Outcome analyses were performed for event-free survival (EFS) and overall survival (OS).

Findings.—HDPEB treatment was associated with significantly improved 6-year EFS rate compared with standard PEB. There was no significant difference in OS. Toxic deaths were more common with HDPEB, as were other treatment-related toxicities.

Conclusions.—The use of HDPEB was associated with a significant improvement in EFS for pediatric patients with high-risk malignant germ cell tumors, but this was not true for OS. The significant toxicity associated with HDPEB limits its usefulness for this pediatric population. Strategies to either improve the effectiveness of standard-dose PEB or reduce the toxicity of HDPEB are being investigated.

▶ These 2 articles (Abstracts 4–7 and 4–8) deal with MGCTs in children and adolescents. Billmire et al (Abstract 4–7) examine the results of 2 large prospective trials of MGCTs specifically in regard to the 131 ovarian GCTs included in these trials. The specific question they addressed concerned whether deviation from standard surgical guidelines (either omissions or more aggressive procedures) had an impact on outcome. They could identify no impact of such deviations on outcome. This underscores the paramount importance of platinum-based chemotherapy in these patients. Cushing et al (Abstract 4–8) report the results of a prospective, randomized, phase III trial comparing bleomycin, etoposide, and either high-dose (40 mg/m^2 per day for 5 days) or low-dose (20 mg/m^2 per day for 5 days) cisplatin for the treatment of 134 patients with advanced MGCTs or either testicular (n = 60) or ovarian (n = 74) origin. This trial shows an advantage for the high-dose cisplatin in regard to EFS at 6 years (89% vs 80%) but not OS. Because of the lack of a difference in OS and the far greater toxicity with the high-dose regimen, the authors conclude that regimen as employed in this trial should not be used.

J. T. Thigpen, MD

▶ The introduction of combination chemotherapy and, particularly, cisplatin-based therapies, have resulted in dramatic improvements in outcome for patients with advanced MGCTs. Several additional studies in adults demonstrated that using high-dose cisplatin further improved outcome. However, a randomized trial in adults comparing high-dose with standard-dose cisplatin showed no significant difference, resulting in the conclusion that standard-dose cisplatin in conjunction with bleomycin and either vinblastine or etoposide represented optimal treatment. The clinical trial described in this report randomly assigned children with MGCTs to receive either high dose (40 mg/m^2 on days 1-5) or standard dose (20 mg/m^2 on days 1-5) along with bleomycin and etoposide. Importantly, groups were balanced for such factors as age, tumor markers, and treatment. Although the results showed an increased EFS for patients with MGCTs, the OS was similar between the 2 regimens because of increased treatment-related toxic deaths in the high-dose cisplatin arm. In addition, hearing deficits were significantly greater in the high-dose cisplatin–treated patients. This is a well-designed randomized trial with important results being reported. Unfortunately, it is one of those circumstances in which the results came after no difference was reported from an adult randomized trial asking essentially the same question with essentially the same tumor types. Hopefully, future work will build on adult studies to develop improved and less-toxic therapies for children rather than performing studies that are confirmatory.

R. J. Arceci, MD, PhD

Outcome of Patients With Residual Germ Cell or Non–Germ Cell Malignancy After Resection of Primary Mediastinal Nonseminomatous Germ Cell Cancer

Schneider BP, Kesler KA, Brooks JA, et al (Indiana Univ, Indianapolis; Walther Cancer Inst, Indianapolis, Ind)

J Clin Oncol 22:1195-1200, 2004 4–9

Background.—The most common origin of extragonadal germ cell tumors (GCT) is the retroperitoneum or anterior mediastinum. Primary mediastinal GCTs are rare and account for approximately 15% of adult anterior mediastinal tumors. Approximately 5% of all GCTs are anterior mediastinal GCTs. The serologic and histologic characteristics of primary mediastinal nonseminomatous GCTs (PMNSGCTs) are similar to their testicular counterparts, but there are significant differences between these tumors in terms of biology and clinical outcomes. Prognostic variables and outcomes were identified in patients with PMNSGCTs with postchemotherapy resection of persistent cancer.

Methods.—A retrospective review was conducted of 47 consecutive patients with residual cancer after resection of PMNSGCT. The mean age of patients was 31 years. The median alpha fetoprotein level was 1595 ng/mL, with a normal range defined as 0 to 25 ng/mL. Mediastinal-only disease was present in 27 patients at presentation, and 20 patients had extramediastinal involvement. All the patients received platinum-based chemotherapy either according to standard therapy at the time or by participation in a clinical trial.

Results.—At diagnosis, serum tumor markers (STMs) were present in 43 patients, and 20 patients had extramediastinal disease. At resection, 21 patients had elevated STMs. After resection, 26 patients had GCTs. Malignant transformation of teratoma with elements of non-GCT were present in 12 patients, and 9 had both GCT and non-GCT. Of the 47 patients, 16 have continuously had no evidence of disease, including 8 of 26 patients with GCT histology and 2 of 12 patients with non-GCT histology. Of the 27 patients with mediastinal-only disease at presentation, 2 have continuously had no evidence of disease. Seven of 21 patients with elevated STMs at time of resection have continuously had no evidence of disease. Overall, 16 of 47 patients have continuously had no evidence of disease, an additional 4 patients have had no evidence of disease with further therapy (currently no evidence of disease), 2 patients are alive with disease, 23 patients died of disease, and 2 patients died postoperatively.

Conclusions.—The presence of elevated STMs at resection does not alter outcome in patients with residual GCT or non-GCT malignancy if residual disease is completely resected. The surgical resection of persistent cancer, even in the presence of elevated STMs, can provide long-term survival in this poor-risk patient population.

► One of the unique aspects of GCTs is that of PMNSGCT. These patients with PMSGCT have a higher association with Klinefelter's syndrome, hematologic disorders (eg, acute megakaryocytic leukemia), and non-GCT malignancies. This is a nicely written review of the experience at Indiana University that clarifies an apparent adverse factor of elevated STMs before resection in patients with PMSGCT. It has been suggested by several authors that such patients who have persistently elevated markers after primary chemotherapy should go on to salvage chemotherapy. In this group, one third of patients with elevated STMs have remained continuously disease free without further therapy. This continues to support the notion that PMNSGCTs fare less well than their gonadal counterparts but nonetheless are potentially curable.

P. J. Loehrer, Sr, MD

Impact of Unnecessary Exploratory Laparotomy on the Treatment of Patients With Metastatic Germ Cell Tumor

Stephenson AJ, Russo P, Kaplinsky R, et al (Mem Sloan-Kettering Cancer, New York)

J Urol 171:1474-1477, 2004 4–10

Introduction.—Germ cell tumors (GCTs) are the most frequently occurring malignancy in men aged 15 to 35 years and the second most common neoplasm in men aged 35 to 39 years. Despite its common occurrence, diagnostic delay is a well-recognized phenomenon of this disease; both patients and physicians contribute to the delay. The impact of unnecessary surgeries in these patients has not been fully explored. The consequences of unnecessary exploratory laparotomy on the treatment of patients with metastatic GCT were evaluated in terms of complications, delays in definitive therapy, intensity of required therapy, and outcome.

Findings.—The medical records of 40 patients who underwent exploratory laparotomy for unsuspected metastatic GCT between 1980 and 2001 were retrospectively reviewed. The mean age at the time of exploratory laparotomy was 34 years. A midline retroperitoneal mass was observed in all patients; 14 had disease at other sites. Abnormalities at the time of physical examination and testicular sonogram were observed in 8 (20%) and 22 (55%) patients, respectively. Elevated serum α-fetoprotein and/or β-human chorionic gonadotropin occurred in 26 patients (65%). Eight patients (22%) had surgical complications. The median interval between laparotomy and chemotherapy was 29 days; the delay in therapy was 30 or more days in 48% of the cohort. In patients with a 30 or more days of delay in therapy, 60% needed intensive chemotherapy (multiple regimens or high-dose or salvage chemotherapy) compared with 26% whose delay was less than 30 days ($P = .01$).

Conclusion.—Exploratory laparotomy contributes to therapeutic delay in a substantial proportion of patients and complicates cancer therapy. At the time of presentation, there was evidence to suggest GCT in all patients. This underscores the importance of physician awareness in making a timely diagnosis.

▶ This is not an uncommon scenario: A young man presents with an abdominal mass and undergoes an exploratory laparotomy. The pathology reveals "a poorly differentiated cancer." Only afterward does the physician obtain serum markers, which suggests a GCT. This report outlines an important syndrome. At the core, good clinical judgment preoperatively can decrease patient morbidity and improves chances for survival.

P. J. Loehrer, Sr, MD

Kidney

Transcriptional Targeting in Renal Cancer Cell Lines via the Human CXCR4 Promoter

Haviv YS, van Houdt WJ, Lu B, et al (Univ of Alabama, Birmingham; Hadassah-Hebrew Univ Med Ctr, Jerusalem)

Mol Cancer Ther 3:687-691, 2004 4–11

Background.—Overall, the rate of response to therapy for metastatic renal cell carcinoma (RCC) is less than 20%. A direct correlation has been noted between the metastatic stage of RCC and death, so the search is underway to identify new agents that address the disease by metastatic stage. Metastases or local invasion for various cancers appears to involve the chemokine SDF-1α/CXCR5 pathway. CXCR4 is highly expressed in breast cancer cells and primary breast cancers, but peak SDF-1α expression is in the tissues where breast cancer tends to metastasize. It was theorized that the CXCR4 promoter could be used to target RCC with gene therapy vectors. An adenoviral vector that encoded a reporter gene controlled by the CXCR4 promoter was constructed to test the hypothesis.

Methods.—Several RCC cell lines (A498, CAKI-1, 786-0, SN12C, and KU-19-20) were investigated to confirm overexpression of CXCR4. Next, an adenoviral vector was constructed in which human CXCR4 promoter regulated the expression of a reporter gene. The activity of the promoter in vitro and in vivo was finally tested by appropriate models.

Results.—The highest mRNA levels of CXCR4 were expressed by the A498 RCC cell line, and the lowest (no expression) was found for the 789-0 RCC line. All cell lines that expressed CXCR4 showed a highly active CXCR4 promoter in the adenoviral backbone. With the highly metastatic SN12C-MMP RCC cell line clone, CXCR4 promoter activity was 10 times higher than the activity of a comparison cytomegalovirus promoter. CXCR4 promoter was also substantially lower in the CXCR4-negative RCC cell line 786-0 than in the CXCR4-positive RCC cells. When normal human cells were examined, CXCR4 promoter was repressed. In mice, the CXCR4 promoter activity was 137-fold lower in the liver than in the kidneys. Mouse kidney showed the highest CXCR4 promoter activity, with lungs showing the next most active pattern.

Conclusions.—Results indicated that the CXCR4 promoter holds promise for transcriptionally targeted transgenic expression. In addition, it was downregulated by the liver, which is a major requirement from potential candidates for transcriptional targeting of cancer. The activity of the CXCR4 promoter in RCC lines and its repression in normal human cells and in the mouse liver were taken as positive indications that it could prove useful in the transcriptional targeting of RCC.

► Clinical science is first beginning to understand the role of cell trafficking in the treatment and management of cancer. The role of chemokines and their interaction with their receptors has long been appreciated in terms of their playing a role in the mitogenic response of immune cells such as neutrophils and lymphocytes. Only recently have investigators begun to assess the role of chemokines and their receptors in the migration of cancer cells. In this study, the authors assessed the presence of CXCR4 on the surface of RCC cell lines and noted that CXCR4 is increased in RCC. The ligand for CXCR4 is SDF-1α, which is expressed in tissues around the body and presumed to be the binding attraction between the ligand and receptor, which results in metastatic lesion development. It is not clear whether the expression of CXCR4 is differentially expressed on early nonmetastatic patients compared with those with metastases, or whether it is the expression of the ligand at distant sites of disease that emerges as the critical factor for the development of metastases. Regardless, it is possible that the CXCR4/SDF-1α pathway may represent a novel target for therapeutic development.

M. S. Gordon, MD

Promoter Hypermethylation Profile of Kidney Cancer

Dulaimi E, Ibanez de Caceres I, Uzzo RG, et al (Fox Chase Cancer Ctr, Philadelphia; Duke Univ, Durham, NC; Univ of Alabama, Birmingham)

Clin Cancer Res 10:3972-3979, 2004 4–12

Background.—In human cancer, DNA methylation is altered. Tumor suppressor genes are inactivated by promoter hypermethylation in cancer cells. Promoter hypermethylation is found frequently, occurs in the tumor suppressor and cancer genes that correspond to various signaling pathways, and follows different patterns with different types of tumors. Approximately 3% of all solid neoplasms found in the United States are cancers of the kidney, most often renal cell carcinomas (RCCs) or transitional cell carcinomas of the renal pelvis. To further the understanding of the inactivation of tumor suppressor and cancer cells in the development of kidney cancer, a hypermethylation profile of kidney cancer was developed.

Methods.—Methylation-specific polymerase chain reaction was used to profile the promoter hypermethylation status in 100 tumors representative of the major kinds of cancers of the kidney. Included were 50 clear cell, 20 papillary, 6 chromophobe, 5 collecting duct, 5 renal cell unclassified, 7 oncocytoma, 6 transitional cell carcinomas of the renal pelvis, and 1 Wilms' tumor. The profile obtained was then correlated with patients' clinicopathologic findings.

Results.—Ninety-three percent of all the tumors had methylation of at least 1 gene; only 7 tumors showed no methylation. Methylation of 1 gene was noted in 33% of cases and methylation of 2 in 34%, with 15% having 3 genes, 8% 4 genes, 2% 5 genes, and 1% 7 genes hypermethylated. Ten normal renal and 5 normal ureteral tissue DNA samples showed no methylation. Gene hypermethylation specific to pathologic findings was noted, with *von Hippel Lindau* methylation only found in clear cell tumors and in men; *RAZ association domain family protein 1A (RASSF1A)* methylation significantly more frequent in papillary renal tumors and higher grade tumors of all cell types; *O⁶-methyl-guanine-DNA-methyltransferase (MGMT)* methylation more often in women and in nonsmokers of both sexes; and *glutathione S-transferase π1 (GSTP1)* methylation found in older patients. A nonsignificant trend in *MGMT* methylation was noted toward high-stage tumors. A negative association was found between the hypermethylation of certain individual genes and that of other individual genes. Gene hypermethylation and survival showed no correlation.

Conclusions.—Aberrant promoter hypermethylation of tumor suppressor and cancer genes was common and widespread by cell type. The process occurred relatively early and involved various pathways in kidney tumorigenesis. Specific associations between the hypermethylation of *von Hippel Lindau*, *RASSF1A*, and *MGMT* and cell type, grade, and stage of cancer, respectively, await confirmation by larger studies but hold promise for use as markers in predicting clinical outcome, differential diagnosis, and prognosis.

▶ Hypermethylation of transcription promoters is a critical pathway related to the inactivation of tumor suppressor genes in cancer. As a result of inactivation of genes such as *PTEN*, tumors may undergo more aggressive proliferative development and progression. Hypermethylation was seen in 1 or more genes in more than 90% of the patient samples studied. Samples consisted of a number of different histologies, including 50 clear cell cancers and 20 papillary cancers. Among the tumor suppressor genes that were inactivated, the *von Hippel Lindau* gene was hypermethylated in 8% of patients. Additional genes involved included the *APC* gene on chromosome 5 and the *GSTP1* gene. Of note is that hypermethylation of the *Timp-3* gene was seen in 58% of samples. This gene is associated with the inhibition of matrix metalloproteinases, which are critical for tumor cell invasion. The understanding of the hypermethylation status of tumors may be valuable in determining the role of new therapies that work by hypomethylating proteins, thereby possibly reactivating previously inactivated proteins.

M. S. Gordon, MD

Genetic Profile of Bone Metastases in Renal Cell Carcinoma

Junker K, Romics I, Szendroi A, et al (Friedrich-Schiller-Univ, Jena, Germany; Semmelweis Univ, Budapest, Hungary; Charles Univ, Hradec Kralove, Czech Republic)

Eur Urol 45:320-324, 2004 4–13

Background.—Up to 30% of patients with renal cell carcinoma (RCC) have bone metastasis develop. Genetic studies have shown histopathologically defined subtypes of RCC have specific genetic patterns. Comparative genomic hybridization (CGH) was performed on primary RCC tumors and related bone metastases to examine whether specific genetic alterations are common to both the primary tumor and the metastasis.

Methods.—DNA from 13 primary tumors and 31 related bone metastases was extracted from paraffin-embedded tissue sections and subjected to degenerate oligonucleotide-primed polymerase chain reaction for amplification. Tumor DNA and normal DNA (isolated from lymphocytes) were labeled by polymerase chain reaction, then examined by CGH. Gains and losses of specific regions were compared in paired primary and metastatic tissues.

Results.—CGH identified genetic alterations in all but 2 of the metastases. A mean of 6.3 genetic alterations was found in each metastasis. The most common changes were losses of chromosomes 3p (76%), 6 (20%), 8p (20%), 9 (34%), 14q (27%), and 18 (20%) and gains of chromosomes 5 (45%), 8q (34%), and 17 (27%). Of the 13 primary tumors, 7 had at least 1 genetic alteration identical to one found in its paired metastatic sample. In these 7 cases, the number of alterations tended to be higher in the primary tumors than in the metastases (4.4 vs 3.7). In 3 other primary tumors, CGH identified no genetic alterations. Finally, in the remaining 3 primary tumors, alterations in the primary tumor were completely different from those in its paired metastatic sample.

Conclusion.—In 7 of 13 primary RCC tumors, the same genetic alteration present in the primary tumor was present in at least 1 bone metastasis, supporting a clonal relation between primary and metastatic tumors in RCC. The failure of CGH to identify any genetic changes in 3 of the primary tumors and 2 of the metastases could be caused by degradation of DNA in the formalin-fixed specimens. Identifying critical regions and genes involved in the metastatic process may lead to novel therapies to prevent bone metastases in patients with RCC.

► A critical question in cancer is what determines the timing and localization of distant metastases in patients with cancer. In this study, the authors assessed the bone metastases and corresponding primary tumors in a series of patients with RCC. By extracting DNA from the paraffin-imbedded tumors, the authors were able to identify specific genetic mutations that were common to both the primary and the metastasis. They noted that in addition to these common abnormalities, there were a series of additional chromosomal abnormalities that were acquired and were hypothesized to be associated with the metastatic potential for the cancer. This study is important because it validates some of the specific issues regarding the differences between primary and metastatic sites and begins to address the issue of not only when tumors metastasize but whether there is a preference to where they metastasize. It has been recognized that different tumors have a propensity to metastasize to bone versus lung versus liver, and if specific changes in the cancer are identified then the ability to develop site-specific therapy to prevent unique metastatic potential could be developed.

M. S. Gordon, MD

Cachexia-Like Symptoms Predict a Worse Prognosis in Localized T1 Renal Cell Carcinoma

Kim HL, Han K-R, Zisman A, et al (Univ of California, Los Angeles)

J Urol 171:1810-1813, 2004 4–14

Background.—For patients with renal cell carcinoma (RCC), cachexia-related findings have been able to independently predict survival. Cachexia-related findings can be a paraneoplastic phenomenon caused by the release of tumor-associated proteins. The prognostic value of cachexia-related findings was assessed in patients with localized stage T1 RCC.

Methods.—Two hundred fifty patients from a kidney cancer database had had partial or radical nephrectomy for T1 RCC. An assessment looked at the prognostic significance of the symptoms found at diagnosis and the results of preoperative laboratory testing. The mean follow-up was 33 months and median follow-up was 43 months.

Results.—At final follow-up, 19% of the patients had died. The cachexia-related findings found to significantly predict a worse disease-specific survival included malaise, weight loss, anorexia, and hypoalbuminemia. Whether the patient had 1 or several cachexia-related findings, the disease-specific survival was not significantly different, so all patients with at least 1 finding were considered to have cachexia. Those with cachexia had a higher tumor grade and a significantly higher risk of recurrence compared with patients with no signs of cachexia.

Conclusions.—Findings related to cachexia, specifically hypoalbuminemia, weight loss, anorexia, and malaise, were predictive of a worse outcome for patients with RCC. When patients with cachexia have high-grade tumors, clinical trials with adjuvant therapy should be considered.

▶ The authors assessed, from their extensive database, an association between symptoms of cachexia and survival in patients with RCC. While such symptoms have been known to be associated with survival in patients with metastatic disease, likely related to the expression of cachexia-inducing cytokines such as interleukin-6 and tumor necrosis factor-α, this study assessed those patients who should have the best prognosis, namely those with early stage T1 tumors who are resected for cure. In reviewing their database, the authors identified 250 patients who underwent primary resection for a T1N0M0 RCC and correlated the survival of these patients with symptoms at presentation. Patients with at least 1 symptom of cachexia had a significantly worse relapse-free as well as overall survival with the worst outcome being seen in patients with high-grade lesions (55% overall survival). Review of the database confirmed that cachexialike symptoms are an independent prognostic factor for outcome and should perhaps be taken into consideration when discussing adjuvant options for patients in this setting.

M. S. Gordon, MD

Robust Classification of Renal Cell Carcinoma Based on Gene Expression Data and Predicted Cytogenetic Profiles

Furge KA, Lucas KA, Takahashi M, et al (Van Andel Research Inst, Grand Rapids, Mich; Univ of Tokyshima, Japan; Iwate Med Univ, Morika, Japan; et al)
Cancer Res 64:4117-4121, 2004 4–15

Background.—The standard subtypes of renal cell carcinoma (RCC) are clear cell, granular cell, papillary, chromophobe, spindle cell, cystic, and collecting duct carcinomas, which are determined by their varying morphologic features. Clear cell, papillary, and chromophobe types are the most common. Classifying RCC on the basis of transcriptional signatures may prove beneficial, but chromosomal alterations are traditionally used to help classify RCC at the molecular level. An attempt was made to differentiate the 3 major RCC subtypes by using gene expression profiles to identify both molecular genetic and cytogenetic classifications.

Methods.—An expression-based RCC classifier was developed by using gene expression profiles for each major RCC subtype. Next, these profiles were evaluated for regional gene expression biases, which are genetic intervals containing a disproportionate number of genes whose upregulation or downregulation is coordinated. Such a finding generally implies a chromosomal abnormality is present. Samples of the 3 major subtypes were then assessed.

Results.—In scanning the gene expression profiles for regional expression biases, these biases were found to correspond well with the traditional cytogenetic profiles of RCC. Papillary samples had frequent upward gene expression biases for chromosomes 7, 16, and 17. Chromophobe samples had frequent downward biases for chromosomes 1, 2, 6, 10q, and 17q. Clear cell samples had frequent downward expression bias for chromosome 13q and frequent upward expression bias for chromosome 5q. These were not previously found in association with chromophobe RCC, but frequent amplifications of chromosomes 20q and 11q were identified with this approach. With the prediction analysis of microarrays, the expression-based RCC classifier correctly identified 100% of the test samples. A cytogenetic classifier was also generated and correctly identified 66% of the clear cell samples, 100% of the papillary samples, and 78% of the chromophobe samples. No significant regional biases were noted in 7 samples that could not be classified. Of 33 additional samples introduced, the expression-based classifier correctly identified 100% of the clear cell samples, 75% of the papillary samples, and 100% of the chromophobe samples. Expression-based classifications were supported by the cytogenetics-based classifier in 82% of the cases. Combining the 2 methods could yield a strong tool for classifying the 3 major types of RCC with a single gene expression profile.

Conclusions.—Transcriptional and cytogenetic features derived from a gene expression profile were used to construct a useful classification model for RCC. The 3 subtypes showed clear differences with this tool. With further study it may be possible to construct a more detailed classification model that will permit the prediction of patient outcomes and other clinical parameters.

► The pathologic review of RCC can be complex. Differences in diagnosis can be associated with significant differences in treatment. Clear cell cancer patients tend to be candidates for primary immunotherapy, while papillary renal cell cancer patients never respond to interleukin-2 or interferon-α therapy and at the present time should never receive immunotherapy. Similarly, chromophobe RCCs tend to have a better survival after resection. In this study, Furge et al performed gene expression profiling of a set of 73 RCC cases. The authors were able to segregate the kidney cancer samples into 3 distinct groups of patients consistent with their clear cell, papillary, and chromophobe histologies. As a result of this work, it is clear that gene expression profiling has the ability to separate the principal histologic subtypes of RCC and may have a role in difficult cases for which histology cannot be confirmed. In addition, this result will allow the identification of various genes that may play a role in prognosis or in prediction of response for those patients with metastatic disease. A molecular classification of RCC may aid in the development of specific therapies in various clinical and pathologic subtypes of RCC.

M. S. Gordon, MD

Prognostic Value of Carbonic Anhydrase IX and Ki67 as Predictors of Survival for Renal Clear Cell Carcinoma

Bui MHT, Visapaa H, Seligson D, et al (Univ of California, Irvine)
J Urol 171:2461-2466, 2004 4–16

Background.—The conventional prognostic factors (grade, stage, and performance status, for example) fail to explain the natural history of renal cell carcinoma (RCC), with wide variations in biologic behavior and clinical outcome. This complex disorder may be better followed through the use of molecular tumor markers. The prognostic value of carbonic anhydrase IX (CAIX) and Ki67, a nuclear antigen present in all cycling human cells, was tested in regard to survival in RCC.

Methods.—Tissue microarrays were constructed from paraffin-embedded specimens obtained from 224 patients who had undergone nephrectomy for clear cell RCC. The samples were subjected to immunohistochemical analysis with a CAIX and a Ki67 monoclonal antibody. The staining associated with CAIX and Ki67 was linked to clinical factors, pathologic features, and survival. Follow-up lasted for 0.3 to 117 months, with a median of 34 months. The primary end point for the study was disease-free survival.

Results.—Ki67 was detected in 75% of the RCC tumors and was localized to the nucleus. High Ki67 staining was positively correlated with the presence of metastasis, increased tumor stage, increased Fuhrman grade, and disease-related death. It was a significant prognostic marker, with a median survival of 21 months and death from RCC significantly linked to high

Ki67 staining. Low Ki67 staining was related to a survival of 101 months. Ninety-three percent of specimens had CAIX expression. The plasma membrane was the most prominent site of CAIX staining, with variations depending on the proportion of target tissue in the core that stained positive. The median survival was 67 months for patients with high CAIX expression and 22 months with low CAIX expression. CAIX labeling correlated significantly with RCC-related death. CAIX expression achieved significance with respect to stratifying the survival of patients with aggressive disease. Thus, both Ki67 and CAIX were identified as independently predictive of survival. Combining the 2 produced a single prognostic index that permitted patients to be stratified according to survival risk (low, intermediate, and high). High Ki67 expression with low CAIX expression carried the worst prognosis for RCC patients. High CAIX and low Ki67 staining was associated with the best outcomes. The combination of these markers displaced grade as a significant factor and was a statistically independent predictor.

Conclusions.—Both Ki67 and CAIX proved to be significant predictors of survival. Ki67 and CAIX labeling correlated inversely, but high Ki67 and low CAIX had the ability to significantly predict survival. Ki67 and CAIX together supplied enough molecular information about the biologic aggressiveness of RCC to develop distinctive prognostic groups. Both the survival prediction and the classification of RCC could be improved by using these biomarkers.

▶ Possibly one of the most significant advances being developed in the management of patients with clear cell RCC is the use of CAIX evaluation in patients with metastatic disease. High expression of CAIX on the tumor surface appears to be associated with a higher rate of response to high-dose interleukin-2–containing regimens. In this article, the authors applied the expression of CAIX and Ki67, the latter a reflection of tumor cell proliferation, to tissue microarrays of patient samples from nephrectomy specimens. The expression of these 2 parameters was gauged as factors for survival with a median follow-up period of nearly 3 years. The results of the assessment reveal that in contrast to its ability to predict immunotherapy response, CAIX expression was inversely correlated with survival. That is, low expression of CAIX was associated with a significantly lower survival rate compared with patients with high CAIX expression. The correlation of CAIX and Ki67 as a single factor correlated strongly with survival as well as Fuhrman grade of the tumor, suggesting that as in other adenocarcinomas, less well-differentiated and more aggressive tumors did more poorly. It should be noted that staining for CAIX is fairly ubiquitous and that less than 5% of the patients had staining of their tumors to a degree of 80% to 90% and overall 20% had staining below the 85% expression cutoff that differentiated high versus low staining. Hence, null staining did no more poorly than intermediate staining. In addition, there was no difference in the survival of patients based on the intensity of the CAIX staining in those with "high" characteristics. CAIX is a surface glycoprotein whose expression appears to be mediated by the expression of hypoxia-inducing factor 1α and may represent a greater degree of dependence on factors such as the expression of vascular endothelial growth factor, another hypoxia-inducing factor–induced protein. Future studies stratifying patients for adjuvant trials on the basis of these factors may be reasonable to consider.

M. S. Gordon, MD

Percutaneous CT-Guided Radiofrequency Ablation of Renal Neoplasms: Factors Influencing Success

Zagoria RJ, Hawkins AD, Clark PE, et al (Wake Forest Univ, Winston-Salem, NC)

AJR 183:201-207, 2004 4–17

Background.—Nearly two thirds of the renal cancers diagnosed in the United States are found incidentally in asymptomatic patients undergoing imaging for other reasons. These tumors tend to be smaller than those in symptomatic patients. Treatment traditionally involves partial or radical nephrectomy, leaving the patient with limited or no functional renal tissue. An alternative approach is radiofrequency ablation. The experience obtained with 22 patients who had radiofrequency ablation for renal neoplasms was reviewed, looking specifically at success rate and risk of serious complications.

Methods.—Treatment was carried out between May 2000 and August 2003. The 22 patients had 24 renal neoplasms and underwent 27 radiofrequency ablation sessions. Renal neoplasms were confirmed at biopsy in 17 cases, and 5 were diagnosed on the basis of CT scans or MRI. Patients ranged in age from 39 to 87 years (mean age, 70 years). Comorbid conditions were noted in 22 patients, a solitary kidney in 2, and metastatic disease in 3, leading to the choice of nonsurgical treatment. CT or MRI studies were obtained 1 to 3 months after ablation. Follow-up extended for 1 to 35 months (mean, 7 months).

Results.—Ninety-one percent of the patients had no residual tumor after either 1 or multiple ablation sessions. Twenty patients had no enhancement of the treated tumors, with 4 having enhancements indicative of residual viable tumor. None had metastases develop during follow-up. Complete ablation of tumor was achieved in 79% of clear cell carcinomas and 100% of papillary carcinomas. Patients with an elevated serum creatinine level had complete ablation in 60% of cases, whereas those with a normal creatinine level had complete ablation in 82% of cases. One hundred percent of tumors less than 3 cm in size were completely ablated; 69% of those measuring more than 3 cm were completely ablated. No complications required intervention or hospitalization, but 4 patients had mild pain, 9 had mild perinephric hematoma, 1 had mild pain and pneumothorax, and 1 had mild pain and perinephric hematoma. No complications were seen in 10 ablation sessions. Only patients with serious comorbid conditions required prolonged hospitalization, and the indications were for other than ablation-related problems. Patients whose immediate contrast-enhanced CT scan indicated no residual viable tumor did not have tumor enhancement on later scans.

Conclusions.—Small renal tumors were safely ablated in 91% of cases with no residual tumor found a mean of 7 months after completing radiofrequency ablation. Contrast-enhanced CT scans taken immediately after the ablation session reliably indicated when residual tumor was present. When none was found immediately, no residual tumor was noted on longer term follow-up. Complications were mild and required no intervention. Patients' comorbid conditions were the determining factor when hospitalization was prolonged.

► The management of incidentally found small renal cell cancers is expanding with regard to options. Patients can undergo invasive surgery including nephrectomy and partial nephrectomy and may or may not undergo these procedures laparoscopically. This report addresses a relatively new method of managing small solitary renal cell cancers by radiofrequency ablation. By this method, patients undergo radiofrequency ablation percutaneously under CT scan guidance. In the first 22 patients in this report, 27 procedures were performed. Twenty of the 22 patients had complete control of their tumors with no evidence of residual tumor detected after the procedure. To achieve this control, 83% of these patients underwent 1 procedure and 8% underwent a second procedure. Two patients with residual tumor on CT scan refused further treatment. Tumors that were less than 3 cm in size (11 patients) achieved total control after 1 procedure in 100% of the cases. Three patients had tumors that were more than 5 cm in size, and all 3 were adequately managed with one procedure. No long-term follow-up exists to determine whether, for these smaller lesions that would otherwise be amenable to less invasive surgery, the cure rate is equal to that of more aggressive surgery. The procedure was performed on an outpatient basis and was well tolerated and represents a possible new option for patients with small, predominantly exophytic renal cell tumors. The downside to this procedure includes the technical difficulty with performing it on centrally located lesions and the absence of available pathologic tissue for further analysis.

M. S. Gordon, MD

The Radiographic Evolution of Radio Frequency Ablated Renal Tumors

Matsumoto ED, Watumull L, Johnson DB, et al (Univ of Texas, Dallas; Univ of Utah, Salt Lake City; Emory Univ, Atlanta, Ga)

J Urol 172:45-48, 2004 4–18

Background.—For small renal neoplasms the treatments chosen tend to be minimally invasive. Radiofrequency ablation (RFA) has produced good short-term results for this application. It can be delivered by laparoscopic or percutaneous routes. After cryoablation, tumors show significant shrinkage and loss of contrast enhancement, but the appearance of tumors treated with RFA has not been well characterized. Contrast-enhanced CT (CE-CT) was used to determine the progressive characteristics of renal tumors undergoing RFA.

Methods.—CE-CT was used to evaluate the appearance of 64 renal tumors in 60 patients who underwent RFA. The scans were assessed after 6 weeks, 3 months, 6 months, and every 6 months thereafter for a median follow-up of 13.7 months (range, 6 weeks to 29 months). The features characteristic of these lesions and their changes with time were noted.

Results.—Thirty-four patients received CT-guided percutaneous RFA, 28 laparoscopic RFA, and 2 open RFA. Contrast enhancement was absent for 62 tumors on all serial imaging. The ablated tumor did not increase in size with time. Seventeen were endophytic lesions, with 75% of the tumor volume within the renal capsule. These initially had a low-density nonenhancing wedge-shaped defect that remained throughout follow-up. With maturity, the wedge gradually retracted from the kidney's perfused portion. Tissue with the density of fat had begun infiltrating between normal and ablated tissue in 50% of cases at 12 months. Forty-seven endophytic tumors maintained the configuration of the original tumor after RFA, evidencing some retraction and minimal shrinkage. Watershed areas where the contrast uptake was diminished occasionally surrounded the ablation defect. A peritumor scar developed around the percutaneous-treated tumors, resembling a halo of fat around the ablated tumor and clearly indicating where the ablated tissue was. One patient had persistent tumor at 6 weeks and required repeat percutaneous RFA, which was successful. One patient had a tumor recurrence at 12 months. The repeat RFA had no enhancement on CE-CT after 6 weeks. One patient died of cerebral vascular accident.

Conclusions.—Renal tumors undergoing RFA demonstrated characteristic features on CE-CT follow-up. Size regression was minimal, with no contrast enhancement found in completely treated tumors. With time, the completely treated lesions may retract from the normal parenchyma and fat infiltration can take place.

▶ RFA is a new approach to the management of small renal cell cancer primary tumors. Methods for performing this procedure include laparoscopic or percutaneous approaches, the latter of which is well tolerated as an outpatient procedure. Unlike surgery, which eliminates the cancer from the radiologic field, RFA results in a residual abnormality that undergoes involution over time but may never completely resolve. The authors of this study report on a series of 64 consecutive renal tumors treated with RFA by laparoscopic (n = 28), percutaneous (n = 34), or open (n = 2) procedures. CE-CT scan was the study of choice after the procedure to determine the likelihood of residual cancer being present afterwards. In general, radiologic abnormalities persisted, whether as an exophytic mass that did not contrast enhance on CT, or as a wedge-shaped, nonenhancing lesion for the endophytic lesions. Residual or recurrent disease, when seen in one patient, demonstrated the expected contrast enhancement seen when cancer is present. These findings provide important information regarding the expected residual abnormalities seen after RFA, which should be appreciated by any practitioner either performing the procedure or seeing patients after the procedure.

M. S. Gordon, MD

Randomized Phase II Study of Multiple Dose Levels of CCI-779, a Novel Mammalian Target of Rapamycin Kinase Inhibitor, in Patients With Advanced Refractory Renal Cell Carcinoma

Atkins MB, Hidalgo M, Stadler WM, et al (Beth Israel Deaconess Med Ctr, Boston; Univ of Texas Health Science Ctr, San Antonio; Univ of Chicago; et al)
J Clin Oncol 22:909-918, 2004 4–19

Background.—Neither interleukin-2 nor interferon-α (IFN-α) are effective for patients with renal cell cancer (RCC) who are refractory to or have a recurrence after standard therapy. CCI-779 is a novel mammalian target of rapamycin (mTOR) kinase inhibitor, and CCI-779-induced inhibition of mTOR significantly reduced tumor size in mice with uterine and adrenal medullary tumors. Activation of mTOR involves a kinase that is regulated by the *PTEN* tumor suppressor gene. Although *PTEN* mutations have not been detected in RCC, *PTEN* expression is often downregulated in RCC. This phase II trial evaluated the effects of 3 doses of CCI-799 in patients with advanced refractory RCC.

Methods.—The subjects were 111 patients (69% men; median age, 57 years) with advanced refractory RCC. Patients were randomly assigned to receive weekly, 30-minute IV infusions of 25 mg (n = 36), 75 mg (n = 38), or 250 mg (n = 37) CCI-779. Treatment continued until disease progressed or unacceptable toxicity developed (median duration of therapy, 5.6 months; median doses, 19). Patients were evaluated at baseline and during therapy to assess tumor size, response to therapy (according to World Health Organization guidelines), time to disease progression, survival, and adverse events.

Results.—One patient with diffuse lung metastases receiving 250 mg CCI-779 had a complete response and is disease free well into his third year of treatment. Partial responses were obtained in 2 patients receiving the 25-mg dose, 3 receiving the 75-mg dose, and 2 receiving the 250-mg dose. Thus, the overall response rate was 7%. Additionally, 29 patients (26%) had a minor response, defined as a decrease in tumor size between 25% and 50%. The median times to tumor progression were 6.3, 6.7, and 5.2 months in the 25-, 75-, and 250-mg groups, respectively. The median survival was 13.8, 11.0, and 17.5 months in the 25-, 75-, and 250-mg groups, respectively. The most common drug-related adverse events (regardless of severity) were maculopapular rash (76%), mucositis (70%), asthenia (50%), and nausea (43%). The most common grades III/IV adverse events were hyperglycemia (17%), hypophosphatemia (13%), anemia (9%), and hypertriglyceridemia (6%). Toxicity did not differ according to CCI-779 dose. In separate analyses based on the patient's response to first-line INF-α therapy, patients with a good response to first-line therapy had a median survival of 18.4 to 23.8 months (depending on CCI-997 dose). Patients with an intermediate response to initial treatment had a median survival of 19.3 to 23.0 months, whereas patients with a poor response to initial therapy had a median survival of 7.1 to 8.6 months.

Conclusion.—CCI-779 has antitumor activity in patients with advanced refractory RCC over the 3 dose levels tested. It appears to be more effective in patients with a good or intermediate response to first-line INF-α therapy than to those with a poor initial response.

▶ The treatment of metastatic RCC remains a difficult problem for clinicians, given the paucity of effective treatments for the broadest number of patients. CCI-779 is a drug that targets mTOR kinase and is believed to be particularly effective in patients with mutations or deletions of *PTEN* tumor suppressor gene. While *PTEN* mutations have not routinely been seen in RCC, the expression of this gene is often downmodulated in RCC. This study assessed patients with refractory metastatic RCC who were treated with CCI-779 at 1 of 3 doses. The doses studied included 25, 75, and 250 mg IV weekly as a 30-minute infusion. Objective responses were seen in 1 patient (7%) and minor responses were seen in 26% of patients. There was no dose relation for either toxicity or response. The common toxicities included rash, mucositis, asthenia, and nausea, which all occurred with a frequency of more than 40%. The median survival of patients treated in the study was 15 months, which was believed to be significantly better than the typical outcome for patients with refractory disease. As a result of a subsequent pilot study of CCI-779 with INF-α, a subsequent randomized front-line trial of INF-α with or without CCI-779 is being performed in previously untreated metastatic RCC.

M. S. Gordon, MD

5 Hematologic Malignancies

Long-term Follow-up of 241 Patients With Monoclonal Gammopathy of Undetermined Significance: The Original Mayo Clinic Series 25 Years Later

Kyle RA, Therneau TM, Rajkumar SV, et al (Mayo Clinic, Rochester, Minn)

Mayo Clin Proc 79:859-866, 2004 5–1

Background.—Monoclonal gammopathy of undetermined significance (MGUS) is characterized by a serum M protein value of 3 g/dL or less; no M protein or only small amounts of monoclonal light chain in the urine; no lytic bone lesions, anemia, hypercalcemia, or renal insufficiency related to the M protein; and 10% of less plasma cells in bone marrow. Long-term follow-up of patients with MGUS seen at the Mayo Clinic was reported.

Methods.—Two hundred forty-one patients seen between 1956 and 1970 were followed up for up to 47 years. Total follow-up in person-years was 3579. The medical records of these patients were analyzed.

Findings.—At the last follow-up, only 6% of the patients were alive with no marked increase in M protein. Fifty-seven percent died with no evidence of multiple myeloma or related disorder. In 27%, a malignant lymphoplasma cell proliferative disorder developed. The median interval from MGUS diagnosis to diagnosis of multiple myeloma or related disorder was 10.4 years, with a range of 1 to 32 years.

Conclusions.—The median survival rate of these patients with MGUS was only slightly shorter than that of a comparable population. The risk of progression from MGUS to lymphoplasma cell malignancy can persist for more than 30 years. No reliable predictors of malignant evolution are known to date.

▶ The authors reviewed the largest single institution experience of patients with MGUS with 25 years of follow-up. The study included 241 patients diagnosed with MGUS 25 years ago or more for whom long-term follow up was available. Overall, 64 patients (27%) had some form of a malignant lymphoplasma cell disorder develop with a median time to diagnosis of 10.4 years. Fifty-seven percent of the patients died without any evidence of a plasma cell malignancy. There was no difference in the median survival rate for the group as a whole compared with the comparable US population and there were no reliable predictive factors that could be used to identify those patients who were destined to have a related malignancy develop. As a result of this study, it is clear that although patients with MGUS require continued observation, there is no need for further aggressive assessment and serial measurements of the serum paraprotein, with modifications of the approach based on changes in its value, is all that is required.

M. S. Gordon, MD

Magnitude of Response With Myeloma Frontline Therapy Does Not Predict Outcome: Importance of Time to Progression in Southwest Oncology Group Chemotherapy Trials

Durie BG, Jacobson J, Barlogie B, et al (Cedar-Sinai Med Ctr, Los Angeles; Cancer Research and Biostatistics, Seattle; Univ or Arkansas, Little Rock)

J Clin Oncol 22:1857-1863, 2004 5–2

Background.—Several trials have suggested the magnitude of the response to treatment does not directly correlate with the duration of survival in patients with multiple myeloma (MM). Members from the Southwest Oncology Group (SWOG) reviewed 4 SWOG trials to determine if the magnitude of the response to standard-dose first-line chemotherapy correlate with median survival in MM.

Methods.—The subjects were 1555 previously untreated patients with MM (61% male; median age, 62 years) enrolled in 4 SWOG phase III trials (S8229, S8624, S9028, and S9210) between 1982 and 1992. Complete remission (CR) was defined as 75% or more reduction in tumor mass and (if Bence-Jones protein was present) either a 90% or more reduction in M-protein levels or a reduction in urine M-protein levels to less than 0.2 g/d. Partial remission (PR) was defined as a 50% to 74% reduction in tumor mass and (if Bence-Jones protein was present) a 50% to 89% reduction in M-protein levels. Progressive disease in nonresponders was defined as a 25% or more increase in tumor size or other signs of disease progression. Progressive disease in responders was defined as a 100% or more increase in tumor mass, increases to greater than the levels defining response, increased lytic bone lesions, or evidence of new disease activity. Stable disease (SD) was defined as a less than 50% reduction or a less than 25% increase in tumor mass and no evidence of new disease. Event-free and overall survival were evaluated according to the magnitude of response at 6 and 12 months after beginning treatment.

Results.—The overall event-free survival was 18 months, and overall survival was 33 months. The median overall survival for patients who did not have disease progression at 6 or 12 months did not differ significantly according to type of response (CR, PR, no response), and was 32 to 34 months at the 6-month landmark and 30 to 35 months at the 12-month landmark. At 6 and 12 months, 85 and 218 patients, respectively, had disease progression. The median overall survival at the 6-month landmark was lower in patients with progressive disease, regardless of the magnitude of their response. The median overall survival was 14 months in nonresponders with disease progression and 4 to 5 months in those with an initial CR or PR whose disease progressed ($P < .0001$). Results were similar at 12 months; the median overall survival at the 12-month landmark was 19 months in nonresponders with disease progression, 11 months in patients with an initial CR whose disease progressed, and 17 months in patients with an initial PR whose disease progressed ($P < .0001$). In Cox proportional hazards regression models, with response and disease progression considered as time-dependent covariates, disease progression had a stronger impact on the duration of survival than the achievement of a response, regardless of the magnitude of response.

Conclusion.—The magnitude of response in patients with MM treated with standard chemotherapy does not predict the duration of overall survival. The strongest predictor of overall survival is the time to disease progression. Patients whose disease progresses within the first year have a poor prognosis, regardless of their initial response to treatment.

▶ Logical in terms of clinical perspective, this study is a large review of the phase III trials conducted by the Southwest Oncology Group (SWOG) myeloma program. More than 1500 patients with myeloma who entered clinical trials were reviewed with regard to the issue of whether the degree of response to primary therapy correlated with median survival. The authors concluded that the most significant parameter for assessment was that the patients actually responded. In fact, there was no difference between those patients with a more than 50% reduction in their paraprotein compared with those with a more than 75% reduction with regard to survival parameters. In contrast, the patients who had progressive disease tended to do the worst with the poorest survival outcome. Even those patients with stable disease tended to do better than the patients with progression. This study highlights the fact that all patients except those with progressive disease should be considered as a single unit with regard to subsequent therapy (eg, stem cell transplant) and that those patients with progressive disease, though a small percentage of the population, have a particularly bad prognosis.

M. S. Gordon, MD

Single Versus Double Autologous Stem-Cell Transplantation for Multiple Myeloma

Attal M, for the InterGroupe Francophone du Myélome (Hôpital Purpan, Toulouse, France; et al)

N Engl J Med 349:2495-2502, 2003 5–3

Introduction.—Stem cell transplantation is recommended in young patients with multiple myeloma as part of initial therapy or at disease progression. The median duration of response after stem cell transplantation does not exceed 3 years, and nearly all patients ultimately relapse. Double-

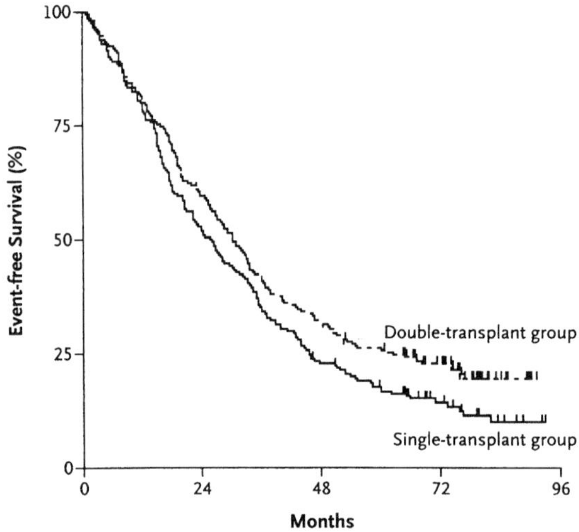

Probability of Event-free Survival (95% CI)			
Single-transplant group	23 (17–29)	14 (10–20)	9 (5–15)
Double-transplant group	32 (26–38)	23 (17–28)	20 (14–26)

FIGURE 1.—Kaplan-Meier estimates of event-free survival. Probabilities of event-free survival are shown with their 95% confidence intervals (*CIs*) below for 3 time points. *Tick marks* indicate patients at risk. (Reprinted by permission of *The New England Journal of Medicine* from Attal M, for the InterGroupe Francophone du Myélome: Single versus double autologous stem-cell transplantation for multiple myeloma. *N Engl J Med* 349:2495-2502, 2003.)

intensive therapy, in which 2 successive autologous stem cell transplantations are performed, has been used to prolong the duration of response in high-risk patients. A direct comparison of double and single transplantation was performed in a randomized trial of patients with multiple myeloma who underwent high-dose chemotherapy, followed by either 1 or 2 successive autologous stem cell transplantations.

Findings.—A total of 399 previously untreated patients younger than 60 years were randomly assigned to treatment with either a single or a double transplant. A complete or very good partial response was observed in 42% of patients in the single-transplant group and 50% of those in the double-transplant group ($P = .01$). The probability of surviving without events for 7 years after diagnosis was 10% and 20%, respectively, in the single- and double-transplant group ($P = .03$) (Fig 1). The estimated overall 7-year survival rate was 21% and 42%, respectively, in the single- and double-transplant group ($P = .01$) (Fig 2). Among those who did not have a very good partial response within 3 months of 1 transplantation, the probability of surviving 7 years was 11% and 43% in the single- and double-transplant group, respectively ($P < .001$) (Fig 3). Four factors were significantly associated with survival: baseline serum levels of β_2-microglobulin ($P < .01$) and lactate dehydrogenase ($P < .01$), age ($P < .05$), and treatment group ($P < .01$).

Conclusion.—Compared with single autologous stem cell transplantation after high-dose chemotherapy, double transplantation improves overall survival among patients with myeloma, particularly those who do not have a

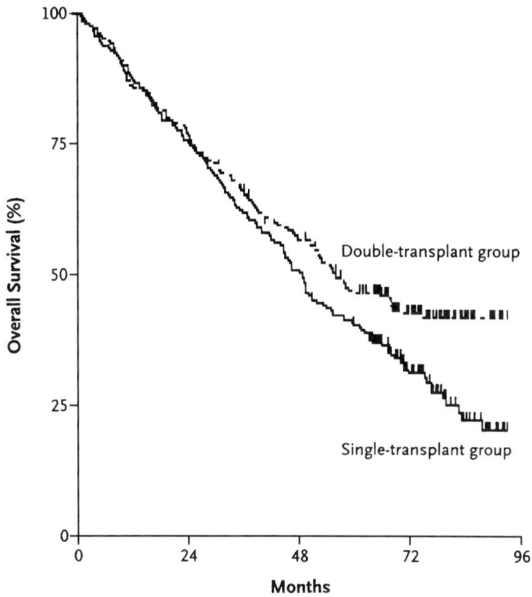

Probability of Overall Survival (95% CI)			
Single-transplant group	50 (43–57)	31 (24–38)	20 (13–29)
Double-transplant group	57 (49–64)	42 (35–50)	42 (34–49)

FIGURE 2.—Kaplan-Meier estimates of overall survival. Probabilities of overall survival are shown with their 95% confidence intervals (*CIs*) below for 3 time points. *Tick marks* indicate patients at risk. (Reprinted by permission of *The New England Journal of Medicine* from Attal M, for the InterGroupe Francophone du Myélome: Single versus double autologous stem-cell transplantation for multiple myeloma. *N Engl J Med* 349:2495-2502, 2003. Copyright 2003, Massachusetts Medical Society. All rights reserved.)

very good partial response after undergoing a single autologous stem cell transplantation.

► In patients younger than 65 years, 2 previously published randomized trials have demonstrated event-free and overall survival advantage when a single course of high-dose chemotherapy with stem cell transplantation is utilized.[1,2] This trial by Attal et al shows that 2 cycles of high-dose chemotherapy with tandem transplants appear to further improve the outcome of therapy with respect to event-free and overall survival. This study was initiated 10 years ago with a long follow-up. It should be noted that the broadest difference in the survival curves seemed to occur at or around 4 years. The best results seemed to occur in those patients who did not have a "very good partial response" after the first transplantation. In more recent years, drugs such as thalidomide and bortezomib have shown activity against myeloma. Ultimately, the incorporation of these agents and the optimal use of transplants will need to be defined. In the interim, it is quite encouraging to see progress in this disease.

P. J. Loehrer, Sr, MD

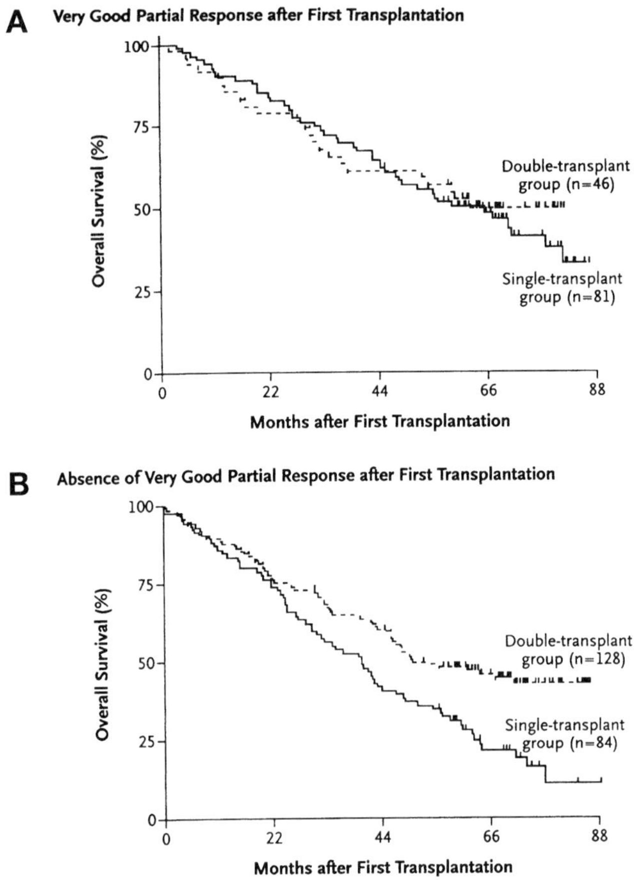

FIGURE 3.—Overall survival according to whether patients had at least a very good partial response after 1 transplantation (**A**) or had no such response (**B**). *Tick marks* indicate patients at risk. (Reprinted by permission of *The New England Journal of Medicine* from Attal M, for the InterGroupe Francophone du Myélome: Single versus double autologous stem-cell transplantation for multiple myeloma. *N Engl J Med* 349:2495-2502, 2003. Copyright 2003, Massachusetts Medical Society. All rights reserved.)

References

1. Attal M, et al for the InterGroupe Francophone du Myélome: A prospective, randomized trial of autologous bone marrow transplantation and chemotherapy in multiple myeloma. *N Engl J Med* 335:91-97, 1996.
2. Child JA, Morgan GJ, Davies FE, et al: High-dose chemotherapy with hematopoietic stem-cell rescue for multiple myeloma. *N Engl J Med* 348:1875-1883, 2003.

► Standard therapy for patients with multiple myeloma typically includes a form of induction therapy, such as the vincristine-doxorubicin-dexamethasone regimen followed by autologous stem cell transplantation (ASCT). The use of ASCT to consolidate induction responses has been shown to prolong survival in patients with myeloma. In this study, the investigators assessed the value of a second tandem transplant in myeloma patients as part of the initial treatment for their myeloma. Patients with newly diagnosed multiple myeloma were randomly assigned to receive either 1 or 2 ASCTs after 3 to 4 cycles of standard vincristine-doxorubicin-dexamethasone induction therapy. Patients in the single-transplant arm were conditioned with high-dose melphalan and total body irradiation (TBI), while the tandem transplant group received high-dose melphalan alone in transplant 1 and the combination of high dose melphalan and TBI in transplant 2. Compliance with the proscribed therapy was good, with 85% of the single-transplant patients undergoing their ASCT and 88% and 78% of the double-transplant patients undergoing 1 and 2 transplants, respectively. Overall, 48% of the single-transplant patients achieved a complete or very good partial response (>90% decrease in the serum paraprotein), whereas only 26% of the double-transplant patients achieved this mark after 1 transplant. The likely difference is accounted for by the absence of the TBI in the first transplant of the double group. In contrast, after the second transplant, the tandem group achieved a complete or very good partial response in 63% of the cases compared with 49% for the single-transplant group for a statistically significant difference ($P < .01$). Compared with the single-transplant group, double transplant improved event-free, relapse-free, and overall survival rates in a statistically significant manner. This study indicates that double transplantation is a superior approach to treatment of multiple myeloma without a significant increase in toxicity (4% and 6% treatment-related mortality rate in the single- and double-transplant groups, respectively) and should be considered for patients who are believed to be able to tolerate this approach.

M. S. Gordon, MD

Durable Responses to Thalidomide-Based Drug Therapy for Myelofibrosis With Myeloid Metaplasia

Mesa RA, Elliott MA, Schroeder G, et al (Mayo Clin, Rochester, Minn)

Mayo Clin Proc 79:883-889, 2004 5–4

Background.—Even with drug therapy, the median overall survival in patients with myelofibrosis with myeloid metaplasia (MMM) is only 5 years. Thalidomide is a cytokine inhibitor that has been effective in a spectrum of hematologic malignancies. The efficacy and safety of thalidomide, with or without prednisone, in the treatment of MMM were investigated in 2 phase II trials.

Methods.—The subjects were 36 patients with symptomatic MMM (67% male; median age, 65 years). The 15 patients in the first trial received oral thalidomide, starting at 2000 mg/d and escalating up to 1000 mg/d if tolerated. The 21 patients in the second trial received a combination of oral thalidomide (50 mg/d) and a tapering dose of prednisone (0.5 mg/kg initially, to 0.125 mg/kg during the third month). Single-agent low-dose thalidomide was continued an additional 3 months in responders. Anemia, thrombocytopenia, splenomegaly, bone marrow microvessel density, and hematopoiesis were assessed at baseline and after treatment.

Results.—Twenty (56%) of the 36 patients had a response to anemia, thrombocytopenia, or splenomegaly. All 20 of these patients responded during the first 3 months after beginning treatment. Specifically, anemia improved in 15 (42%) of 36 patients, thrombocytopenia improved in 10 (77%) of 13 patients, and splenomegaly improved in 5 (17%) of 30 patients. Combined low-dose thalidomide and prednisone was more effective than thalidomide monotherapy (overall initial response rates of 62% and 47%, respectively). During a median follow-up of 25 months, 10 patients (28%) had an ongoing response, including 8 patients who had stopped treatment 16 to 31 months earlier. A durable response, however, was seen only for anemia and thrombocytopenia, not splenomegaly. Neither bone marrow fibrosis, angiogenesis, osteosclerosis, cytogenetics, nor circulating myeloid progenitor (CD34) cell counts at baseline affected the response to treatment. Toxicity was lower with combined low-dose thalidomide and prednisone; none of these patients discontinued therapy because of adverse events compared with 53% of patients receiving thalidomide monotherapy. Unusual drug-related adverse events included marked leukocytosis in 8 patients, thrombocytosis in 6 patients, marked increase in blood CD34 count in 5 patients, and deep venous thrombosis in 1 patient. All these effects were reversible.

Conclusion.—Thalidomide, alone or in combination with prednisone, provides long-lasting improvements in anemia and thrombocytopenia in patients with MMM. The combination was more effective and better tolerated than thalidomide monotherapy. More than one fourth of patients who initially responded maintained a durable response well after therapy had been discontinued.

► The immunomodulatory agent thalidomide is being used in a variety of diseases. One recent area of investigation has been in patients with MMM. Because this disease is characterized by varying degrees of cytopenias as well as splenomegaly, in many individuals the specific criteria for assessing response is complex. This report summarizes the results of 2 separate phase II trials for thalidomide alone and thalidomide plus prednisone. Overall, patients with cytopenias, including anemia and thrombocytopenia, responded with improvements in 42% and 77%, respectively. Responses in splenomegaly were seen in 5 of 30 patients. The therapy was generally well tolerated, though the combination of thalidomide and prednisone was better tolerated than thalidomide alone. With a median follow-up of 25 months, ongoing responses were seen in 28% of the patients primarily consisting of those with anemia and thrombocytopenia. None of the classic features of myelofibrosis predicted for response to therapy. In a disease with limited options, the use of thalidomide and prednisone represents a reasonable option for patients with myelofibrosis.

M. S. Gordon, MD

Frequency of Major Molecular Responses to Imatinib or Interferon Alfa Plus Cytarabine in Newly Diagnosed Chronic Myeloid Leukemia

Hughes TP, for the International Randomised Study of Interferon Versus STI571 (IRIS) Study Group (Inst of Med and Veterinary Science, Adelaide, Australia; et al)

N Engl J Med 349:1423-1432, 2003 5–5

Background.—Chronic myeloid leukemia (CML) is a clonal disease of the hematopoietic stem cell in which a reciprocal translocation between chromosomes 9 and 22 forms the Philadelphia chromosome (Ph) with a novel fusion gene, BCR-ABL. An activated tyrosine kinase expressed by the BCR-ABL gene is central to the pathogenesis of CML. Imatinib mesylate is a tyrosine kinase inhibitor that blocks the kinase activity of BCR-ABL, which inhibits the proliferation of Ph-positive progenitors. Imatinib has demonstrated activity against all phases of CML, yet responses have been most durable and substantial in patients in the chronic phase of disease. In a previous study, 1106 patients in the chronic phase of CML were assigned to imatinib or interferon alfa plus cytarabine as initial therapy. Levels of BCR-ABL transcripts were measured in all patients in this trial who had a complete cytogenetic remission.

Methods.—Levels of BCR-ABL transcripts were measured by a quantitative real-time polymerase chain reaction (RT-PCR) assay. The results were expressed in relation to the median level of BCR-ABL transcripts in the blood of 30 patients with untreated CML in the chronic phase.

Results.—In the patients who experienced a complete cytogenic remission, levels of BCR-ABL transcripts had dropped after 12 months of treatment by at least 3 log in 57% of those in the imatinib group and in 24% of patients in the group that received interferon alfa plus cytarabine. An estimated 39% of all patients treated with imatinib but only 2% of all patients given interferon alfa plus cytarabine had a reduction in BCR-ABL transcript levels of at least 3 log. For patients who had a complete cytogenetic remission and a reduction in transcript levels of at least 3 log at 12 months, the probability of remaining progression-free was 100% at 24 months, compared with 95% for patients with a reduction of less than 3 log and 85% for patients who were not in complete cytogenetic remission at 12 months.

Conclusions.—The proportion of patients with chronic myeloid leukemia who had a reduction in BCR-ABL transcript level of at least 3 log after 12 months of therapy was much greater among those treated with imatinib than among those who received interferon alfa plus cytarabine. Patients in the imatinib group who attained this level of molecular response had a negligible risk of disease progression during the subsequent 12 months.

▶ The use of targeted therapy designed to inhibit the tyrosine kinase activity of the *BCR-ABL* gene mutation has been proven to improve overall survival compared with more standard interferon-alpha–containing regimens in a randomized trial. While cytogenetic responses can be assessed by standard techniques, the use of more sensitive technologies such as RT-PCR has the ability to identify 1:100,000 residual cells molecularly. As an extension of the randomized trial, the investigators in this study performed molecular RT-PCR studies on all patients with a complete cytogenetic response (CCR) to determine the true rate of clearance of the malignant clone. Overall, 57% of the imatinib patients who achieved a CCR achieved the gold standard of a 3-log decrease in transcript expression compared with only 24% of the interferon-treated patients. Given the relative infrequency of CCR in interferon-treated patients (this translated into 68% in the imatinib group compared with 7% in the interferon-treated group), only 2% of the interferon-treated patients achieved this important benchmark at the 12-month time point compared with 39% of the imatinib patients. Because molecular CCR appears to be associated with a failure-free rate of between 95% and 100% at 2 years, this is a potentially critical end point to achieve. It is not yet clear how imatinib-treated patients who do not achieve this end point should be treated, though clearly those patients achieving this end point should not be considered for other alternative therapies until their cytogenetic response relapses.

M. S. Gordon, MD

Proteomic Patterns of Tumour Subsets in Non–Small-Cell Lung Cancer

Yanagisawa K, Shyr Y, Xu BJ, et al (Vanderbilt Univ, Nashville, Tenn)

Lancet 362:433-439, 2003 5–6

Background.—Prognosis is difficult in patients with non–small cell lung cancer (NSCLC). Whether matrix-assisted laser desorption/ionization time-of-flight mass spectroscopy (MALDI-TOF MS) comprehensive analysis of protein expression patterns in lung tissue could be used to classify lung tumors was investigated.

Study Design.—MALDI-TOF MS peaks were aligned across samples by a custom genetic algorithm parallel search strategy. Important proteins that were differentially expressed were selected. The weighted flexible compound covariate method (WFCCM) was used for the class prediction model to verify that these proteomic proteins could be used to classify tissue samples into normal versus tumor tissue. A prediction model was generated from 50 tissue samples and was then applied to 43 validation samples in a blinded cohort.

Findings.—MALDI-TOF MS revealed more than 1600 protein peaks from small pieces of frozen lung sections. Differential expression enabled lung cancers to be classified by histologic analysis, to distinguish primary tumors from metastases, and to classify nodal involvement with 85% accuracy in the prediction model samples. Samples were well classified when these same criteria were applied to the blinded validation cohort. A set of 15 protein peaks distinguished between patients with NSCLC with poor prognosis and those with good prognosis.

Conclusions.—Protein profiles obtained from nanogram amounts of tissue can be used to accurately classify lung cancers, determine prognosis, and predict risk of nodal involvement. This technology may have important clinical implications for the management of patients with NSCLC and, potentially, other cancers.

▶ NSCLC is a very heterogeneous disease, comprising several histopathologic subtypes. Within these varying subtypes, significant clinical variation exists. Some tumors behave in an indolent fashion, and others are more aggressive. Some spread to certain organs, and others spare these sites. Some respond to standard chemotherapy, and others are entirely resistant. Proteomic-based approaches are being evaluated to help better understand the biological behavior of many cancers, including NSCLC. This study from Vanderbilt reports on MALDI-TOF MS to assess protein expression profiles in surgically resected lung cancer. The investigators were able to distinguish primary tumors from metastases, classify histologies, and predict those who had a good versus poor long-term outcome. This technology may form the basis on which future trial design is carried out and has the potential to aid physicians in individualizing patient care.

N. H Hanna, MD

Activating Mutations in the Epidermal Growth Factor Receptor Underlying Responsiveness of Non–Small-Cell Lung Cancer to Gefitinib

Lynch TJ, Bell DW, Sordella R, et al (Harvard Med School, Boston; Harvard School of Public Health, Boston)

N Engl J Med 350:2129-2139, 2004 5–7

Introduction.—Most patients with non–small cell lung cancer (NSCLC) do not respond to the tyrosine kinase inhibitor gefitinib, which targets the epidermal growth factor receptor (EGFR). About 10% of patients experience a rapid and frequently dramatic clinical response. The molecular mechanisms underlying the sensitivity to gefitinib in patients with NSCLC are not understood. Tumors from patients with NSCLC who had dramatic responses to treatment with gefitinib were examined to ascertain the underlying mechanisms.

Methods.—A search was performed for the *EGFR* gene in primary tumors from patients with NSCLC who had a response to gefitinib, those with no response, and those who had not been exposed to gefitinib. The functional consequences of identified mutations were assessed after the mutant proteins were expressed in cultured cells.

Results.—Heterozygous mutations were detected in the tyrosine kinase domain of the *EGFR* gene in 8 of 9 patients with gefitinib-responsive lung cancer, compared with none of the 7 with no response ($P < .001$). Mutations were either small, in-frame deletions or amino acid substitutions that were clustered around the adenosine triphosphate–binding pocket of the tyrosine kinase domain. Similar mutations were identified in tumors from 2 of 25 (8%) patients with primary NSCLC who were not exposed to gefitinib.

All mutations were heterozygous. Identical mutations were seen in multiple patients, indicating an additive specific gain or function. In vitro, *EGFR* mutations revealed enhanced tyrosine kinase activity in response to epidermal growth factor and increased sensitivity to inhibition by gefitinib.

Conclusion.—A subgroup of patients with NSCLC have specific mutations in the *EGFR* gene, which correlate with clinical responsiveness to gefitinib. These mutations produce increased growth factor signaling and bestow susceptibility to the inhibitor. Screening for these mutations in lung cancers may identify patients who will respond to gefitinib.

EGFR Mutations in Lung Cancer: Correlation With Clinical Response to Gefitinib Therapy

Paez JG, Jänne PA, Lee JC, et al (Dana-Farber Cancer Inst, Boston; Harvard Med School, Boston; Massachusetts Inst of Technology, Cambridge; et al)
Science 304:1497-1500, 2004 5–8

Background.—Chemotherapy is only marginally effective for the treatment of non–small cell lung carcinoma (NSCLC). Gefitinib, an epidermal growth factor receptor (EGFR) tyrosine kinase inhibitor, was recently approved for NSCLC treatment in the United States and Japan. Whether mutation of receptor tyrosine kinases plays a causal role in NSCLC was determined.

Methods.—Somatic genetic changes were sought in 119 primary NSCLC tumors. The tumors included 58 samples from a center in Japan and 61 from a US center. Seventy samples were lung adenocarcinomas, and 49 were other NSCLCs. None of the patients had been treated with gefitinib. Receptor tyrosine kinase genes were sequenced in the tumors and in matched normal tissue.

Findings.—Somatic mutations of the *EGFR* gene were identified in 15 tumors from the Japanese center and in 1 tumor from the US center. Such mutations were also found in other lung cancer samples from US patients who had responded to gefitinib, as well as in a lung adenocarcinoma cell line hypersensitive to growth inhibition by gefitinib. However, *EGFR* mutations were not found in gefitinib-insensitive tumors or cell lines.

Conclusions.—Mutations in *EGFR* may predict sensitivity to gefitinib. The striking differences in Japanese and US patients' frequency of *EGFR* mutations and responses to gefitinib raise questions about variations in the molecular pathogenesis of cancer in different ethnic groups, cultures, and geographic areas.

▶ These 2 important articles (Abstracts 5–7 and 5–8) report consistent results, identifying a specific mutation of the EGFR, which predicts responsiveness to gefitinib. The mutation appears to be located in the tyrosine kinase domain of the *EGFR* gene, precisely the targeted site of gefitinib. The mutations were small in-frame deletions or amino acid substitutions, and appear to confer an enhanced tyrosine kinase activity in response to the epdiermal growth factor and, therefore, increased sensitivity to inhibition by gefitinib. It has been observed that subsets of patients appear to benefit more with gefitinib, based on clinical and pathologic variables. More specifically, female patients, Japanese ancestry, adenocarcinoma histology (particularly with bronchioloalveolar features), and never-smoking status predict a higher likelihood of response to gefitinib. Interestingly, this clinical observation may be validated with the findings by Lynch (Abstract 5–7) and Paez (Abstract 5–8), in that these subsets of patients appear to have a higher incidence of the somatic mutation in the *EGFR* gene. This information on the molecular basis for response to gefitinib has important scientific and clinical implications; however, several questions remain unanswered. First, in the Lynch series, one responding patient in his cohort did not have the presence of the mutation, which begs the question: is there an alternative mechanism of action or alternate mutation that has not yet been identified? Second, is the gene mutation present or absent in the population of patients with stable disease radiographically but with symptom improvement? Third, should patients with early stage disease undergoing surgery be treated with gefitinib in the adjuvant setting, and is there a role for gefitinib in the treatment of patients with locally advanced disease treated with chemoradiation?

N. H. Hanna, MD

Expression of Hepatoma-Derived Growth Factor Is a Strong Prognostic Predictor for Patients With Early-Stage Non–Small-Cell Lung Cancer

Ren H, Tang X, Lee JJ, et al (Univ of Texas, Houston; Johns Hopkins Univ, Baltimore, Md)

J Clin Oncol 22:3230-3237, 2004 5–9

Background.—Lung cancer prognosis is correlated with disease stage at diagnosis. Among patients with stage I non–small cell lung cancer (NSCLC), 40% will die within 5 years after potentially curative surgery. Adjuvant chemotherapy may be useful for those patients with disease progression, but it is also associated with serious side effects. Therefore, identification of prognostic factors would be extremely beneficial. Hepatoma-derived growth factor (HDGF) is overexpressed in NSCLC. HDGF expression was investigated in NSCLC tumor specimens to determine whether any association exists with the biological behavior of NSCLC.

Study Design.—The study included 98 patients with stage I NSCLC who had complete resection of primary tumor at M. D. Anderson Cancer Center from 1975 to 1990, did not have adjuvant therapy, had at least 5 years of follow-up data, and had tissue sections available. The median follow-up was 10.1 years among the 27 patients who were still alive. The presence of HDGF was determined by immunohistochemical analysis. The HDGF labeling index was defined as the weighted mean of percentage of tumor cells with nuclear immunoreactivity multiplied by the degree of staining intensity. The prognostic effect of HDGF expression levels in tumors was analyzed.

Findings.—Virtually all NSCLC tumors expressed HDGF. Patients whose tumors had higher HDGF indexes had significantly worse 5-year overall survival, disease-specific, and disease-free survival probabilities than those of patients with lower HDGF indexes. Multivariate analysis confirmed that

HDGF levels were an independent predictor of overall, disease-specific, and disease-free survival probabilities for patients with NSCLC.

Conclusions.—These findings indicate that high levels of HDGF expression are correlated with poor prognosis in patients with NSCLC. This suggests that HDGF is a potentially useful marker for disease-management planning and may be useful in the search for novel molecular therapies.

Upregulation of the Tissue Inhibitor of Metalloproteinase-1 Protein Is Associated With Progression of Human Non–Small-Cell Lung Cancer

Aljada IS, Ramnath N, Donohue K, et al (State Univ of New York, Buffalo; Univ of Pennsylvania, Philadelphia; H Lee Moffitt Cancer Ctr, Tampa, Fla; et al)

J Clin Oncol 22:3218-3229, 2004 5–10

Background.—The 5-year survival rate for patients with non–small cell lung cancer (NSCLC) remains poor. Reliable prognostic factors are needed to optimize treatment. Tissue inhibitors of metalloproteinases (TIMP) appear to have paradoxical effects on tumor progression. The expression of TIMP-1 and its association with the prognosis for patients with NSCLC were assessed retrospectively.

Study Design.—The study data included 160 patients diagnosed at Roswell Park Cancer Center between March 1995 and September 1999 with primary NSCLC, stage IA to IIIA, who had been treated with surgery and for whom complete clinicopathologic data were available. Patients were observed through March 2002. Lung cancer was the cause of death in 88% of these patients. Surgical specimens were analyzed by immunohistochemistry for TIMP-1, metalloproteinases (MMP-2, MMP-9) and Bcl-2.

Findings.—Increased expression of TIMP-1 was detected in 27% of these NSCLC tumors. Overexpression of TIMP-1 in NSCLC was associated with poor overall survival compared with that of those patients whose tumors did not overexpress TIMP-1. Disease stage, patient age, and performance status were also all significantly related to patient survival probability. Multivariate analysis demonstrated that patients who overexpressed TIMP-1 had a 90% increased risk of death compared to the risk of those with low tumor expression of TIMP-1. TIMP-1 expression was not correlated with metalloproteinase expression.

Conclusions.—TIMP-1 appears to be overexpressed in a subgroup of NSCLC patients. This overexpression is associated with poor clinical outcome, suggesting that TIMP-1 overexpression may serve as a prognostic marker for primary NSCLC and may be useful for clinical decision making. TIMP-1 may also be useful as a novel therapeutic target.

▶ The majority of patients with stage I NSCLC who undergo a complete surgical resection will be cured of their disease. Despite this success, 10% to 45% of patients will still die within 5 years. While surgery alone remains the standard of care for patients with stage Ia disease, adjuvant chemotherapy has recently proven to improve survival in patients with stage Ib disease. Discovering predictive markers for relapse is exceedingly important. Patients with a "low risk" of relapse may be spared the risk and side effects of adjuvant therapy. Hepatoma-derived growth factor (HDGF) is overexpressed in NSCLC cell lines, but its importance in the pathogenesis and biological behavior of NSCLC is undefined (Abstract 5–9). Aljada et al (Abstract 5–10) report worse outcome for patients whose tumors had higher HDGF indices. Similarly, the upregulation of tissue inhibitors of metalloproteinase-1 protein appears to increase the risk of death in surgically resected patients. Further study of these markers is warranted, and future randomized trials may need to stratify for these markers, if validated in future studies.

N. H. Hanna, MD

The Role of Radiotherapy in Treatment of Stage I Non–Small Cell Lung Cancer

Qiao X, Tullgren O, Lax I, et al (Karolinska Hosp, Stockholm)

Lung Cancer 41:1-11, 2003 5–11

Background.—The role of radiotherapy (RT) as a curative modality in patients with stage I non–small cell lung cancer (NSCLC) has not been established definitively. A literature search was conducted to better define the role of RT in this setting.

Methods and Findings.—The review included 18 studies of RT alone in the treatment of stage I NSCLC published between 1988 and 2000 (Table 1). Most patients were treated with RT because they were medically inoperable. The primary contraindications for surgery were grave pulmonary function impairment and serious cardiovascular disease. The most common reason for treatment failure was local recurrence. However, this varied greatly among studies, ranging from 6.4% to 70%. Regional node failure alone was reported in only 0 to 3.2% of the cases. In general, smaller tumor size, low T stage, and increased dose had a favorable impact on local control. Better local control generally led to increased survival. In most of the studies reviewed, no serious treatment complications occurred. However, the overall treatment outcomes were disappointing, with median survival ranging from 18 to 33 months. The mean overall survival rate was 34% at 3 years and 21% at 5 years (Fig 1 and Table 2). Cause-specific survival was 39% at 3 years and 25% at 5 years (Figs 2 and 4).

Conclusions.—In these studies, the use of RT alone in patients with stage I NSCLC yielded disappointing outcomes. To improve local control and survival, dose escalation, with conformal RT using field or stereotactic RT, should be the focus of developmental treatment strategies in patients with inoperable stage I NSCLC.

▶ This article from the Karolinska Hospital in Stockholm reviews the literature on definitive radiation therapy alone for stage I NSCLC in 18 articles published between 1988 and 2000. As might be expected, the reason that most of the patients received definitive radiation therapy reflected their medical inopera-

TABLE 1.

Author (Year)	Age (Years)		Number of Patients		Medically Inoperable Patients (%)
	Mean/Median	Range	Stage 1	All	
(A) Patients characteristics					
Slotman et al., 1996 [9]	75/–	54-85	31	31	81
Zhang et al., 1989 [7]	57.1/–	37-70	35	44	72.7
Hayakawa et al., 1999 [8]	n.s.	n.s.	36	36	88.9
Haffty et al., 1988 [19]	64/–	51-83	43	43	86
Kupelian et al., 1996 [10]	n.s.	n.s.	45	71	100
Slotman et al., 1994 [17]	75	57-93	47	47	n.s.
Jeremic et al., 1997 [4]	–/63	51-70	49	49	59.2
Noordijk et al, 1988 [13]	74/–	n.s.	50	50	84
Kaskowitz et al., 1993 [16]	–/73	44-86	53	53	81.8
Talton et al., 1990 [11]	65/–	40-89	60	77	n.s.
Sandler et al., 1990 [18]	–/72	n.s.	77	77	78
Cheung et al., 2000 [6]	–/71.5	45-86	92	102	76.5
Graham et al., 1995 [22]	–/67	43-89	93	103	70
Dosoretz et al., 1992 [12]	–/74	51-88	106	152	88.8
Krol et al., 1996 [15]	74.2/–	58-88	108	108	88
Sibley et al., 1998 [20]	–/70	46-95	141	141	100
Morita et al., 1997 [14]	74.2/74.6	50-89	149	149	83
Gauden et al., 1995 [5]	–/70	34-90	347	347	64
Total			1562	1680	
	Total dose (Gy)	Fractions (F)	Acute BED (Gy)	D2	Prophylactic node irradiation yes/no

(Continued)

bility. This was usually because of a major compromise of pulmonary function or serious coexistent cardiovascular disease. The 3- and 5-year overall survival figures were 34% and 21%, respectively, which is not particularly shocking since the patients were treated with radiation because they were deemed not medically operable in the first place. There was a significant rate of local recur-

TABLE 1 (cont.)

Author (Year)	Age (Years) Mean/Median	Age (Years) Range	Number of Patients Stage 1	Number of Patients All	Medically Inoperable Patients (%)
(B) Compilation of publications on treatment of early stage NSCLC by RT alone					
Slotman et al., 1996 [9]	48	12 F	76.4		0/31
Zhang et al., 1989 [7]	55-70	2 Gy/F	62.8		44/0
Hayakawa et al., 1999 [8]	60-81	2 Gy/F	68.1	67.1	10/26
Haffty et al., 1988 [19]	54	6 weeks/split course	59	62.2	38/5
	59	6-7 weeks/continuous			
Kupelian et al., 1996 [10]	63.23		65	60	51/20
Slotman et al., 1994 [17]	32 Gy/6 F, 40 Gy/ 10 F 48 Gy/ 12 F, 56 Gy/20 F	28/19			
Jeremic et al., 1997 [4]	69.6	1.2 Gy bid	71	58.5	49/0
Noordijk et al., 1988 [13]	60	Split course, 3 Gy/F	63.4	72	0/50
Kaskowitz et al., 1993 [16]	63.2*	2 Gy/F	65.1	63	n.s.
Talton et al., 1990 [11]	60	30 F	62.8	60	77/0
Sandler et al., 1990 [18]	60*	2 Gy/F	62.8	60	69/8
Cheung et al., 2000 [6]	52.5	20 F	67.8	59	0/102
Graham et al., 1995 [22]	60	30F	62.8	60	82/21
Dosoretz et al., 1992 [12]	45-75	1.8-2 Gy/F	62.8	60	n.s.
Krol et al., 1996 [15]	60	7 weeks, 3 Gy bid 65/5.2 weeks, 2.5 qd	63.4/74.3	72	0/108
Sibley et al., 1998 [20]	64*	1.2 bid, 3 qd			103/38
Morita et al., 1997 [14]	64.7*	2 Gy/F	65.3	64.7	66/88
Gauden et al., 1995 [5]	50	20 F/4 weeks	62.5	55	347/0

*Median, D2 is the total dose given with 2 Gy per fraction, calculated with the BED formalism.

(Reprinted by permission of the publisher from Qiao X, Tullgren O, Lax I, et al: The role of radiotherapy in treatment of stage I non–small cell lung cancer. *Lung Cancer* 41:1-11, 2003. Copyright 2003 by Elsevier Science Inc.)

rence, although it was highly variable from one series to the next. The authors seem more optimistic about dose escalation than I am. They seem to assume that an improvement in local control will be translated into an improvement in survival. I believe that is wishful thinking and remains to be seen, since the

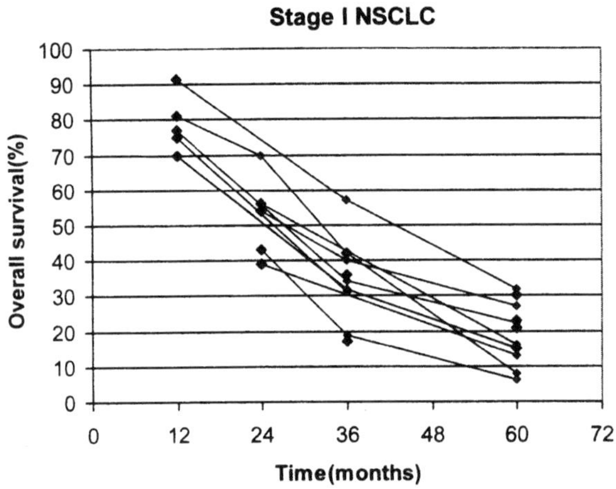

FIGURE 1.—Overall survival of stage I NSCLC (the estimated 3, 5-year overall survival rate is 34 ± 9 and 21 ± 8%, respectively). The data were extracted from the studies presented in Table 2. (Reprinted by permission of the publisher from Qiao X, Tullgren O, Lax I, et al: The role of radiotherapy in treatment of stage I non–small cell lung cancer. *Lung Cancer* 41:1-11, 2003. Copyright 2003 by Elsevier Science Inc.)

stage I category is a clinical stage and not a pathologic stage (as is true for most surgical series). Incidentally, there is no statement in this article that details what, if any, staging procedures were carried out in these patients.

In any event, this is a helpful review of the literature.

E. Glatstein, MD

TABLE 2.—Survival After RT for Stage I NSCLC

Authors	Median Survial (Month)	Overall Survival (%)				Cause-Specific Survival (%)				Disease-Free Survival (%)		
		1	2	3	5-Year	1	2	3	5-Year	2	3	5-Year
Zhang et al. [7]		91.4		57.1	31.4							
Krol et al. [15]		75		31	15	81		42	31			
Hayakawa et al. [8]				42	23			56	39			
Kaskowitz et al. [16]	20.9		43	19	6		54	33	13		33	
Slotman et al. [9]	33	81	72	42	8		93					
Jeremic et al. [4]	33				30							41
Sibley et al. [20]	18		39		13		60		32	48		28
Slotman et al. [17]	20	70		33	15	90		53	32			
Sandler et al. [18]	20			17				22				
Haffty et al. [19]	28			36	21							
Noordijk et al. [13]	27		56		16							
Morita et al. [14]	27.2	77.9		34.2	22.2							
Gauden et al. [5]	27.9		54	40	27					41	32	23

(Reprinted by permission of the publisher from Qiao X, Tullgren O, Lax I, et al: The role of radiotherapy in treatment of stage I non–small cell lung cancer. *Lung Cancer* 41:1-11, 2003. Copyright 2003 by Elsevier Science Inc.)

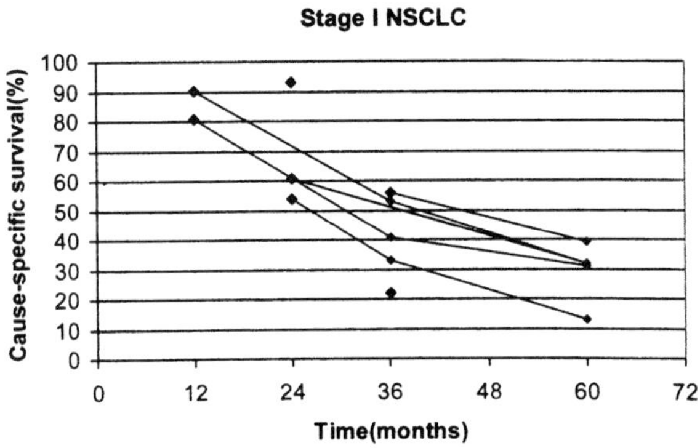

FIGURE 2.—Cause-specific survival of stage I NSCLC (the estimated 3, 5-year cause-specific survival is 39 ± 10 and 25 ± 9%, respectively). The data were extracted from the studies presented in Table 2. (Reprinted by permission of the publisher from Qiao X, Tullgren O, Lax I, et al: The role of radiotherapy in treatment of stage I non–small cell lung cancer. *Lung Cancer* 41:1-11, 2003. Copyright 2003 by Elsevier Science Inc.)

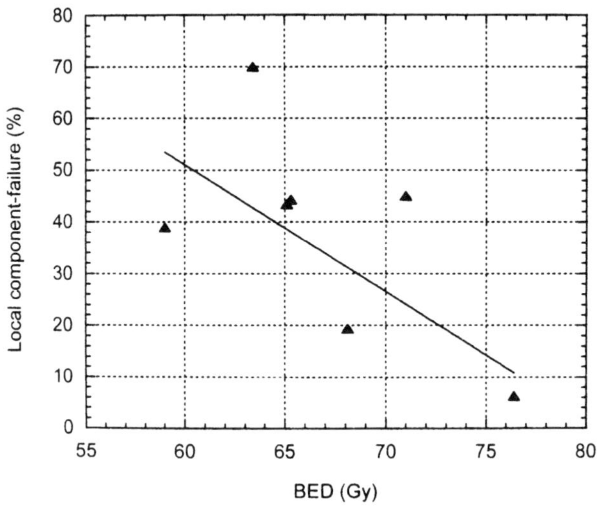

FIGURE 4.—Local-component failure (including local failure alone, local plus regional failure, and local plus distant failure) vs. biologically effective dose (*BED*). (Reprinted by permission of the publisher from Qiao X, Tullgren O, Lax I, et al: The role of radiotherapy in treatment of stage I non–small cell lung cancer. *Lung Cancer* 41:1-11, 2003. Copyright 2003 by Elsevier Science Inc.)

Unresectable Pulmonary Malignancies: CT-guided Percutaneous Radiofrequency Ablation—Preliminary Results

Suh RD, Wallace AB, Sheehan RE, et al (University of California, Los Angeles)
Radiology 229:821-829, 2003 5–12

Background.—Percutaneous radiofrequency (RF) ablation, an established technique for treating various cardiac and neurologic conditions, involves the use of heat to produce tissue necrosis. The current study investigated whether RF ablation of unresectable pulmonary malignancies is safe and technically feasible. The utility of CT nodule densitometry as a tool for following up tumors after ablation was also studied.

Methods.—Twelve patients (mean age, 60.6 years) with unresectable disease were included in the study. All underwent nodule CT densitometry and CT-guided percutaneous RF ablation of a total of 19 lung tumors. Thirty-two percent of the tumors were adenocarcinoma; 32%, sarcoma less than 50 cm^2 in area; 21%, colorectal carcinoma; 10%, bronchoalveolar carcinoma; and 5%, large cell carcinoma. None of the patients had symptoms before RF ablation. Follow-up CT densitometry was planned at 1, 3, 6, and 12 months after the initial procedure.

Findings.—All patients tolerated RF ablation well. Complications during the procedure included 12 pneumothoraces, 2 cases of pleural effusion, and 2 of moderate pain. In the 8 patients with 3 months of follow-up, lesion size remained stable in 6 and increased in 2. However, mean contrast enhancement in these patients declined from 46.8 HU at baseline to 9.6 HU in the 1

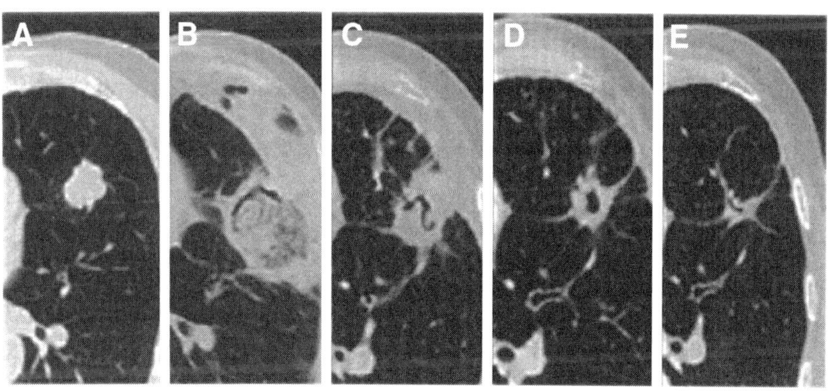

FIGURE 2.—Transverse contrast-enhanced thin-section CT scans obtained with the patient in prone position show lingual segment nodule before and at follow-up after RF ablation. (**A**) Baseline CT scan obtained before RF ablation shows 2.2 × 2.8 cm nodule with enhancement of 35.9 HU. (**B**) Follow-up 1-month CT scan depicts marked interval increase in nodule size, with early formation of thick-walled cavity and adjacent anterolateral complicated hydropneumothorax. Lesion enhancement increase from baseline was 0.0 HU. (**C**) Follow-up 3-month CT scan depicts interval regression of cavitary lesion, with enhancement increase from baseline of 4.0 HU and resolution of adjacent hydropneumothorax. (**D**) Follow-up 6-month CT scan shows further interval regression of cavitary lesion with enhancement increase from baseline of 26 HU. (**E**) Follow-up 12-month CT scan shows interval regression of lesion with scarring and enhancement increase from baseline of 15 HU. (Courtesy of Suh RD, Wallace AB, Sheehan RE, et al: Unresectable pulmonary malignancies: CT-guided percutaneous radiofrequency ablation—Preliminary results. *Radiology* 229:821-829, 2003. Radiological Society of North America.)

to 2 months after the procedure. The 1 patient with 12 months of follow up had lesion enhancement on CT densitometry less than 50% that at baseline (Fig 2). Lesion diameter remained stable in this patient.

Conclusions.—Percutaneous RF ablation appears to be safe and technically feasible in patients with unresectable pulmonary malignancies. These preliminary data also indicate that CT densitometry may have potential as a noninvasive technique for following up tumors after RF ablation.

▶ This group of investigators from UCLA reports on 12 patients with CT diagnosed malignant lesions in the lungs. These patients were thought to have unresectable disease because of either poor pulmonary function or multifocal lesions. What they show is that percutaneous radiofrequency ablation technology can be applied to pulmonary lesions, although there is a size limitation. Nonetheless, lesions of limited size appear to be amenable to this treatment in the lungs and in the liver. This treatment appears to be extremely well tolerated and for the appropriate peripheral lesion it is probably useful. Like many treatments, its usefulness depends to a major degree on how patients are selected for this kind of treatment. This is not going to be useful for all patients.

E. Glatstein, MD

Randomized Study of Adjuvant Chemotherapy for Completely Resected Stage I, II, or IIIA Non–Small-Cell Lung Cancer

Scagliotti GV, for the Adjuvant Lung Project Italy/European Organisation for Research and Treatment of Cancer–Lung Cancer Cooperative Group Investigators (Univ of Torino, Italy; et al)

J Natl Cancer Inst 95:1453-1461, 2003 5–13

Introduction.—Surgery is the main treatment option for patients with stage I, II, or IIIA non–small cell lung cancer (NSCLC). The long-term survival of patients with NSCLC treated with surgery only is greatly unsatisfactory. The role of adjuvant chemotherapy in patient survival has yet to be determined. The Adjuvant Lung Project Italy, a randomized trial to evaluate the mitomycin C, vindesine, and cisplatin (MVP) regimen, was conducted in patients with radically resected stages I, II, or IIIA NSCLC.

Methods.—Between January 1994 and January 1999, 1209 patients with stage I, II, or IIIA NSCLC were randomly assigned to treatment with mitomycin C (8 mg/m^2 on day 1), vindesine (3 mg/m^2 on days 1 and 8), and cisplatin (100 mg/m^2 on day 1) every 3 weeks for 3 cycles (MVP group; 606 patients) or no treatment (control group, 603 patients) after complete resection. Randomization was stratified by investigational center, tumor size, lymph-node involvement, and the intention to treat with radiotherapy. The major end point was overall survival. The secondary end points were progression-free survival and toxicity linked with adjuvant treatment.

Results.—At a median follow-up of 64.5 months, there were no statistically significant differences between the active treatment and control groups in overall survival (hazard ratio, 0.96; 95% confidence interval, 0.81-1.13; *P* = .589) or progression-free survival (hazard ratio, 0.89; 95% confidence interval, 0.76-1.03; *P* = .128). Only 69% of patients underwent all 3 planned cycles of MVP. Grades 3 and 4 neutropenia were observed in 16% and 12%, respectively, of patients in the MVP arm. Radiotherapy was completed by 65% and 82% of patients in the MVP and control groups, respectively. Multivariate analysis revealed that only disease stage and gender were associated with survival.

Conclusion.—These data do not prospectively verify a significant role for adjuvant chemotherapy in completely resected NSCLC.

Cisplatin-Based Adjuvant Chemotherapy in Patients With Completely Resected Non–Small-Cell Lung Cancer

Arriagada R, and The International Adjuvant Lung Cancer Trial Collaborative Group (Instituto de Radiomedicina, Santiago, Chile; et al)

N Engl J Med 350:351-360, 2004 5–14

Introduction.—Despite several randomized trials, adjuvant treatment in patients with completely resected non–small cell lung cancer (NSCLC) is not advantageous for patients who had prolonged adjuvant treatment with alkylating agents. Radiotherapy for patients with early stage disease has had deleterious effects on long-term survival. The International Adjuvant Lung Cancer Trial was performed to compare the effect on overall survival of adjuvant chemotherapy consisting of cisplatin plus a vinca alkaloid or etoposide with that of no adjuvant chemotherapy in patients with completely resected NSCLC.

Methods.—Patients were randomly assigned to either 3 or 4 cycles of cisplatin-based chemotherapy or to observation. Before randomization, every center determined the pathologic stages to include both its policy for chemotherapy (the dose of cisplatin and the drug to be combined with cisplatin) and its postoperative radiotherapy policy. The primary end point was overall survival.

Results.—Of 1867 patients who underwent randomization, 36.5% had pathologic stage I disease, 24.2% had stage II, and 39.3% had stage III. The drug allocated with cisplatin was etoposide in 56.5% of patients, vinorelbine in 26.8%, vinblastine in 11.0%, and vindesine in 5.8%. Of 932 patients assigned to chemotherapy, 73.8% received at least 240 mg cisplatin/meter^2 of body-surface area. The median follow-up was 56 months.

Patients assigned to chemotherapy had a significantly higher rate of survival than those in the observation group (44.5% vs 40.4% at 5 years [469 vs 504 deaths; hazard ratio for death, 0.86; 95% confidence interval, 0.76-0.98; *P* < .03). Patients in the chemotherapy group also had a significantly higher disease-free survival rate than those in the observation group (39.4% vs 34.3% at 5 years [518 vs 577 events]; hazard ratio, 0.83; 95% confidence interval, 0.74-0.94; *P* < .003) (Fig 1). There were no significant interactions

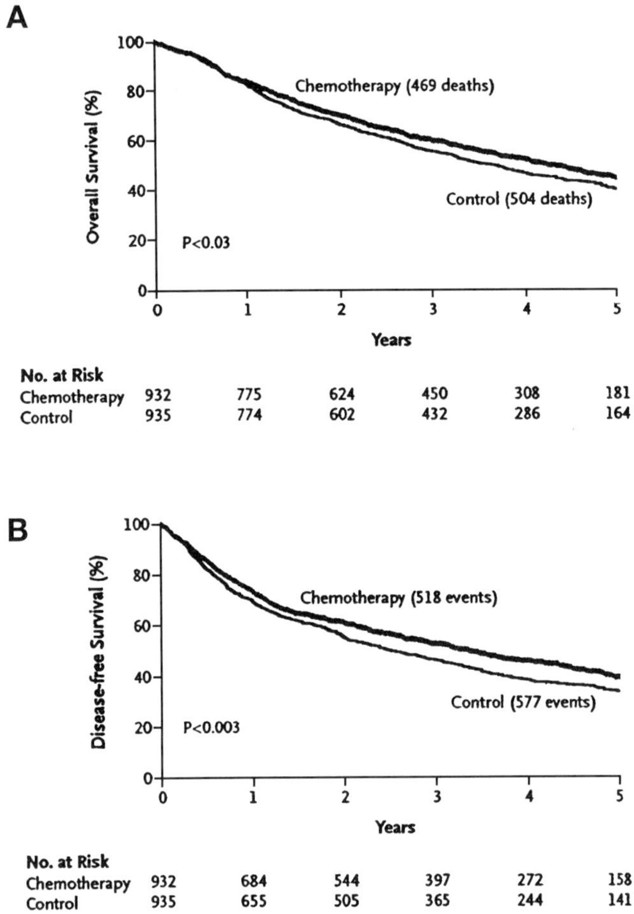

FIGURE 1.—Overall survival (A) and disease-free survival (B). The hazard ratio for death in the chemotherapy group as compared with the control group was 0.86 (95% confidence interval, 0.76-0.98), and the hazard ratio for disease progression or death was 0.83 (95% confidence interval, 0.74-0.94). (Reprinted by permission of *The New England Journal of Medicine* from Arriagada R, and The International Adjuvant Lung Cancer Trial Collaborative Group: Cisplatin-based adjuvant chemotherapy in patients with completely resected non–small-cell lung cancer. *N Engl J Med* 350:351-360, 2004. Copyright 2004, Massachusetts Medical Society. All rights reserved.)

with prespecified components. Chemotherapy-induced toxic effects caused 7 deaths (0.8%).

Conclusion.—Cisplatin-based adjuvant chemotherapy improves survival in patients who have undergone complete resection for NSCLC.

▶ Adjuvant cisplatin-based chemotherapy was reported to offer a small survival advantage, which did not reach statistical significance, over no chemotherapy in a meta-analysis published in 1995.[1] These 2 large phase III trials evaluating the role of adjuvant chemotherapy after surgical resection for patients with stage I, II, and III NSCLC provide contradicting results.

The trial reported from the Adjuvant Lung Project of Italy (ALPI) by Scagliotti et al (Abstract 5–13) used a uniform regimen of MPV every 3 weeks for 3 cycles, while the International Adjuvant Lung Trial (IALT) (Abstract 5–14) allowed physicians to choose between various cisplatin-based chemotherapy regimens. What might account for the different results on these 2 large trials? In both trials, adjuvant radiation therapy was allowed (given sequentially to chemotherapy for those patients randomized on the chemotherapy arm). The results of the postoperative radiation therapy (PORT) meta-analysis indicated that radiation therapy may have a detrimental effect on survival for those patients with stage I or II disease.[2] However, given the equal distribution of patients receiving PORT on both arms of both trials, it is unlikely that this would account for the difference.

Perhaps the use of mitomycin in the postoperative setting results in more toxicity and therefore a decrement in survival. In addition, the IALT trial was designed to detect a smaller difference in survival compared with the ALPI trial, and therefore enrolled more patients. Indeed, the tail of the survival curve on the ALPI trial appears to be separating, suggesting that with more patients and longer follow-up, chemotherapy may have demonstrated a small advantage. The role of adjuvant chemotherapy will remain the subject of some debate until more clinical trials evaluating adjuvant therapy are fully reported.

N. H. Hanna, MD

References

1. Non-small cell lung cancer collaborative group: Chemotherapy in non-small cell lung cancer: A meta-analysis using updated data on individual patients from 52 randomised clinical trials. *BMJ* 311:899-909, 1995.
2. PORT Meta-analysis Trialist Group: Postoperative radiotherapy in non-small cell lung cancer: Systematic review and meta-analysis of individual patient data from nine randomised controlled trials. *Lancet* 352:257-263, 1998.

6 Lymphoproliferative and Lymphoma

Involved-Field Radiotherapy Is Equally Effective and Less Toxic Compared With Extended-Field Radiotherapy After Four Cycles of Chemotherapy in Patients With Early-Stage Unfavorable Hodgkin's Lymphoma: Results of the HD8 Trial of the German Hodgkin's Lymphoma Study Group

Engert A, Schiller P, Josting A, et al (Univ Hosp of Cologne, Germany; Univ Clinic Münster, Germany; Univ Clinic Nürnberg, Germany; et al)

J Clin Oncol 21:3601-3608, 2003 6–1

Background.—Most clinical studies of early stage unfavorable Hodgkin's disease (HD) have attempted to improve chemotherapy and radiotherapy to reduce toxicity, maintaining response rates and overall survival. Whether radiotherapy can be decreased without losing efficacy from extended field (EF) to involved field (IF) after 4 cycles of chemotherapy was determined.

Methods.—Between 1993 and 1998, 1204 patients with newly diagnosed early-stage unfavorable HD were randomly assigned to cyclophosphamide, vincristine, procarbazine, and prednisone (COPP) plus doxorubicin, bleomycin, vincristine, and dacarbazine (ABVD) for 2 cycles, followed by radiotherapy consisting of 30 Gy EF plus 10 Gy to bulky disease (arm A) or 30 Gy IF plus 10 Gy to bulky disease (arm B). Final arm comparison included 1064 eligible patients. Patients were followed up for a median 54 months.

Findings.—At 5 years after randomization, the overall survival rate was 91%, with an 83% freedom from treatment failure rate. These rates did not differ between arms A and B. In addition, the arms did not differ in complete remission (at 98.5% and 97.2%, respectively), progressive disease (0.8% and 1.9%), relapse (6.4% and 7.7%), death rate (8.1% and 6.4%), or secondary neoplasia (4.5% and 2.8%). However, acute side effects, including leukopenia, thrombocytopenia, nausea, gastrointestinal toxicity, and pharyngeal toxicity, occurred more frequently in the EF arm.

Conclusions.—A reduction in radiotherapy volume size from EF to IF after COPP plus ABVD chemotherapy for 2 cycles in patients with early stage unfavorable HD is less toxic than the EF regimen. Reducing the volume size does not compromise long-term outcomes.

▶ This trial represents 1 of the largest clinical trials in HD to date. The study in question randomly assigned more than 1200 patients with early stage unfavorable HD to either EF radiation therapy or IF radiation therapy after completing 4 cycles of standard combination chemotherapy. The patient population included those patients with stages I or II disease with 1 or more high-risk features as well as patients with stage IIIA disease with no high-risk features. After completing chemotherapy, patients received identical doses of radiation (30 Gy with a 10 Gy boost to bulky disease) to either the EF or IF depending on the site of disease. The primary end point of the study was overall survival and the study was designed as an equivalence study to identify an 8% or greater difference in survival for the EF group. With a median observation period of 54 months, there was no difference between the 2 groups with regard to overall or disease-free survival. There was a slight but statistically insignificant increase in the incidence of secondary malignancies between the EF group (4.5%) and the IF group (2.8%). In contrast, acute toxicities such as nausea and vomiting, pharyngitis, leukopenia, thrombocytopenia, and gastrointestinal toxicities were statistically significantly greater in the EF group. As a result, it is reasonable to adapt the IF radiation plan for this patient population after induction chemotherapy with 4 cycles of therapy.

M. S. Gordon, MD

In Vitro Evaluation of ^{213}Bi-rituximab Versus External Gamma Irradiation for the Treatment of B-CLL Patients: Relative Biological Efficacy With Respect to Apoptosis Induction and Chromosomal Damage

Vandenbulcke K, De Vos F, Offner F, et al (Ghent Univ, Gent, Belgium; Inst for Transuranium Elements, Karlsruhe, Germany)

Eur J Nucl Med Mol Imaging 30:1357-1364, 2003 6–2

Introduction.—External source radiotherapy and β radioimmunotherapy (RIT) are both effective in the treatment of lymphoid malignancies. The development of RIT with alpha emitters is appealing due to the high linear energy transfer (LET) and short path length, permitting higher tumor cell kill and lower toxicity to healthy tissues. The relative biological efficacy (RBE) of alpha-emitting RIT (in vitro) was compared with external photon irradiation with respect to apoptosis in B chronic lymphocytic leukemia (B-CLL) and induction of chromosomal damage in healthy donor B and T lymphocytes.

Methods.—Healthy donor T lymphocytes were measured via a micronucleus assay. ^{213}Bi was eluted from a ^{225}Ac generator and conjugated to CD20 antibody (rituximab) using CHX-A''-DTPA as a chelator. In 5 patients, B-CLL cells were cultured for 24 hours in RPMI/10% FCS while exposed to ^{213}Bi conjugated to CD20 antibody or after external ^{60}Co gamma irradiation.

Binding assays were conducted in samples from all patients to determine the total absorbed dose. Apoptosis was scored via flow cytometric analyses of cells stained with annexin V-FITC and 7-AAD. and expressed as percent excess over spontaneous apoptosis in controls.

Results.—Full dose range experiments showed that ^{213}Bi-conjugated CD20 antibody was more effective than equivalent doses of external photon irradiation. Similar plateau values were achieved at 10 Gy. The RBE for induction of apoptosis in B-CLL ranged between 1.5 and 7 Gy.

The micronucleus yield in lymphocytes of healthy volunteers was measured to evaluate the late toxicity caused by induction of chromosomal instability. Photon irradiation induced a steady increase in micronucleus yields in B and T cells. The damage induced by ^{213}Bi was more dramatic with RBE and ranged between 5 and 2 with 0.1 Gy and 2 Gy, respectively. ^{213}Bi inhibited mitogen-stimulated mitosis nearly completely at 2 Gy.

Conclusion.—High-LET–targeted alpha particle exposure killed B-CLL cells more effectively than did external photon irradiation at low dose (RBE = 2). A plateau was observed at a high dose. Long-term toxicity on healthy B and T lymphocytes was systematically higher for the α emitter (RBE = 5 to 2).

▶ These investigators have carried out an in vitro study evaluating the antibody rituxan made radioactive with ^{213}Bi, an alpha emitter, and compared the effects of external photon beam in tissue culture on cells with B-CLL. Theoretically, an alpha emitter requires only 1 nuclear hit to kill a cell, but it does not penetrate very deeply due to its mass. Not very surprisingly, the authors show that high-LET labeled rituximab was more efficient at killing B-CLL cells in tissue culture than a modest dose of external beam gamma radiation.

Of course, because the ^{213}Bi actually represents high-LET radiation, the fundamental issue is its impact on nonmalignant cells. In tissue culture using a micronucleus assay, it appears as though the B cells and T cells from healthy donors are significantly more likely to be destroyed by the α-emitting antibody.

These are interesting studies evaluating a variety of cells, but they really do not add a great deal to what would be predicted on the basis of information that we have had for decades. Alpha emitters should be more effective at killing cells. The major issue is what kinds of long-term morbidity will be achieved. The ^{213}Bi has a modest half-life of a few days. The RBE for inducing apoptosis appeared to be 2, which is a significant increase over what could be expected with external beam. The problem is that RBE of 2 does not appear to be restricted to tumor but probably can be extrapolated to a variety of other cells that get exposure.

I believe it was Alexander Pope who said, "The proper study of mankind is man."

E. Glatstein, MD

Substantial Impact of FDG PET Imaging on the Therapy Decision in Patients With Early-Stage Hodgkin's Lymphoma

Naumann R, Beuthien-Baumann B, Reiß A, et al (Dresden Univ of Technology, Germany; Chemnitz Med Ctr, Germany)

Br J Cancer 90:620-625, 2004 6–3

Background.—Accurate staging is crucial to selecting appropriate therapy for patients with Hodgkin's lymphoma (HL). Conventional staging involves chest radiography; US; and contrast-enhanced CT of the neck, chest, abdomen, and pelvis. Whether ^{18}F-fluorodeoxyglucose (FDG) positron emission tomography (PET) would be useful in staging and managing patients with HL was examined.

Methods.—The subjects were 88 patients (65% men; median age, 34 years) with primary (n = 77) or recurrent (n = 11) HL. All patients underwent FDG PET in addition to conventional staging of disease. Treatment strategies were based only on the results of conventional staging. The possible effects of PET findings on clinical staging or management were assessed.

Results.—Results of FDG PET were in agreement with those of conventional staging in 70 patients (80%). Of the remaining 18 patients, FDG PET found additional lymphoma sites in 11 patients and correctly identified a false-positive cervical site found on US in 1 patient. There were no false-positive FDG PET findings, but FDG PET failed to identify retroperitoneal nodal involvement in 3 patients, inguinal and cervical nodal involvement in 2 patients, and biopsy-proven liver involvement in 1 patient. All these findings would have resulted in a change in staging in these 18 patients (20%), with 11 patients (13%) being upstaged and 7 patients (8%) being downstaged. Consequently, had FDG PET findings been considered, treatment would have been changed in 16 patients (18%), including an intensification of treatment in 9 patients (10%) and a minimization of treatment in 7 patients (8%). In particular, among the 44 patients with early (stage IA-IIB) disease, treatment would have been intensified in 9 of them (20%).

Conclusion.—FDG PET is a noninvasive complement to conventional methods for staging patients with HL and can have a substantial impact on treatment, especially in patients with early disease.

► Optimal staging of HL continues to be a significant issue for clinicians. The more frequent use of chemotherapy has rendered the role of the staging laparotomy inconsequential, and as a result better clinical staging techniques have been sought. CT scans represented a major advance over prior studies such as lymphangiography, and the current study addressed the role of PET scanning in this patient population. In addition to providing anatomic information, especially with current techniques for CT colocalization, the use of PET scanning to assess the physiologic state of residual masses could prove important in decision making. The authors studied 88 consecutive patients with HL who underwent an FDG PET scan in addition to conventional staging studies. PET scanning was concordant with conventional staging studies in 80% of the patients studied. The PET scan suggested a change in stage in 20% of the patients, with a predicted management change in 18% of the patients (10% with treatment intensification and 8% with treatment minimization). In the 44 patients with early stage disease (stages IA-IIB), treatment would have been intensified in 9 of the 44 patients, suggesting that for early stage patients valuable information may be derived from PET scans that may have a clinically significant impact on outcome. This study did not address the role of subsequent PET scans after therapy in determining the frequency of occult residual disease. Overall, the most appropriate use of PET scanning remains to be determined. In patients with more advanced disease where it will not affect treatment decision-making, there is little defined value in performing this study, whereas in early stage disease where upstaging might play a significant role in therapeutic decision-making, there may be a role for PET scanning on a routine basis.

M. S. Gordon, MD

Prediction of Survival in Diffuse Large-B-Cell Lymphoma Based on the Expression of Six Genes

Lossos IS, Czerwinski DK, Alizadeh AA, et al (Stanford Univ, Calif; Univ of Miami, Fla; Applied Biosystems, Foster City, Calif)

N Engl J Med 350:1828-1837, 2004 6–4

Background.—Several gene expression signatures have been found useful for predicting prognosis in patients with diffuse large-B-cell lymphoma. However, the lack of practical tests for a genome-scale analysis has limited the use of this technique. The authors sought to create a predictive model based on the genes correlated with overall survival, positively or negatively, that would be simple and applicable for routine clinical use.

Methods.—Thirty-six genes whose expression has been shown to predict survival in patients with diffuse large-B-cell lymphoma were studied. The expression of each gene was measured in independent samples of lymphoma from 66 patients. Quantitative real-time polymerase chain reaction (RT-PCR) analysis was used. Findings were then related to overall survival. Genes were ranked on the basis of their ability to predict survival in univariate and multivariate analyses.

Findings.—Univariate analysis indicated that *LM02, BCL6, FN1, CCND2, SCYA3*, and *BCL2* were the strongest predictors. A multivariate model based on the expression of these 6 genes was developed and validated with the use of 2 independent microarray data sets. The model was found to be independent of the International Prognostic Index (IPI), contributing to its predictive value.

Conclusions.—Overall survival in patients with diffuse large-B-cell lymphoma can be predicted by measuring the expression of 6 genes. This 6-gene model and quantitative RT-PCR can probably be used to identify patients who would benefit from new treatments.

▶ The use of genomics in cancer is being extensively explored in terms of determining new targets for therapy, prediction of response to therapy, and/or resistance as well as the prediction of survival in patients being uniformly treated. One of the valued benefits of the use of such a technology is the ability to characterize various subgroups of histologically similar cancers based on gene expression patterns. In this study, Lossos et al have assessed the impact of gene expression patterns on the survival of a cohort of patients with histologically similar non-Hodgkin's lymphoma. Thirty-six genes were selected from a series of microarray studies performed on previous samples. These genes appeared to be those that were most significantly altered in terms of expression in the pilot samples. RT-PCR for these genes was performed on RNA isolated from the 66 patients who participated in this study. As a result of the expression patterns, 6 specific genes were combined into a profile that predicts overall survival. This approach was applied not only to the investigators' 66 patients but to 2 other large previously published series of patients and indicated that these 6 genes predicted for survival in a manner that was independent of the classical IPI scores. The potential use of this 6-gene model to separate patients with diffuse large cell lymphoma into varying prognostic groups has the benefit of possibly identifying patients who should be considered for more aggressive or varying therapeutic options, based on their scoring thus initiating a process wherein patients' therapy will be determined, not exclusively by their diagnosis or clinical presentation but by the biology of their cancer.

M. S. Gordon, MD

Randomized Phase 2 Study of Fludarabine With Concurrent Versus Sequential Treatment With Rituximab in Symptomatic, Untreated Patients With B-cell Chronic Lymphocytic Leukemia: Results From Cancer and Leukemia Group B 9712 (CALGB 9712)

Byrd JC, Peterson BL, Morrison VA, et al (Ohio State Univ, Columbus; Duke Univ, Durham, NC; Minneapolis Veterans Affairs Med Ctr; et al)

Blood 101:6-14, 2003 6–5

Background.—Recent research suggests that rituximab can modulate antiapoptotic proteins associated with drug resistance in patients with chronic lymphocytic leukemia (CLL). This randomized phase 2 trial was initiated to establish the efficacy, safety, and optimal administration schedule of rituximab with fludarabine in previously untreated patients with CLL.

Methods and Findings.—One hundred four patients were assigned randomly to 6 monthly courses of fludarabine concurrently with rituximab, followed 2 months later by 4 weekly doses of rituximab for consolidation therapy, or to sequential fludarabine alone followed 2 months later by rituximab consolidation therapy). During induction, 74% of patients assigned to the concurrent regimen and 41% assigned to the sequential arm had grade 3 or 4 neutropenia. In addition, grade 3 or 4 infusion-related toxicity occurred in 20% of patients in the concurrent arm, compared with none in the sequential arm. In both arms, patients tolerated consolidation rituximab treatment well. All other toxicities were comparable between groups. The overall response rates were 90% in the concurrent arm and 77% in the sequential arm. In the concurrent regimen, complete response rate was 47%, and the partial response rate was 43%. In the sequential regimen, complete and partial response rates were 28% and 49%, respectively. At a median 23-month follow-up, the median response duration and survival have not been reached in either group.

Conclusions.—Rituximab given concurrently with fludarabine in previously untreated patients with CLL is clinically effective with acceptable toxicity. Phase 3 studies are now warranted.

► CLL remains a frustrating disease for treatment. This article from members of the CALGB randomized 104 patients on a phase 2 study by giving all patients fludarabine and half the patients receiving concurrent rituximab and the other half receiving sequential rituximab after completion of the fludarabine treatment. Response rates with the concurrent regimen were 90% and about half of those were complete responders. On the other hand, the frequency of toxicity was greater, as was its severity, a finding that should not be considered to be surprising. These are pretty good figures for CLL, and suggest that concurrent rituximab in conjunction with fludarabine has excellent potential for further aggressive treatment strategies, although physicians need to be attentive to the potential morbidities.

E. Glatstein, MD

Fludarabine Plus Mitoxantrone With and Without Rituximab Versus CHOP With and Without Rituximab as Front-Line Treatment for Patients With Follicular Lymphoma

Zinzani PL, Pulsoni A, Perrotti A, et al (Univ of Bologna, Italy; Univ of La Sapienza, Rome; Univ of Rome; et al)

J Clin Oncol 22:2654-2661, 2004 6–6

Background.—Fludarabine plus mitoxantrone (FM) and the mouse/human anti-CD20 antibody rituximab are promising new treatments for follicular lymphoma (FL). The current randomized trial compared FM with cyclophosphamide, doxorubicin, vincristine, and prednisone (CHOP) front-line chemotherapy with and without sequential rituximab.

Methods.—All 151 previously untreated patients with $CD20^+$ FL seen at 15 Italian centers were randomly assigned beginning in 1999. After clinical or molecular restaging, patients in complete remission with *bcl-2/IgH* negativity (CR^-) received no further treatment. Patients in complete remission with *bcl-2/IgH* positivity (CR^+) and negative or positive partial responders received rituximab. The final analysis included 72 patients assigned to FM and 68 assigned to CHOP.

Findings.—After chemotherapy, the rate of CR was higher in the FM arm than in the CHOP arm, at 68% and 42%, respectively. The CR^- rate was also greater in the FM arm, at 39% compared with 19%. Fifty-eight percent of patients treated with rituximab achieved CR^- status. Final CR rates were 71% in the FM arm and 51% in the CHOP arm. However, at a median follow-up of 19 months, differences between study arms in progression-free and overall survival rates were not significant.

Conclusions.—Front-line treatment with FM appears to be superior to CHOP in patients with FL. Also, rituximab is an effective sequential treatment option. However, the efficacies of these treatments are not likely to translate into improved progression-free or overall survival.

▶ Follicular non-Hodgkin's lymphoma is an incurable disease for which treatment has been focused on an approach of either watchful waiting or aggressive chemotherapy. Regardless, with time, all patients relapse and require subsequent therapy. Various chemotherapy regimens have been used and range from oral single alkylating agents to combination chemotherapy. The combination of fludarabine and mitoxantrone is one that has garnered a significant degree of interest because of the high response rates associated with high complete response rates and long durations of freedom from progression. In this study, the investigators randomly assigned 140 patients to receive either standard CHOP or FM for a total of 6 cycles. At the end of the 6 cycles of therapy, patients were evaluated molecularly for the *bcl-2/IgH* gene rearrangement that is characteristics of this disease. Overall, the CR rate for the FM patients was statistically superior to that of CHOP (68% vs 42%, $P = .003$). When molecular analysis was performed on the patients with CR, the rate of molecular negativity was also significantly higher in the FM arms (39% vs 19%, $P = .001$). This strongly suggests that the FM regimen is a preferred regimen in terms of outcome. There were no significant differences in the toxicity of the regimens, though the FM regimen was associated with less alopecia, peripheral neuropathy, and constipation although the frequencies of these events are small enough to not allow statistical analysis. In a second phase of the study, all patients with molecularly positive CR and all those with partial remission were treated with sequential rituximab antibody therapy. Of the 41 patients in the FM arm who were treated with rituximab, 23 achieved a molecularly negative CR compared with 22 of 54 patients in the CHOP arm. Overall, a greater percentage of patients achieved a molecularly negative CR with FM + rituximab (71%) compared with CHOP + rituximab (51%). Whether because of the small numbers in the trial or because of the possibility that rituximab is an excellent consolidative therapy, there is no difference in progression-free or overall survival between the 2 arms. This study demonstrates the superiority and better tolerability of FM compared with CHOP and suggests that the former regimen should be used for those low-grade lymphoma patients who are to be treated with combination chemotherapy. The use of sequential rituximab as opposed to relayed immunotherapy at the time of relapse cannot be assessed without a randomized controlled trial.

M. S. Gordon, MD

Rapid Mobilization of CD34+ Cells Following Administration of the CXCR4 Antagonist AMD3100 to Patients With Multiple Myeloma and Non-Hodgkin's Lymphoma

Devine SM, Flomenberg N, Vesole DH, et al (Washington Univ, St Louis; Thomas Jefferson Univ, Philadelphia; Med College of Wisconsin, Milwaukee; et al)

J Clin Oncol 22:1095-1102, 2004 6–7

Background.—When the CXC chemokine receptor CXCR4 binds to its only known ligand stromal derived factor-1 (SDF-1), multiple signal transduction pathways are activated and ultimately trigger chemotaxis. The interaction between CXCR4 and SDF-1 has an important role in stem cell mobilization. If either molecule is disrupted, the result is lethal in mice, with no migration of hematopoietic stem cells (HCS) from the liver to bone marrow, defects in B-lymphopoiesis, and cerebellar dysgenesis. The bicyclam molecule AMD3100 has a potent and selective inhibition of HIV types 1 and 2 replication by binding to the chemokine receptor CXCR4. It also reversibly inhibits binding between CXCR4 and SDF-1 without affecting other cell surface chemokine receptors. Some data suggest that AMD3100 may be able to increase the yield of CD34+ cells collected when it is combined with granulocyte colony-stimulating factor. A phase I investigation looked at the effects of AMD3100 alone in patients who had multiple myeloma (MM) or non-Hodgkin's lymphoma (NHL).

Methods.—Seven patients with MM and 6 with NHL were given AMD3100 in a dose of 160 or 240 µg/kg. Four and 6 hours after injection, white blood cells (WBC) and peripheral blood (PB) CD34+ cell counts were determined.

Results.—The WBC count was increased from a baseline value of 4732/µL to 12,366/µL after 4 hours and 13,568/µL after 6 hours, which were significant increases regardless of the dose of AMD3100 used. The mean WBC count was still significantly elevated on the second day after injection. The frequency of CD34+ cells in PB was 0.06% at baseline and increased to 0.13% at both 4 and 6 hours after injection. The mean PB absolute CD34+ cell count increased from a baseline value of 2.6/µL to 15.6/µL after 4 hours and 16.2/µL after 6 hours. These were significant increases. Compared with those given the 160-µg/kg dose, patients given the 240-µg/kg dose had a greater increase in absolute CD34+ cell count and a greater increase at 4 and 6 hours. No significant toxic reactions occurred with either dose.

Conclusions.—Both WBC count and PB CD34+ count increased significantly after a single injection of AMD3100 in patients with MM and NHL. The effect was greater with the larger dose. All the adverse reactions were mild and transient, so AMD3100 was well tolerated. Further study of

AMD3100 alone and in combination with granulocyte colony-stimulating factor for patients with hematologic malignancies is indicated.

▶ The chemokines/chemokine receptor pathway is a complex system that is poorly understood. Responsible primarily for the trafficking of cells, chemokine receptors are commonly expressed. CXCR4 is a well-recognized chemokine receptor responsible for the migration of various cells. It appears to play a role not only in the mobilization of hematopoietic precursors, but possibly also tumor cells, where the expression of CXCR4 is frequently expressed on tumor cells. It is believed that the ligand for CXCR4, SDF-1, may be expressed in sites of metastatic disease and that this interaction may be responsible for the site-specific migration of tumor cells to specific organs. This study assessed the role of a CXCR4 antagonist AMD3100 to mobilize hematopoietic precursors. The mechanism of action appears to be competitive binding to the CXCR4 receptor, thereby disengaging the progenitor cells from the bone marrow cavity. AMD3100 was administered in a single subcutaneous dose at 1 of 2 different dosages, including 160 μg/kg or 240 μg/kg. The study drug was well tolerated without dose-limiting toxicity. All adverse events were grade 1 in severity. The hematologic effects of AMD3100 were characterized by assessment of circulating WBCs and their subsets as well as by flow cytometric assessment of circulating CD34+ progenitor cells. Within 4 hours of dosing, both doses produced significant elevations of WBCs and peripheral blood CD34+ cells. A mean 7-fold increase in circulating CD34+ cells was seen 6 hours after the 240 μg/kg dose. Further evaluation of AMD3100 is warranted as a stem cell mobilizing agent and in other possible settings where CXCR4 blockade may be of value, such as in primary cancer therapy.

M. S. Gordon, MD

Nonablative Allogeneic Stem-Cell Transplantation for Advanced/Recurrent Mantle-Cell Lymphoma

Khouri IF, Lee M-S, Saliba RM, et al (Univ of Texas, Houston)
J Clin Oncol 21:4407-4412, 2003 6–8

Background.—Despite combination chemotherapy, the median survival in patients with mantle-cell lymphoma (MCL) is only approximately 3 years. High-dose therapy and allogeneic transplantation can be effective but are associated with high mortality rates (approximately 40%) and are contraindicated in many patients because of age. A nonablative conditioning regimen with allogeneic stem-cell transplantation has recently been developed to encourage engraftment and to reduce treatment-related toxicity, and results of this approach in patients with low-grade MCL are encouraging. The efficacy and safety of nonablative allogeneic stem-cell transplantation in patients with relapsed MCL were investigated.

Methods.—The subjects were 18 patients (83% male; aged 46-64 years) with diffuse MCL who did not respond to as many as 10 previous trials of conventional chemotherapy or autologous stem-cell transplantation. Two different regimens were tested. The first 5 patients received cisplatin (25 mg/m^2 per day on days 6-3 before transplantation), fludarabine (30 mg/m^2 per day on days 4-3 before transplantation), and cytarabine (1000 mg/m^2 per day on days 4-3 before transplantation). Because of concerns about nephrotoxicity with cisplatin, the remaining 13 patients received fludarabine (30 mg/m^2 per day on days 5-3 before transplantation), cyclophosphamide (750 mg/m^2 per day on days 5-3 before transplantation), and rituximab (375 mg/m^2 on day 13 before transplantation, 1000 mg/m^2 on day 6 before transplantation, and 1000 mg/m^2 on days 1 and 8 after transplantation). Patients with a mismatched sibling donor or a matched unrelated donor received 15 mg/kg equine antithymocyte globulin on days 5 to 3 before transplantation, and they received granulocyte colony-stimulating factor-mobilized stem cells at transplantation. After transplantation, all patients also received tacrolimus and methotrexate as prophylaxis against graft-versus-host disease (GVHD). Patients were followed up for a median of 26 months to determine response rates, progression-free survival, and overall survival.

Results.—Sixteen of the 18 patients had chemosensitive disease. Donor cell engraftment occurred in all 18 patients, and none had grade 3/4 acute GVHD or nonhematologic toxicity. All but 1 patient (94.4%) achieved a complete response; the 1 patient who did not respond had received 10 previous trials of chemotherapy. Remission occurred in 3 patients at 2, 3, and 12 months after transplantation, and 2 underwent donor lymphocyte infusion. Infusion was able to reinduce a complete response in 1 patient (which has continued for >45 months), whereas the other patient has stable disease. All patients were still alive at 100 days after transplantation. Three patients died: 1 from GVHD, 1 from progressive disease, and 1 from an event not related to treatment (patient with a history of deep vein thrombosis had a pulmonary embolism 15 months after transplantation). Kaplan-Meier estimated current progression-free survival at 3 years was 82% and 3-year survival was 85.5%.

Conclusion.—These promising results suggest nonablative allogeneic stem-cell transplantation is safe and effective in patients with relapsed and chemosensitive MCL.

▶ The treatment of MCL is generally poor, with few long-term survivors in the population of patients with advanced or recurrent disease. Previously studied therapies include autologous stem-cell transplantation and immunotherapy. The authors of this study report on their limited experience with nonablative allogeneic stem-cell transplantation (otherwise known as minitransplants or "transplant lite"). In 2 consecutive studies with different conditioning regimens, 18 patients with advanced or recurrent MCL underwent a minitransplant from predominantly matched sibling donors. The day 100 treatment-related mortality rate was 0%, reinforcing the safety of this therapy in patients with cancer. Engraftment was rapid and little cytopenia-related toxicity was seen. None of the patients had greater than grade 2 GVHD, and a complete remission was attained in 17 of the 18 patients. Only 3 patients relapsed, and 1 was successfully treated with donor lymphocyte infusions. The 3-year event-free survival was 82%. This early experience highlights the fact that patients with advanced or relapsed MCL have options that should be considered, though treatments such as those described should be performed at specialized centers. Additional studies in this patient population are necessary to ensure that the validity of these early results is confirmed.

M. S. Gordon, MD

Initial Treatment of Aggressive Lymphoma With High-Dose Chemotherapy and Autologous Stem-Cell Support

Milpied N, for the Groupe Ouest-Est des Leucémies et des Autres Maladies du Sang (Univ of Hosp of Nantes, France; et al)

N Engl J Med 350:1287-1295, 2004 6–9

Background.—Adult patients with disseminated aggressive lymphoma generally receive a regimen of cyclophosphamide, doxorubicin, vincristine, and prednisone (CHOP). An alternative approach involving short-term conventional chemotherapy followed by high-dose chemotherapy and transplantation of autologous hematopoietic stem cells has proved highly effective in phase II trials. These 2 approaches were compared in patients with disseminated aggressive lymphoma who had a low, low-intermediate, or high-intermediate risk, as determined by the age-adjusted International Prognostic Index.

Methods.—Patients ranging in age from 15 to 60 years were randomly assigned to receive 8 courses of CHOP or high-dose chemotherapy plus autologous stem-cell support when they were diagnosed. None of the patients had received previous treatment, and all had histologically proved aggressive lymphoma. Event-free survival at 5 years was the primary outcome sought.

Results.—Seventy-two percent of the CHOP group and 85% of the high-dose group completed their assigned treatments. After 4 courses of CHOP the response rate was 84%, and after 2 courses of high-dose therapy the response rate was 86%. By the end of treatment, 62% of the CHOP group and 81% of the high-dose group responded. Complete remission rates were 57% and 76% for the CHOP and high-dose groups, respectively. Elevated lactate dehydrogenase level was the only adverse factor that had a significant effect on the response rate. The overall survival was 63.4% and the event-free survival was 46.4% after 4 years. A significant difference was found between groups regarding the event-free survival rates at 5 years. The CHOP group had an event-free survival at 5 years of 37%, and the high-dose group's was 55%. Overall survival did not differ significantly between the 2 groups, with a trend toward a higher rate for the high-dose group (71%) than for the CHOP group (56%). Patients with a high-intermediate risk had significantly higher event-free survival rates (56% vs 28%) and overall survival rates (74% vs 44%) when given the high-dose therapy compared with the CHOP therapy. Event-free survival was independently influenced by the type of treatment received. Disease progression or relapse occurred during treatment in 96 patients, 58 of whom were receiving CHOP and 38 the high-dose therapy. Of those patients with a complete, unconfirmed complete, or partial response at intermediate evaluation, the 5-year disease-free survival was 65% for the high-dose group and 45% for the CHOP group, with no significant difference in overall survival at 5 years. When disease progressed or relapse occurred, patients had a 5-year survival of 26% in the CHOP group and 36% in the high-dose group. Severe infections developed in 14 patients and interstitial pneumonitis in 7. Nausea and vomiting was reported by 15 patients and diarrhea by 11. One patient in the CHOP group and 3 in the high-dose group died from treatment.

Conclusions.—The event-free survival rate for these never-before treated patients with aggressive lymphoma was higher after high-dose chemotherapy plus stem-cell support than after the CHOP regimen. The overall survival at 5 years was comparable. Among patients whose risk of death was high intermediate, intensive chemotherapy with autologous stem-cell support achieved significantly better results than CHOP.

▶ The optimal treatment for high-risk aggressive non-Hodgkin's lymphoma is somewhat controversial with regard to the timing of the use of high-dose chemotherapy with stem-cell transplantation. The use of high-dose chemotherapy has been shown to have the ability to cure approximately 30% of patients with primary relapsed/refractory disease and hence has a significant place in the management strategy for patients with intermediate and high-grade disease. The use of such aggressive therapy in de novo, previously untreated high-risk patients remains controversial. In this study, the authors performed a randomized trial in 207 patients with previously untreated aggressive (intermediate or high-grade) non-Hodgkin's lymphoma. All patients demonstrated at least 2 adverse prognostic factors as defined by the International Prognostic Index. Overall, 197 patients were randomly assigned to receive either standard CHOP chemotherapy for 8 courses or a more dose-intense regimen of cyclophosphamide, epirubicin, vindesine, and prednisone (CEEP) followed by high-dose chemotherapy (HDC) and stem cell transplantation (the latter for those patients with at least a partial response to induction therapy). Nearly 80% of patients were able to complete all planned therapy per protocol. The rates of complete remission after the completion of all planned therapy was 57% in the CHOP arm and 76% in the CEEP/HDC arm. After a median of 4 years of follow-up, the intent-to-treat event-free survival was 37% in the CHOP arm and 55% in the CEEP/HDC arm (P = .037). The 5-year overall survival rate did not differ statistically, though there was a trend toward the CEEP/HDC arm being superior (56% vs 71%, P = .076). This benefit appeared to be most significantly visible for the subset of patients with high-intermediate risk according to the index where the overall survival favored the CEEP/HDC arm significantly (74% vs 44%, P = .001). This study indicates that high-dose chemotherapy as a part of the primary therapy for patients with high-risk non-Hodgkin's lymphoma has a role and should be considered, especially for the subgroup of individuals with high-intermediate risk prognostic features. While HDC can be used in the salvage setting, it appears to be most effective when used up front in this subgroup of patients.

M. S. Gordon, MD

Syngeneic Hematopoietic Stem-Cell Transplantation for Non-Hodgkin's Lymphoma: A Comparison With Allogeneic and Autologous Transplantation—The Lymphoma Working Committee of the International Bone Marrow Transplant Registry and the European Group for Blood and Marrow Transplantation

Bierman PJ, Sweetenham JW, Loberiza FR Jr, et al (Univ of Nebraska, Omaha; Univ of Colorado, Denver; Intl Bone Marrow Transplant Registry, Milwaukee, Wis; et al)

J Clin Oncol 21:3744-3753, 2003 6–10

Background.—Several studies have shown that allogeneic transplantation can provide lower relapse rates than autologous transplantation in the treatment of non-Hodgkin's lymphoma (NHL). These results could be attributed to a lack of tumor contamination or to selection bias favoring patients with better prognostic characteristics. However, many investigators have hypothesized that the most likely explanation for this finding is a graft-versus-lymphoma effect. Comparisons of syngeneic and allogeneic bone marrow transplantation for leukemia are supportive of the existence of a graft-versus-leukemia effect. It has been proposed that a comparison of syngeneic and allogeneic NHL transplants could also provide insights into whether a similar graft-versus-lymphoma effect exists. The results of syngeneic, allogeneic, and autologous hematopoietic stem-cell transplantation were compared for the treatment of NHL.

Methods.—A search was conducted of the databases of the International Bone Marrow Transplant Registry and the European Group for Blood and Marrow Transplantation to identify 89 NHL patients who received syngeneic transplants (Table 1). These patients were compared with NHL patients identified from a search of the International Bone Marrow Transplant Registry and the Autologous Blood and Marrow Transplant Registry who received allogeneic (T-cell depleted and T-cell replete) and autologous (purged and unpurged) transplants.

Results.—There were no significant differences in relapse rates when the results of allogeneic transplantation were compared with syngeneic transplantation for any histology (Fig 1). The T-cell depletion of allografts was not associated with a higher risk of relapse, but it was associated with an improvement of overall survival for patients with low-grade and intermediate-grade histology. The patients who received unpurged autografts for low-grade NHL had a 5-fold greater risk of relapse than patients who received syngeneic transplants, and patients who received unpurged autografts had a 2-fold greater risk of relapse than patients who received purged autografts. Among the low-grade NHL patients, the use of purging was associated with significantly better disease-free survival and overall survival in comparison with patients who received unpurged autografts (Fig 3).

Conclusions.—This analysis did not find evidence of a graft-versus-lymphoma effect, but it did provide indirect evidence to support the hypothesis that tumor contamination may contribute to lymphoma relapse, and

TABLE 1.—Patient Characteristics

Characteristic	Syngeneic No.	Syngeneic %	Autologous Unpurged No.	Autologous Unpurged %	Autologous Purged No.	Autologous Purged %	Allogeneic T-Cell–Replete No.	Allogeneic T-Cell–Replete %	Allogeneic T-Cell–Depleted No.	Allogeneic T-Cell–Depleted %
No. of patients	89		2,018		376		774		119	
Age										
Median	42		48		47		33		37	
Range	4-68		11-68		6-71		2-62		5-62	
Male	51	57	1,232	61	230	61	495	64	69	58
Karnofsky performance status										
≥ 90%	30	34	1,203	60	272	72	440	57	92	77
< 90%	27	30	712	35	55	15	313	40	16	13
Unknown	32	36	103	5	49	13	21	3	11	10
Histology										
Low-grade	30	34	427	21	160	42	189	24	36	30
Intermediate-grade	31	35	1,417	70	180	48	194	25	26	22
High-grade	28	31	174	9	36	10	391	51	57	48
"B" symptoms at diagnosis										
Absent	39	44	1,191	59	244	65	402	52	55	46
Present	24	27	787	39	124	33	255	33	39	33
Unknown	26	29	40	2	8	2	117	15	25	21
Stage at diagnosis										
I to II	18	20	578	29	97	26	137	18	25	21
III to IV	57	64	1,417	70	277	73	566	73	73	61
Unknown	14	16	23	1	2	<1	71	9	21	8
Bone marrow involvement at diagnosis or transplantation										
Absent	57	64	1,816	90	285	76	255	33	32	27
Present	9	10	121	6	20	5	186	24	16	13
Unknown	23	26	81	4	71	19	333	43	71	60
Sensitivity to chemotherapy										
Sensitive	50	56	1,464	72	280	74	308	40	31	26
Resistant	13	15	316	16	63	17	110	14	13	11
Untreated or unknown	26	29	238	12	33	9	356	46	75	63

(Continued)

TABLE (cont.)

Characteristic	Syngeneic No.	Syngeneic %	Autologous Unpurged No.	Autologous Unpurged %	Autologous Purged No.	Autologous Purged %	Allogeneic T-Cell–Replete No.	Allogeneic T-Cell–Replete %	Allogeneic T-Cell–Depleted No.	Allogeneic T-Cell–Depleted %
Disease status at transplantation										
Primary induction failure	22	25	449	22	64	17	194	25	27	23
CR1	18	20	238	12	53	14	150	19	32	27
≥ CR2	14	16	319	16	74	20	140	18	19	16
Rel 1	24	27	650	32	82	22	168	22	14	12
Rel 2	6	7	171	8	30	8	53	7	11	9
Not assessable	5	5	191	10	73	19	69	9	16	13
TBI for conditioning	25	28	557	28	225	60	559	72	107	90
Type of graft										
Peripheral stem cell	23	26	1,359	67	48	13	92	12	—	—
Bone marrow	66	74	659	33	328	87	682	88	119	100
Grown factor given within 7 days posttransplantation	26	30	1,155	61	146	44	246	33	24	22
Year of transplantation										
1985-1989	17	19	86	5	31	9	177	23	36	30
1990-1992	23	26	392	19	137	36	255	33	20	17
1993-1995	22	25	884	44	145	38	193	25	56	47
1996-1998	27	30	656	32	63	17	149	19	7	6

Abbreviations: CR, Complete remission; *Rel*, relapse; *TBI*, total-body irradiation.

(Courtesy of Bierman PJ, Sweetenham JW, Loberiza FR Jr, et al: Syngeneic hematopoietic stem-cell transplantation for non-Hodgkin's lymphoma: A comparison with allogeneic and autologous transplantation—The Lymphoma Working Committee of the International Bone Marrow Transplant Registry and the European Group for Blood and Marrow Transplantation. *J Clin Oncol* 21[20]:3744-3753, 2003. Reprinted with permission from the American Society for Clinical Oncology.)

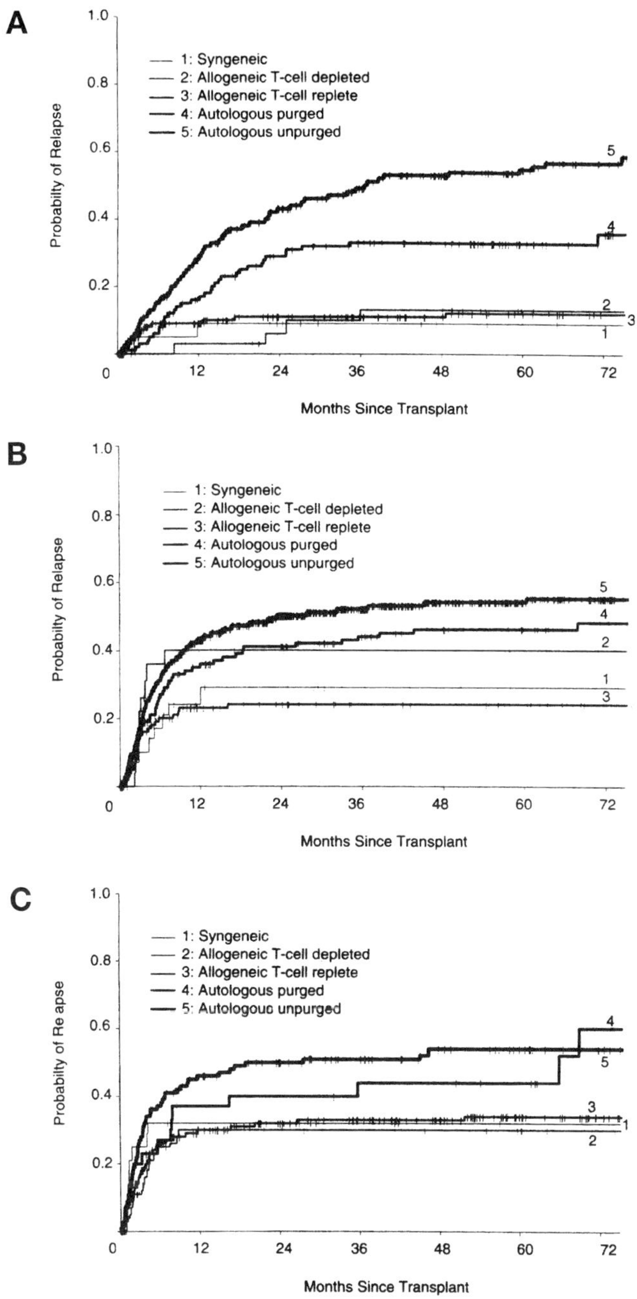

FIGURE 1.—Cumulative incidence of relapse after transplantation for all patients according to type of transplant. A, Low-grade histology. B, Intermediate-grade histology. C, High-grade histology. (Courtesy of Bierman PJ, Sweetenham JW, Loberiza FR Jr, et al: Syngeneic hematopoietic stem-cell transplantation for non-Hodgkin's lymphoma: A comparison with allogeneic and autologous transplantation—The Lymphoma Working Committee of the International Bone Marrow Transplant Registry and the European Group for Blood and Marrow Transplantation. *J Clin Oncol* 21[20]:3744-3753, 2003. Reprinted with permission from the American Society for Clinical Oncology.)

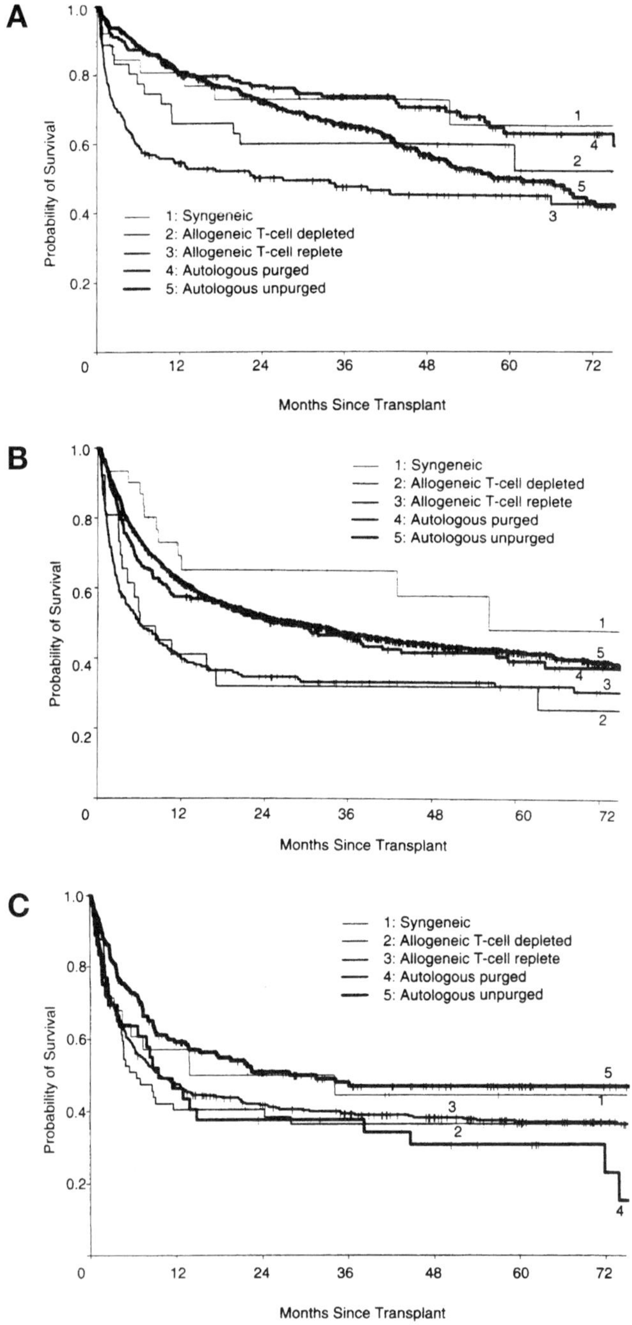

FIGURE 3.—Actuarial probability of overall survival after transplantation for all patients according to type of transplant. **A**, Low-grade histology. **B**, Intermediate-grade histology. **C**, High-grade histology. (Courtesy of Bierman PJ, Sweetenham JW, Loberiza FR Jr, et al: Syngeneic hematopoietic stem-cell transplantation for non-Hodgkin's lymphoma: A comparison with allogeneic and autologous transplantation—The Lymphoma Working Committee of the International Bone Marrow Transplant Registry and the European Group for Blood and Marrow Transplantation. *J Clin Oncol* 21[20]:3744-3753, 2003. Reprinted with permission from the American Society for Clinical Oncology.)

that purging may benefit patients undergoing autologous hematopoietic stem-cell transplantation for the treatment of low-grade NHL.

► The problem of interpreting the results of bone marrow transplantation for NHLs is complex. There are several different types of transplant (syngeneic, allogeneic, and autologous, the latter of which is probably best thought of not as a true transplant, but as a replant). There is also an enormous selection factor in terms of who actually receives the transplant. Typically, older patients are eliminated, persons who are sick with poor performance status or a variety of other medical diseases are excluded, and most patients must have achieved a good pretransplant response to their chemotherapy, which is usually second line, since most of these patients have had a relapse already.

This is a group of solid investigators reporting on 89 syngeneic patients, more than 2000 autologous unpurged patients, another 376 autologous purged patients, and almost 900 patients who underwent allogeneic transplants, with more than 100 of those patients having T-cell depletion as part of their allograft. The data here are not commonly available, and it is valuable that they go out to 72 months, since so many transplant articles stop the curves at about 36 months. The data look good for syngeneic or allogeneic transplants for low-grade histologies, although it is not clear how well the patients are followed up for relapse, since relapse can be very subtle in that group of patients. It can be very humbling to get marrow samples in asymptomatic patients who have lymphoma with indolent histologies. In any event, the data that the authors have generated do not show any clear evidence of a graft-versus-lymphoma effect. Within the low-grade category, there is a suggestion that purging improved outcome, implying that tumor cell contamination with the transplanted cells may contribute to relapse. In any event, this is an important article not only for the transplant team but also for the lymphoma doctor.

E. Glatstein, MD

7 Thoracic Cancer

Miscellaneous Topics

Randomized, Multinational, Phase III Study of Docetaxel Plus Platinum Combinations Versus Vinorelbine Plus Cisplatin for Advanced Non–Small-Cell Lung Cancer: The TAX 326 Study Group

Fossella F, Pereira JR, von Pawel J, et al (MD Anderson Cancer Ctr, Houston; Instituto do Câncer Arnaldo Vieira de Carvalho, Sao Paulo, Brazil; Asklepios Fachkliniken München-Gauting, Germany; et al)

J Clin Oncol 21:3016-3024, 2003 7–1

Background.—Non–small cell lung cancer (NSCLC) is the leading cause of cancer deaths in men and women. Most patients are not diagnosed until they have locally advanced stage III or metastatic stage IV disease. The survival and quality of life associated with docetaxel plus platinum regimens were compared with those associated with vinorelbine plus cisplatin for use as first-line chemotherapy in patients with advanced NSCLC.

Methods.—The study included 1218 patients with stage IIB to IV NSCLC who were assigned randomly to docetaxel 75 mg/m^2 and cisplatin 75 mg/m^2 every 3 weeks (DC group); docetaxel 75 mg/m^2 and carboplatin area under the curve of 6 mg/mL min every 3 weeks (DCb group); or vinorelbine 25 mg/m^2 plus cisplatin 100 mg/m^2 every 4 weeks (VC group).

Findings.—The median survival was 11.3 months for the DC group and 10.1 months for the VC group. Survival rates at 2 years for the DC and VC groups were 21% and 14%, respectively. Overall response rates were 31.6% and 24.5% for the DC and VC groups, respectively. Patients in the DCb group had a similar median survival and response rate to those in the VC group. The 3 treatment groups were similar in neutropenia, thrombocytopenia, infection, and febrile neutropenia. However, grades 3 to 4 anemia, nausea, and vomiting were more common in the VC group than in the DC or DCb groups. The quality of life was superior for patients in the DC and DCb groups than for patients in the VC group. In the latter group, quality of life deteriorated.

Conclusions.—Patients treated with DC had more favorable overall response and survival rates than those treated with VC. Both DC and DCb were more tolerable than VC, consistently improving quality of life. A docetaxel plus platinum combination is a good treatment option for first-line therapy in patients with advanced or metastatic NSCLC.

► The late 1980s and early 1990s were noteworthy in that a number of new agents were introduced for the treatment of patients with advanced NSCLC. These so-called third generation drugs were subsequently combined and compared with "first-generation" (cisplatin, vinblastine, mitomycin) and "second" generation (carboplatin, etoposide) drugs, to result in a plethora of combinations. In general, third-generation, platin-based doublets tended to be better tolerated and somewhat more effective than their first-generation cousins. The last half of the 1990s was spent comparing many of these third-generation doublets to determine if any particular combination was more effective or less toxic.

The study reported by Fossella et al compared DC and DCb with VC. The median survival for the DC combination was 11.3 months compared with 10.1 months in the VC arm ($P = .044$), and 9.4 months in the DCb arm compared with 9.9 months in the VC arm ($P = .657$).

This study is unique in that it is the first to demonstrate a difference in survival with 1 third-generation combination over another. Numerous other studies have also compared third-generation doublets (for review, see Reference 1), but almost all have been negative in demonstrating a survival improvement with any 1 combination, although all have reported differences in toxicities. Why was this one positive? Although VC has been compared to cisplatin,[2] vindesine/cisplatin,[3] and paclitaxel/carboplatin,[4] it had not been compared to the doublet of DC. It should also be noted that in the Fossella study, the authors failed to meet their original end point; superiority was not demonstrated using a significance level of 0.028, although clearly there was a strong trend favoring DC. Although the study was not designed to compare DC with DCb, the differences in survival and response between the 2 are intriguing.

In addition to survival outcomes, however, one must not forget another end point of crucial importance to NSCLC patients—reduction of symptoms and improvement in quality of life. In this study, patients treated with either docetaxel regimen had consistently improved quality of life compared to the vinorelbine/cisplatin-treated patients, who experienced a deterioration in quality of life.

Based on the strong trend toward improved survival with docetaxel/cisplatin, and improved quality of life with both docetaxel regimens, one must conclude that DC is probably the preferred combination over VC.

J. H. Schiller, MD

References

1. Traynor AM, Schiller JH: First line therapy in the treatment of advanced lung cancer, in Pass HI, Johnson DH, Mitchell JB, et al: *Lung Cancer: Principles and Practice*, 2003. New York: Lippincott Williams & Wilkins, pp 1-16.
2. Wozniak AJ, Crowley JJ, Balcerzak SP, et al: Randomized trial comparing cisplatin with cisplatin plus vinorelbine in the treatment of advanced non–small-cell lung cancer: A southwest oncology group study. *J Clin Oncol* 16:2459-2465, 1998.

3. Le Chevalier T, Brisgand D, Douillard J, et al: Randomized study of vinorelbine and cisplatin versus vindesine and cisplatin versus vinorelbine alone in advanced non–small-cell lung cancer: Results of a European multicenter trial including 612 patients. *J Clin Oncol* 12:360-367, 1994.
4. Kelly K, Crowley J, Bunn P, et al: Randomized phase III trial of paclitaxel plus carboplatin versus vinorelbine plus cisplatin in the treatment of patients with advanced non–small-cell lung cancer: A Southwest Oncology Group trial. *J Clin Oncol* 19:3210-3218, 2001.

Bronchioloalveolar Pathologic Subtype and Smoking History Predict Sensitivity to Gefitinib in Advanced Non–Small-Cell Lung Cancer

Miller VA, Kris MG, Shah N, et al (Mem Sloan-Kettering Cancer Ctr, New York)

J Clin Oncol 22:1103-1109, 2004 7–2

Introduction.—Gefitinib is an inhibitor of the epidermal growth factor receptor tyrosine kinase. It induces radiographic regressions and symptomatic improvement in patients with non–small cell lung cancer (NSCLC). Phase II trials indicate that female gender and adenocarcinoma are linked with response. Additional pathologic characteristics associated with sensitivity to gefitinib were examined.

Methods.—The medical records, pathologic material, and imaging studies were reviewed for 139 patients with NSCLC treated in 1 of 3 consecutive trials of gefitinib monotherapy at a single institution. Patients experiencing a major objective response were identified. Their clinical and pathologic features were compared with those of patients not having a major objective response. Univariate and multivariate analyses were performed on potential predictive characteristics linked with sensitivity to gefitinib.

Results.—Twenty-one patients (15%; 95% confidence interval, 9%-21%) had a partial radiographic response. Variables determined to be significant in univariate analysis included adenocarcinoma versus other NSCLCs (19% vs 0%; $P = .004$), adenocarcinoma with bronchioloalveolar features versus other adenocarcinomas (38% vs 14%; $P < .001$), never-smoker status versus former/current smoker (36% vs 8%; $P < .001$), and Karnofsky performance status 80% or greater versus 70% or greater (22% vs 8%; $P = .03$). Multivariate analysis showed that the presence of adenocarcinoma with any bronchioloalveolar features ($P = .004$) and never smoking ($P = .006$) were independently predictive of response.

Conclusion.—Patients in whom gefitinib is efficacious are more likely to have adenocarcinomas of the bronchioloalveolar subtype and to have never smoked. It may be that NSCLC has a different biology in individuals who never smoked and those with bronchioloalveolar carcinoma.

► This article summarizes the results of a retrospective review of patients treated with gefitinib at a single institution and correlates efficacy with clinical and pathologic features of disease. While the overall response rate with gefitinib in previously treated patients with NSCLC is low, it appears that certain subsets of patients are more likely to benefit than others. Namely, in a univariate analysis, adenocarcinoma (especially those with bronchioloalveolar features), never-smoker status, and higher performance status, were associated with improved outcomes compared with nonadenocarcinoma histology, current smokers, and lower performance status.

These data are consistent with subset analyses reported on other trials with gefitinib.[1,2] In addition, female gender appears associated with response, compared with males. These observations may reflect the biological differences in NSCLC within these subgroups. Future clinical trials should take into account these variables when assigning patient treatment and determining the optimal way to utilize this new class of drugs.

N. H. Hanna, MD

References

1. Fukuoka M, Yano S, Giaccone G, et al: Multi-institutional randomized phase II trial of gefitinib for previously treated patients with advanced non-small cell lung cancer. *J Clin Oncol* 21:2237-2246, 2003.
2. Kris M, Natale R, Herbst R, et al: Efficacy of gefitinib, an inhibitor of the epidermal growth factor receptor tyrosine kinase, in symptomatic patients with non-small cell lung cancer. *JAMA* 290:2149-2158, 2003.

► Gefitinib was approved by the Food and Drug Administration for therapy in recurrent NSCLC last year. Overall, only 15% of patients will respond, but a subgroup of patients seen has a much greater probability for response. These patients include those with adenocarcinoma containing bronchioloalveolar features and those who never smoked. The survival curve of responders had a striking difference compared to nonresponders. This points to a unique biology in these patients with bronchioloalveolar carcinoma, perhaps related to a less heterogenic gene mutation. This is an important syndrome of which internists should be aware.

P. J. Loehrer, Sr, MD

Gefitinib in Combination With Paclitaxel and Carboplatin in Advanced Non–Small-Cell Lung Cancer: A Phase III Trial—INTACT 2

Herbst RS, Giaccone G, Schiller JH, et al (Univ of Texas, Houston; Univ of Wisconsin, Madison; Cedars-Sinai Comprehensive Cancer Ctr, Beverly Hills, Calif; et al)

J Clin Oncol 22:785-794, 2004 7–3

Introduction.—Preclinical trials suggest that gefitinib may enhance the antitumor efficacy of cytotoxics. In combination with paclitaxel and carboplatin, it has demonstrated acceptable tolerability in a phase I trial. Gefitinib monotherapy has shown unparalleled antitumor activity for a biological agent, with lower toxicity levels versus docetaxel in phase II trials in patients with refractory, advanced non–small cell lung cancer (NSCLC). A phase III randomized, placebo-controlled, double-blind trial was performed to assess gefitinib plus paclitaxel and carboplatin in chemotherapy-naïve patients with advanced NSCLC.

Methods.—IV paclitaxel 225 mg/m^2 and IV carboplatin area under concentration/time curve of 6 mg/min/mL (day 1 every 3 weeks) plus gefitinib 500 mg/d, gefitinib 250 mg/d, or placebo was administered. After a maximum of 6 cycles, daily gefitinib or placebo was continued until disease progression. The end points included overall survival, time to progression (TTP), response rate (RR), and safety assessment.

Results.—The baseline characteristics were well balanced in the 1037 patients who were recruited. No difference was observed in overall survival (median, 8.7, 9.8, and 9.9 months for gefitinib 500 mg/d, 250 mg/d, and placebo, respectively; $P = .64$), TTP, or RR between treatment arms. Expected dose-associated diarrhea and skin toxicity were seen in patients in the gefitinib group, with no new significant or unexpected safety findings from combination with chemotherapy. Subset analysis of patients with adenocarcinoma who received more than 90 days of chemotherapy showed statistically significant prolonged survival, indicating a gefitinib maintenance effect.

Conclusion.—The use of gefitinib offered no added benefit to survival, TTP, or RR, compared with standard chemotherapy alone. This large placebo-controlled trial verified the favorable gefitinib safety profile seen in phase I and II monotherapy trials.

▶ In this article, Herbst et al report the negative results of a large, multi-institutional phase III trial that failed to demonstrate an improvement in RR, TTP, or overall survival when empirically adding gefitinib to carboplatin and paclitaxel in chemotherapy-naïve patients with advanced NSCLC. A subset of patients with adenocarcinoma who received 90 days or more of treatment appeared to have prolonged survival when utilizing gefitinib. The trial design allowed patients to enter, regardless of their tumor epidermal growth factor receptor (EGFR) status. However, the majority of NSCLCs express the EGFR, and it is therefore unlikely that selecting only patients with EGFR expression would have resulted in a positive survival outcome. The results of a similar trial performed in Europe with cisplatin plus gemcitabine with/without gefitinib were nearly identical.[1]

Why were the results of these trials negative? One could speculate on several reasons, namely, gefitinib is targeting the same treatment-sensitive tumor cell population as chemotherapy, there may have been an antagonism between the agents given in this schedule, or perhaps the inability to select a more targeted patient population which would be susceptible to the effects of gefitinib resulted in this negative trial result.

It should not be surprising, however, that empirically adding a third active agent to a platinum-based doublet would not result in a positive result, as many 3-drug combinations have failed to improve survival over 2-drug combinations. Future trials of targeted agents such as gefitinib will take into account both patient and tumor characteristics which have been observed to result in a higher likelihood of responding to this agent.

N. H. Hanna, MD

Reference

1. Giaccone G, Herbst R, Manegold C, et al: Gefitinib in combination with gemcitabine and cisplatin in advanced non–small-cell lung cancer: A phase III trial-INTACT 1. *J Clin Oncol* 22:777-784, 2004.

Determinants of Tumor Response and Survival With Erlotinib in Patients With Non–Small-Cell Lung Cancer

Pérez-Soler R, Chachoua A, Hammond LA, et al (Albert Einstein College of Medicine, Bronx, NY; New York Univ; Inst for Drug Development, San Antonio, Tex; et al)

J Clin Oncol 22:3238-3247, 2004 7–4

Introduction.—Erlotinib is a highly specific epidermal growth factor receptor (HER1/EGFR) tyrosine kinase inhibitor that is a direct and reversible enzyme inhibitor in vitro, with a median inhibitory concentration of 2 nmol/L (0.79 ng/mL). The objective tumor response rate of erlotinib administered as a single agent in patients with advanced (stage IIIB or IV) or recurrent metastatic HER1/EGFR-positive non–small cell lung cancer (NSCLC) previously treated with platinum-based combination therapy was examined in a phase II investigation.

Methods.—An oral, continuous daily dose of 150 mg erlotinib was administered to 57 patients. Objective response was measured by World Health Organization and Response Evaluation Criteria in Solid Tumors. The European Organization for Research and Treatment of Cancer Quality of Life Questionnaire C30, supplemented with a lung cancer module, Quality of Life Questionnaire LC13, was used to assess health-related quality of life.

Results.—Treatment with oral erlotinib yielded a response rate of 12.3% (95% confidence interval [CI], 5.1%-23.7%). Responses were seen regardless of type or number of previous chemotherapy regimens. The median survival was 8.4 months (95% CI, 4.8-13.9 months). One-year survival was 40% (95% CI, 28%-54%). Erlotinib therapy was linked with tumor-associated symptom improvement. It was well tolerated. Drug-related cutaneous rash and diarrhea occurred in 75% and 56% of the cohort, respectively. Toxicity consisting of severe grade 3 rash and diarrhea occurred in 1 patient. Time since diagnosis and good performance status were significant predictors of survival by a multivariate Cox proportional hazards model; HER1/EGFR staining intensity was not predictive of survival. Survival was associated with the occurrence and severity of rash.

Conclusion.—Erlotinib was active and well tolerated in patients with advanced or recurrent HER1/EGFR-expressing NSCLC. Cutaneous rash appears to be a surrogate marker of clinical benefit.

▶ This is a phase II study evaluating the EGFR tyrosine kinase inhibitor, erlotinib, in previously treated patients with advanced NSCLC. The overall response rate, stable disease rate, and quality of life scores with erlotinib on this trial are similar to those seen with another EGFR tyrosine kinase inhibitor, gefitinib. While patients were allowed to dose escalate, the majority received the standard 150-mg daily dose. Patient selection included a large percentage whose diagnosis of lung cancer was more than 12 months before study entry and who were receiving erlotinib as third- or fourth-line therapy and had a performance status (PS) of 0 or 1. Response seemed to correlate with skin rash, an observation seen on other studies with EGFR inhibitors. Response to erlotinib was independent of PS or the number of prior regimens received, although overall survival time significantly favored those with a good PS. This study adds to the body of evidence that EGFR inhibitors play an important role in some patients with NSCLC.

N. H. Hanna, MD

Early Stage and Adjuvant Therapy

Estimate of Lung Cancer Mortality From Low-Dose Spiral Computed Tomography Screening Trials: Implications for Current Mass Screening Recommendations

Patz EF Jr, Swensen SJ, Herndon JE II (Duke Univ, Durham, NC; Mayo Clinic, Rochester, Minn)

J Clin Oncol 22:2202-2206, 2004 7–5

Background.—Low-dose helical CT has been suggested for lung cancer screening, as it can detect small pulmonary nodules in asymptomatic individuals. Data from 2 published trials were reanalyzed to determine the effect of CT screening on lung cancer mortality rates.

Study Design.—A comprehensive literature review found only 2 CT screening trials that had published the lung cancer prevalence at initial screening and at least the first annual examination: the Mayo Clinic Study and the Early Lung Cancer Action Program (ELCAP). Previously published 5-year survival data were used to calculate the number of predicted lung cancer deaths. The actual mortality rate was calculated for each study, and these were compared with the data in the previously published Mayo Lung Project, which used chest radiographs and sputum cytology for screening.

Findings.—The lung cancer mortality rate was 4.1 deaths per 1000 person-years in the Mayo Clinic CT screening trial, 5.5 per 1000 person-years in the ELCAP study, 4.4 per 1,000 person-years in the interventional arm and 3.9 per 1000 person-years in the standard-care arm of the Mayo Lung Project.

Conclusions.—This reanalysis of published data found that CT screening did not improve lung cancer mortality rates above standard screening methods and that standard screening was not better than usual care controls. Mass screening for lung cancer should not be recommended to the general public until randomized clinical trials demonstrate benefit.

► The majority of patients diagnosed with non–small cell lung cancer will succumb to the disease within 5 years. The vast majority of those surviving more than 5 years after the diagnosis are found to have stage I or II disease. While prevention is the ultimate goal to reduce the incidence of death due to lung cancer, early detection remains an important population-based strategy. Unfortunately, earlier efforts to reduce lung cancer mortality with chest radiograph (CXR) screening and sputum evaluation have not proven effective, even though earlier detection was achieved. Spiral CTs are able to image smaller lung tumors than CXR and more accurately image the mediastinum as well. Several randomized trials are under way evaluating the ability of spiral CTs in reducing lung cancer mortality rate. This study by Patz et al reports similar lung cancer mortality rate with screening CXR and earlier reports on screening CT scans. These data suggest that CT screening studies may produce similar outcomes to those with CXR screening studies.

N. H. Hanna, MD

[18F]FLT PET for Diagnosis and Staging of Thoracic Tumours

Dittmann H, Dohmen BM, Paulsen F, et al (Eberhard-Karls-Univ Tübingen, Germany)

Eur J Nucl Med Mol Imaging 30:1407-1412, 2003 7–6

Background.—For non–small cell lung cancer (NSCLC), the ultimate goal of treatment is the arrest of tumor cell proliferation. An accumulation of 3'-deoxy-3'-[^{18}F]fluorothymidine (FLT) is noted after phosphorylation by cellular thymidine kinase-1. The uptake of FLT depends on cell proliferation, with increased levels in tumor tissue and other rapidly proliferating normal tissue, such as bone marrow. Positron emission tomography (PET) with FLT was used to detect untreated malignant thoracic tumors and metastases in patients with NSCLC and esophageal cancer. Because of the high sensitivity of fluorine-18 fluorodeoxyglucose (FDG) PET in evaluating thoracic nodules and staging lung cancer, FDG PET was used for direct comparison with FLT in all patients except those with esophageal cancer. Verification of the PET findings was based on conventional morphologic imaging, histology, and follow-up data.

Methods.—Sixteen patients with 18 tumors underwent whole-body FLT PET before beginning treatment. The 12 tumors that were not esophageal cancers were also studied with FDG PET. Measurements included the calculation of average and maximum standardized uptake values.

Results.—Both the hematopoietic bone marrow and the liver had intense FLT uptake, and the kidneys and urinary bladder were regularly seen because they are involved with renal excretion of the FLT. Minor tracer accumulation was found in all other organs. Significant FLT and FDG uptake was found in all primary NSCLCs (Fig 1). Neither of these methods detected a small renal carcinoma in one patient. All the esophageal tumors were clearly indicated by the high FLT uptake. Tumors of the squamous cell type had higher FLT uptake than adenocarcinomatous tumors. Six patients had metastases, and regional and distant metastases both showed high uptake. Brain metastases were clearly differentiated from normal brain tissue by FLT. FDG detected 1 of the 2 brain metastases. A bone metastasis in the cer-

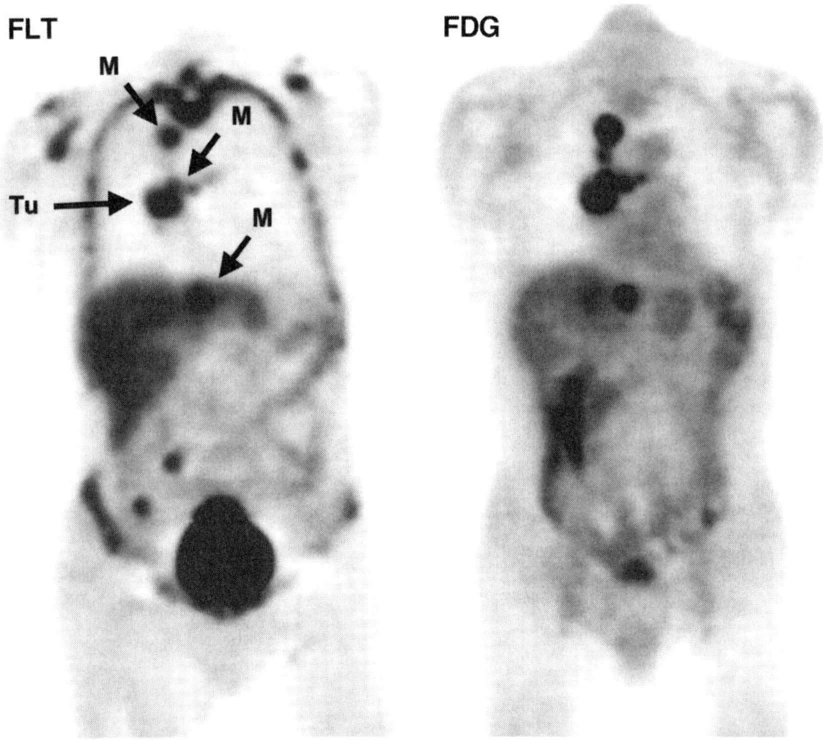

FIGURE 1.—PET findings with FLT (**left**) and FDG (**right**) in a patient (no. 5) presenting with NSCLC and locoregional, mediastinal, and distant metastases in the liver. *Abbreviations: M*, Metastasis; *Tu*, primary tumor. (Courtesy of Dittmann H, Dohmen BM, Paulsen F, et al: [^{18}F]FLT PET for diagnosis and staging of thoracic tumours. *Eur J Nucl Med Mol Imaging* 30:1407-1412, 2003. Copyright 2003, Springer-Verlag.)

vical spine was missed by FLT; in another patient, a bone lesion displayed intense FLT accumulation. FDG PET was able to detect both lesions. Increased FLT uptake in the upper abdomen in the absence of any physiologic abnormality was attributed to radioactivity accumulated in the colon wall. In comparison with the uptake of FDG, the uptake of FLT was significantly less at most primary or metastatic sites. One case suspected to have rapid cell proliferation had preferential FLT accumulation. The average and maximum standardized uptake values for FLT and for FDG were moderately but significantly correlated. Neither of the PET tracers yielded any false-positive results.

Conclusions.—FLT PET was highly sensitive for detecting untreated malignant tumors of the thorax. High physiologic FLT uptake in the liver and bone marrow tends to lessen the effectiveness of FLT. For brain lesions, FLT may be more sensitive than FDG.

► With the advent of PET scanning, diagnosis and staging based on FDG has been common and highly touted for patients with malignant diseases, particularly lymphomas and lung cancer. These investigators from Germany have looked at FLT and have some impressive pictures to suggest that FLT PET scanning may actually be superior to FDG. Certainly, the FDG has major problems distinguishing inflammation from neoplasm. It remains to be seen just how important this step is, but I believe this approach is certainly worth evaluating prospectively.

E. Glatstein, MD

Randomized Controlled Trial of the Role of Positron Emission Tomography in the Management of Stage I and II Non–Small-Cell Lung Cancer

Viney RC, Boyer MJ, King MT (Univ of Technology, Sydney, Australia; Sydney Cancer Centre, Australia; Royal Prince Alfred Hosp, Sydney, Australia; et al)

J Clin Oncol 22:2357-2362, 2004 7–7

Introduction.—Positron emission tomography (PET) is a costly new technology that has the potential to improve preoperative assessments in patients with non–small cell lung cancer (NSCLC). Pressure is increasing to include PET in the standard diagnostic workup of these patients before making decisions regarding the surgical management of NSCLC. The influence of PET on clinical management and surgical outcomes was evaluated in patients with stage I-II NSCLC in a randomized controlled trial.

Methods.—The study included 184 patients with stage I-II NSCLC (92% had stage I disease) who were assigned randomly to either PET or no PET (conventional staging). Patients in the PET group underwent preoperative [^{18}F]fluorodeoxyglucose (FDG) PET. On the basis of PET results, the provisional diagnosis and planned management were reviewed. Local or distant metastatic disease was verified by biopsy. When abnormalities identified by PET were unable to be confirmed, thoracotomy was performed.

Results.—Compared with the results of conventional staging, PET upstaged 22 patients, verified staging in 61, and staged 2 patients as benign. Stage IV disease was rarely identified (n = 2). In 13% of patients, PET led to further investigation or a change in clinical management; it provided information that could have impacted management in an additional 13% of patients. The sensitivity and specificity of PET for diagnosis of mediastinal disease was 73% and 90%, respectively. No significant between-group differences were noted in the number of thoracotomies avoided (P = .2).

Conclusion.—In patients who are carefully and appropriately staged with stage I-II disease, PET provides potential for more appropriate stage-specific therapy but may not lead to a significant decrease in the number of thoracotomies avoided.

► Staging of NSCLC now routinely involves the use of PET imaging. Accurate staging of the mediastinum remains a fundamental problem as therapeutic decisions will vary significantly, based upon the extent of tumor involvement in the mediastinum. The study by Viney et al. poses an interesting question: Does PET imaging, which results in an additional cost in the preoperative workup, reduce the number of patients who undergo "futile" thoracotomies?

Compared to conventional staging, PET suggested a different stage in 24 patients and no change in stage in 61 patients. In this study, PET imaging detected only 3 patients with stage IV disease. There was no significant difference in the number of thoracotomies avoided between the PET arm and the non-PET arm. The utility of PET appears to be in the more accurate staging of the mediastinum; however, the optimal management of patients with stage III disease remains controversial, including the role of surgery altogether. If PET detects mediastinal lymph node involvement in apparent "normal" lymph nodes, does therapeutic management change? Furthermore, other factors that may be important should also be considered in interpreting the results of PET-positive mediastinal disease, such as the type of surgery necessary for a "rule out" resection, the size and location of the primary tumor, the number of mediastinal nodal stations involved, and the number of nodes involved at each station.

N. H. Hanna, MD

Detecting Lung Cancer in Plasma With the Use of Multiple Genetic Markers

Andriani F, Conte D, Mastrangelo T, et al (Istituto Nazionale Tumori, Milan, Italy; European Inst of Oncology, Milan, Italy; Royal Brompton Hosp, London)
Int J Cancer 108:91-96, 2004 7–8

Background.—Recent research has shown that detecting genetic changes in the plasma DNA of patients with cancer is possible. A panel of molecular markers for lung cancer detection in plasma DNA was validated.

Methods.—The study included 64 patients with stage I through III non–small-cell lung cancer. Three markers were used to identify mutations in tumor and plasma DNA. These were p53, *FHIT*, and microsatellite changes at loci on chromosome 3. Direct sequencing of exons 5 through 8 in tumor DNA was used to determine p53 mutations. Plaque hybridization assay and sequencing were done in plasma DNA. Allelic losses were assessed using fluorescent polymerase chain reaction (PCR) in tumor and plasma DNA.

Findings.—Genomic mutations on p53 were found in 40.6% of tumor DNA samples. The identical mutation was identified in the plasma of 73.1% of the samples. Microsatellite changes at *FHIT* and 3p loci were documented in 62.5% of tumors and in 35.9% of plasma samples. The same change in plasma DNA was identified in 47.5% of the 40 patients with microsatellite changes in tumors. One or more of the genetic markers studied was altered in the plasma of 51.6% of the group overall and in 60.7% of patients with stage I disease. Genetic markers in plasma identified 64.4% of all stages and 68.2% of stage I cases with an alteration.

Conclusions.—These data support the hypothesis that alterations in plasma DNA are tumor specific in most patients. Blood testing should be considered as a noninvasive strategy for early detection.

▶ Lung cancer is a common disease in both men and women in the United States and around the world and remains the No. 1 cause of cancer-related death. Cures are possible for patients with early stage lung cancer, particularly those with stage I and II; however, the majority of patients are diagnosed with advanced stage disease at clinical presentation. Early detection of lung cancer is possible with routine chest x-ray (CXR) screening; however, early detection does not necessarily translate into reduced lung cancer–specific mortality rates. Modern CT imaging provides a tool to detect tumors that are undetectable on CXR; therefore, it is possible that more patients will be diagnosed with even smaller stage I lung cancers with CT screening compared with CXR screening. Unfortunately, as the resolution of our studies improves, more "innocent" nodules are detected as well and are subsequently biopsied. Therefore, a noninvasive manner to discriminate between benign and malignant nodules is desirable. Andriani et al report the results of their work evaluating plasma DNA of cancer patients. The goal was to validate a panel of genetic markers that predict for lung cancer detection. P53 mutations, *FHIT*, and microsatellite alterations in chromosome 3 were used. Their research reported that a high percentage of patients with lung cancer had detectable levels of one or more of these markers. Further study, including prospective trials, is needed to further validate this data. Sensitivity of these assays remains an obstacle for use of this in routine practice.

N. H. Hanna, MD

Protein Expression Profiles in Adenocarcinomas and Squamous Cell Carcinomas of the Lung Generated Using Tissue Microarrays

Ullmann R, Morbini P, Halbwedl I, et al (Univ Med School of Graz, Austria; Univ of Pavia, Italy; Univ of Torino, Italy)

J Pathol 203:798-807, 2004 7–9

Introduction.—Tissue microarrays (TMAs) permit the simultaneous and cost-efficient analysis of a large number of tumors for alterations in DNA, RNA, and proteins. A broad spectrum of antibodies identifying proteins engaged in apoptosis, genome surveillance, cell adhesion, and other cellular activities was examined by using TMAs to establish protein profiles for adenocarcinomas (ACs) and squamous cell carcinoma (SQCC).

Methods.—Two TMAs were generated: 1 that included 75 primary ACs and 1 that was composed of 67 primary SQCCs. On both arrays, every tumor was represented by an average of 5 cores. Additionally, 1 punch of normal lung parenchyma adjacent to each tumor was included. Immunohistochemical expression of 86 proteins was evaluated; the results were analyzed by nonparametric tests, hierarchical clustering, and principal component analysis.

Results.—For both AC and SQCC, parenchyma and tumors were clearly separated by hierarchical clustering. By using the same statistical approach, it was possible to distinguish ACs from SQCCs with 98% accuracy and to distinguish parenchyma adjacent to the ACs from those adjacent to SQCCs with 96% accuracy. It was possible to separate ACs into 3 groups that significantly varied in survival. Cathepsin E and hsp10 were recognized as previously unknown predictors of survival in lung AC.

Conclusion.—Protein profiles are feasible tools for predicting biologic behavior. The approach of individualized therapeutic strategies based on the new, defect-targeted drugs will alter the way tumors need to be assessed, thanks to the creation of tumor profiles based on analysis of molecular defects.

▶ This interesting study by Ullmann et al evaluates a broad spectrum of antibodies detecting proteins engaged in apoptosis, genome surveillance, cell adhesion, and other cellular activities by using TMAs. The authors detected some shared protein expressions in SQCCs and ACs but also reported that they differed in approximately 50% of other proteins. Furthermore, ACs could be further divided into 3 main clusters according to clinical outcome. Specific proteins, such as cathepsin E and hsp 105 were identified as predictors of survival. This study demonstrated that protein profiles are feasible tools to predict clinical behavior. Future study of these protein pathways and their corresponding genes is needed.

N. H. Hanna, MD

Prognostic Model of Pulmonary Adenocarcinoma by Expression Profiling of Eight Genes As Determined by Quantitative Real-Time Reverse Transcriptase Polymerase Chain Reaction

Endoh H, Tomida S, Yatabe Y, et al (Aichi Cancer Ctr Hosp, Japan; Gunma Univ, Maebashi, Japan)

J Clin Oncol 22:811-819, 2004 7–10

Introduction.—Several expression-profiling investigations have revealed that adenocarcinoma can be classified into subgroups that also reflect patient survival. Forty-four genes were investigated to test whether their expression patterns were relevant to prognosis. A prognostic model applicable to clinical practice was created.

Methods.—Expression levels were determined in patients by quantitative reverse transcriptase polymerase chain reaction in 85 consecutive patients who underwent pulmonary resection between December 1995 through May 1998. Cluster analyses were performed. The prognostic model was created by the proportional hazards model by using a stepwise method.

Results.—Hierarchical clustering divided cases into 3 main prognostic groups that were independent of pathologic stage, differentiation, or extent of tumor content. One of the subgroups (group B; 21 cases) demonstrated significantly poorer overall survival compared with the other 2 subgroups and included preferentially more male, more elderly, and more smoking patients. In an attempt to identify a smaller number of genes of predictive value, 8 genes were selected (*PTK7, CIT, SCNN1A, PGES, ERO1L, ZWINT*, and 2 *ESTs*). A risk index was calculated that was defined as a linear combination of gene expression values weighted by their estimated regression coefficients. The risk index was a significant independent prognostic factor on multivariate analysis ($P = .0021$). The robustness of the model was verified by using an independent set of 21 patients ($P = .085$).

Conclusion.—By analyzing a relatively small number of genes, patients with adenocarcinoma could be stratified by prognosis. This prognostic model can be applied to future decisions regarding treatment.

► Adenocarcinoma is the most common histology of lung cancer in Japan and the United States. Optimal treatment planning requires identifying patients with a good prognosis after surgery with those who have a poor prognosis. This study used real-time reverse transcriptase polymerase chain reaction to evaluate 44 genes as prognostic markers for adenocarcinoma of the lung. Endoh et al reports 3 major clusters of adenocarcinoma that were independent of stage, differentiation, or tumor content. In addition, 8 genes (of the 44 studied) were selected to calculate a risk index predictive of outcome.

N. H. Hanna, MD

Preoperative F-18 Fluorodeoxyglucose–Positron Emission Tomography Maximal Standardized Uptake Value Predicts Survival After Lung Cancer Resection

Downey RJ, Akhurst T, Gonen M, et al (Mem Sloan-Kettering Cancer Ctr, New York)

J Clin Oncol 22:3255-3260, 2004 7–11

Introduction.—The rate of F-18 fluorodeoxyglucose [^{18}F]FDG) in the primary site of non–small cell lung cancer (NSCLC) has been linked with doubling time and proliferation rates, which are known to be correlated with tumor aggressiveness. On the basis of these findings, it has been suggested that the intensity of [^{18}F]FDG uptake, as measured by positron emission tomography (PET) imaging (the maximal standardized uptake value [SUV_{MAX}]) in the primary tumor may be predictive of survival. A retrospective review of surgically treated patients imaged preoperatively with [^{18}F]FDG-PET was performed to ascertain whether the primary tumor SUV is predictive of patient survival.

Methods.—Patients with NSCLC or carcinoid pT1-4, NO-4 disease treated with surgical resection alone underwent CT scan and PET within 90 days preoperatively. Prognostic variables were assessed by log-rank test and survival was calculated by Kaplan-Meier analysis.

Results.—The medical records of 100 consecutive patients (48 male, 52 female) were reviewed. The median follow-up of survivors was 28 months (range, 16-81 months). The median SUV_{MAX} was 9. The 2-year survival for patients with SUV_{MAX} greater than 9 and less than 9 was 68% and 96%, respectively ($P < .01$). Multivariate analysis that included pathologic tumor size, involved nodes, histology, and SUV_{MAX}, showed only tumor size greater than 3 cm and SUV_{MAX} greater than 9 and their interaction were significantly predictive of survival ($P = .01$, $P = .02$, and $P < .01$, respectively). The 3-year survival rate among patients with both tumor size smaller than 3 cm and SUV_{MAX} less than 9 was 97%; for those with tumor size smaller than 3 cm and SUV_{MAX} greater than 9, it was 94%; for those with tumor size larger than 3 cm and SUV_{MAX} less than 9, it was 93%; and for patients with tumor size larger than 3 cm and SUV_{MAX} greater than 9, survival was 47% ($P < .01$).

Conclusion.—In patients with NSCLC who are surgically managed, SUV is predictive of overall survival after resection. The addition of SUV_{MAX} to pathologic size identifies a subgroup of patients at highest risk of death of recurrent disease after resection.

▶ The treatment of early stage NSCLC in patients who are medically operable with surgically resectable disease is undertaken with curative intent. Recent evidence suggests that adjuvant chemotherapy improves survival for patients with completely surgically resected stage Ib-IIIa disease. However, outcomes vary significantly depending on the stage of disease, size of primary tumor, and presence of mediastinal nodal involvement, including the number of nodes and levels involved. Because of this heterogeneity of disease, treatment decisions can be difficult for an individual patient. This report from the Thoracic Surgery Service of Memorial Sloan-Kettering Cancer Center reports that the SUV of FDG-PET is a predictor of overall survival after surgical resection. Although this is a retrospective review, these data suggest a significantly lower survival rate for patients with SUV greater than 9 compared with those less than 9 (2-year survival, 68% vs 98%). Further evaluation of this preoperative variable is warranted and may lead to the need for future randomized trials to stratify based on preoperative SUV.

N. H. Hanna, MD

Positron Emission Tomography in Limited-Stage Small-Cell Lung Cancer: A Prospective Study

Bradley JD, Dehdashti F, Mintun MA, et al (Washington Univ, St Louis)

J Clin Oncol 22:3248-3254, 2004 7–12

Background.—Accurate staging of small cell lung cancer (SCLC) is important for both prognosis and treatment planning. SCLC staging usually involves CT and bone scintigraphy. To determine the utility of fluorodeoxyglucose positron emission tomography (FDG-PET) in the staging of SCLC and in treatment planning, a prospective study was done.

Study Design.—Pretreatment FDG-PET was performed on 24 patients with newly diagnosed SCLC, who were determined to have limited disease by standard staging techniques. The utility of FDG-PET in staging and treatment planning was assessed.

Results.—FDG-PET had findings consistent with extensive stage SCLC in 3 of these 24 patients considered to have limited stage disease by conventional staging. PET correctly identified tumor in each SCLC mass. PET detected previously unsuspected regional node metastases in 6 of 24 patients. The therapy plan of these patients was significantly altered to include these PET-identified nodes within the high-dose radiation therapy region.

Conclusions.—FDG-PET has a high sensitivity for SCLC. This technique appears to be a useful adjunct for both staging and treatment planning of patients with SCLC.

▶ This article reports the sensitivity of FDG-PET for staging SCLC. Currently, all patients with SCLC are divided into 2 stages: limited versus extensive. All patients are treated with chemotherapy; however, chest radiation is usually used for those with limited stage disease. Chest radiation significantly increases the toxicity (including toxic death) and, thus, accurate staging is vital. Given the high proliferate rates of SCLC, FDG-PET ranging would be a logical staging modality. The author from Washington University in St Louis reports a high degree of sensitivity for FDG-PET staging of SCLC, including upstaging 2 patients and discovering unsuspected nodal disease in 25% of patients. FDG-PET may have value, therefore, in treatment planning for patients with SCLC. Further studies are certainly warranted.

N. H. Hanna, MD

Advanced Diseases

Long-term Survival in SCLC After Treatment With Paclitaxel, Carboplatin and Etoposide: A Phase II Study

Reck M, Jagos U, Grunwald F, et al (Hosp Grosshansdorf, Hamburg, Germany; Community Hosp, Hamburg-Harburg, Germany; Hosp Gauting, Munich)

Lung Cancer 39:63-69, 2003 7–13

Background.—In the treatment of small cell lung cancer (SCLC), standard chemotherapy regimens achieve complete response rates of 65% to 90% when there is limited disease (LD), and 20% to 30% with extensive disease (ED). Carboplatin can be substituted for cisplatin to minimize the nephrotoxicity and neurotoxicity accompanying cisplatin while maintaining a good response. Paclitaxel has proved promising in patients with extensive SCLC when combined with etoposide. The addition of paclitaxel to a carboplatin/etoposide regimen was evaluated to determine the resulting toxicity profile and activity as first-line treatment for patients with limited and extensive SCLC.

Methods.—For the 89 patients (median age, 61 years; age range, 36-76 years) who participated, paclitaxel 175 mg/m^2 was given by a 1-hour IV infusion immediately before a 30-minute infusion of carboplatin at an area under the concentration time curve of 5 on day 1, and etoposide, 50 mg orally twice a day, was given on days 2 through 8. The courses were repeated every 21 days, with patients who had objective responses undergoing a maximum of 6 courses. On completing chemotherapy, LD patients who responded had consolidative radiotherapy (total dose, 50-56 Gy) in standard fractions of 1.8 to 2 Gy over 6 weeks. Those with complete remission (CR) also had adjuvant cranial irradiation in single doses of 2 to 2.5 Gy up to a total dose of 30 Gy. LD was defined as local tumor disease with ipsilateral or contralateral mediastinal or hilar lymph node metastases. ED I was defined as local advanced tumor with infiltration of the surrounding organ systems or pleural/pericardial effusion, or ipsilateral/contralateral supraclavical lymph node metastases.

Results.—Fifteen patients had CR, 54 had partial response (PR), 13 had stable disease, and 2 had disease progression. The overall response rate was 82.1%. Among those with LD, CR was noted in 20.4% and PR in 66.6%. In the patients with ED, 13.3% had CR and 60.0% had PR. Neutropenia developed in 44.9% of all courses, with infrequent episodes of thrombocytopenia and anemia. Moderate nonhematologic toxic reactions developed, principally gastrointestinal symptoms and myalgia. Alopecia developed in 51% of all courses. The median overall survival was 18.1 months. One-year survival was 56.8% and 3-year survival was 14.8%. LD patients had a 20.5-month median survival, a 71.4% survival rate at 1 year, and a 21.4% survival rate at 3 years. ED I patients had a median survival of 11 months, 1-year survival rate of 31.3%, and a 3-year survival rate of 3.1% (Fig 1). The median progression-free interval for LD patients was 12.3 months; that for ED I patients was 8 months. The overall median progression-free interval was 10.3 months.

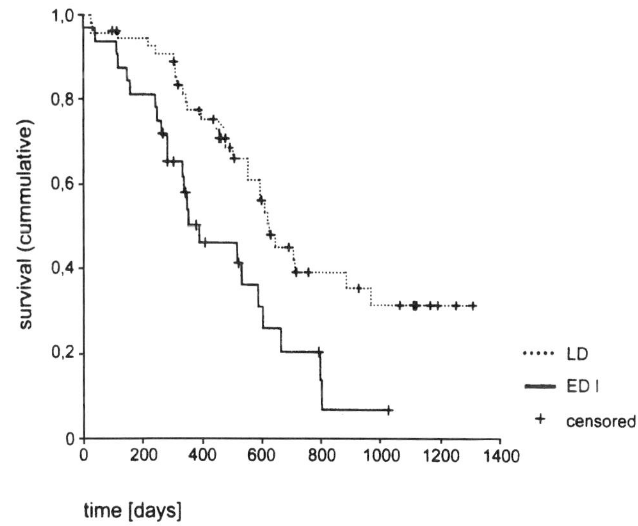

FIGURE 1.—Kaplan-Meier analysis: Overall survival (stages LD + ED I). Stage LD: Median survival: 618 days = 20.5 months (95% confidence interval: 495-741 days). Mean survival: 750 days = 24.7 months (95% confidence interval: 626-875 days) 27 of 56 cases censored. One-year survival: 71.4%. Three-year survival: 21.4%. Stage ED I: Median survival: 330 days = 11.0 months (95% confidence interval: 163-497 days). Mean survival: 390 days = 12.0 months (95% confidence interval: 301-479 days) 9 of 32 cases censored. One-year survival: 31-3%. Three-year survival: 3.1%. (Reprinted by permission of the publisher from Reck M, Jagos U, Grunwald F, et al: Long-term survival in SCLC after treatment with paclitaxel, carboplatin and etoposide: A phase II study. *Lung Cancer* 39:63-69, 2003. Copyright 2003 by Elsevier Science Inc.)

Conclusions.—The combination of paclitaxel, carboplatin, and etoposide proved to be effective and well tolerated in these patients with SCLC.

► These German investigators present a phase II study on SCLC, treating such patients with paclitaxel, carboplatin, and etoposide. You can read the title and the abstract and not know that LD patients who responded received consolidative thoracic radiotherapy as well as prophylactic cranial irradiation. Looking at Fig 1, there is no particular reason to get excited about the results in ED, and the results that they report in LD patients are not obviously better than what has been reported in several large cooperative study settings.

It would have been nice to have seen the words "radiation treatment" somewhere in the abstract or in the title of this article. For those who only read the abstract, they would take away an erroneous conclusion.

E. Glatstein, MD

Phase II Study of Imatinib in Patients With Small Cell Lung Cancer

Johnson BE, Fischer T, Fischer B, et al (Dana Farber Cancer Inst, Boston; Universitaets-Klinikum, Mainz, Germany; Glasgow Royal Infirmary, Scotland; et al)

Clin Cancer Res 9:5880-5887, 2003 7–14

Introduction.—Small cell lung cancer (SCLC) is rarely cured by currently available therapy. Chemotherapy has improved survival during the past 20 years, but the 5-year survival rate in patients with extensive-stage SCLC remains only 2%. Additional effective anticancer therapies are needed. Both autocrine and paracrine growth mechanisms can stimulate the growth of SCLC. Bombesin-like peptides are produced and secreted by SCLC cells, bind to 1 of 3 bombesin receptors, and stimulate their own growth. An antibody that binds to the bombesin-like peptides has demonstrated antitumor activity. The objective response to imatinib was assessed in previously treated and untreated patients with extensive-stage SCLC.

Methods.—All patients were treated with 600 mg daily imatinib for up to 12 months. The response was evaluated at 3 and 6 weeks with the use of Southwest Oncology Group criteria. Tumor specimens were analyzed by immunohistochemistry for the KIT receptor.

Results.—Of 19 participants (16 men, 3 women), 9 had previously untreated extensive-stage disease and 10 had sensitive relapse. A central pathology review verified SCLC in 14 patients. There were no objective responses, but 1 patient with sensitive-relapse disease experienced prolonged stabilization of disease (more than 3 months) while receiving imatinib therapy. The median time to disease progression was 0.8 months (range, 0.6-1.3 months) and 1.2 months (range, 0.2-4.1 months) in the previously untreated and sensitive-relapse groups, respectively. The KIT receptor (CD117) was detected in tumor tissue samples from 4 (21%) patients.

Conclusion.—No antitumor activity was observed in this limited phase II trial of patients with SCLC, in which only a few tumors demonstrated expression of the imatinib target. These findings are regarded as inconclusive concerning the antitumor activity of imatinib against SCLC with the targeted KIT receptor (CD117).

▶ Imatinib is an orally bioavailable small molecule that inhibits not only the Bcr-Abl fusion protein, found in chronic myeloid leukemia, but also PDGF and *c*-Kit, the latter being found in the rare gastrointestinal stromal tumor. Based upon reports showing that up to 70% of SCLCs express the KIT receptor and/or its ligand SCF, Johnson and co-workers conducted a phase II study of imatinib in chemotherapy-naive extensive stage SCLC or SCLC in a sensitive relapse.

No responses were observed. However, only 4 of the 19 patients had tumor samples which were positive for the KIT receptor. This study is inconclusive regarding the activity of imatinib in SCLC, given that only 4 patients had the target of interest. It also demonstrates, however, that KIT expression is much lower in SCLC than originally believed.

J. H. Schiller, MD

The Outcome of Combined-Modality Therapy for Stage III Non–Small-Cell Lung Cancer in the Elderly

Schild SE, Stella PJ, Geyer SM, et al (Mayo Clinic, Rochester, Minn; Michigan Cancer Consortium Community Clinical Oncology Program (CCOP), Ann Arbor, Mich; Univ of Alabama, Birmingham; et al)

J Clin Oncol 21:3201-3206, 2003 7–15

Background.—In a recent phase III trial, the North Central Cancer Treatment Group found no survival difference between chemotherapy plus twice-a day radiation therapy (RT) or daily RT in patients with stage III non–small cell lung cancer (NSCLC). A secondary analysis was done to investigate the possible association between patient age and outcome.

Methods.—The original study randomly assigned 246 patients to etoposide plus cisplatin and RT daily or in a split-course twice-daily regimen. Outcomes of elderly patients (70 years or older) were compared with those younger than 70. Of the 244 assessable patients, 26% were elderly, and 74% were younger.

Findings.—Among younger patients, survival rates were 39% at 2 years and 18% at 5 years. Among the elderly group, these rates were 36% and 13%, respectively. Rates of toxicity of grade 4 or higher were 62% in younger patients and 81% in elderly patients. Of the younger patients, 56% had grade 4 or higher hematologic toxicity, compared with that of 78% of elderly patients. Grade 4 or higher pneumonitis occurred in 1% of the younger group and in 6% of the elderly group.

Conclusions.—The elderly patients receiving combined-modality treatment for locally advanced NSCLC had more pronounced toxicity, especially myelosuppression and pneumonitis. However, elderly patients had survival rates comparable to those of younger patients. Otherwise healthy elderly persons with locally advanced NSCLC should be encouraged to undergo combined-modality treatment, preferably in clinical studies with careful monitoring.

The Impact of Age on Toxicity, Response Rate, Quality of Life, and Survival in Patients With Advanced, Stage IIIB or IV Nonsmall Cell Lung Carcinoma Treated With Carboplatin and Paclitaxel

Hensing TA, Peterman AH, Schell MJ, et al (Univ of North Carolina, Chapel Hill; Northwestern Univ, Chicago)

Cancer 98:779-788, 2003 7–16

Background.—The best strategy for treating advanced non–small cell lung carcinoma (NSCLC) in elderly patients is unclear. A retrospective analysis of a phase III trial was conducted to determine the impact of age on response rate, survival, toxicity, and quality of life associated with a carboplatin plus paclitaxel regimen.

Methods.—The study included 230 patients with stage IIIB or IV NSCLC who were assigned randomly to either 4 cycles of carboplatin at an area under the curve (AUC) of 6 and paclitaxel 100 mg/m^2 every 21 days or carboplatin plus paclitaxel (C/P) until disease progression was noted. At disease progression, patients in both groups were given second-line weekly paclitaxel 80 mg/m^2 per week. Twenty-nine percent of the patients enrolled were 70 years or older.

Findings.—Both younger and older patients had a median 4 cycles of treatment delivered. Survival rates were comparable in the 2 age groups. In addition, progression of quality-of-life outcomes did not differ. None of the most common toxicities associated with C/P differed significantly between the younger and older groups, including neutropenia, neuropathy, leukopenia, myalgia/arthralgia, malaise, anemia, thrombocytopenia, anorexia, and nausea/emesis.

Conclusions.—The survival rates and toxicity profiles associated with C/P were similar in elderly patients and younger patients. Thus, C/P appears to be a reasonable standard treatment regimen in elderly persons with stage IIIB or IV NSCLC.

► Lung cancer is a disease of the elderly: the incidence increases with age and peaks in the eighth decade of life. As treatments become more effective, the question of how to treat elderly patients with lung cancer remains. Concerns arise regarding the physiologic and functional changes that accompanying aging, and the comorbidities often experienced by elderly patients, and the ability to tolerate chemotherapy.

The retrospective study reported by Hensing et al (Abstract 7–16) found no difference in survival between patients 70 years or older compared to those younger than 70 who were treated with C/P. Similarly, the retrospective analysis of a North Central Cancer Treatment Group (NCCTG) study, reported by Schild and coworkers (Abstract 7–15), of combined-modality therapy for stage

III patients also failed to observe a difference in survival between those younger and older than 70. These studies contribute to the growing body of evidence that elderly patients have survival rates similar to younger individuals (for review, see Reference 1).

However, the issue of toxicities in the elderly individuals is less certain. The Hensing study reported no difference in toxicity with C/P, whereas the NCCTG study observed an increase in myelosuppression and pneumonitis with combined-modality therapy. Other retrospective analyses have also reported enhanced toxicity in patients over the age of 70, despite similar survival rates.[2,3] Thus, further studies need to be done to identify and define the "fit" elderly patients and to identify ways to decrease toxicity of therapy.

J. H. Schiller, MD

References

1. Traynor AM, Schiller JH: First line therapy in the treatment of advanced lung cancer, in Pass HI, Johnson DH, Mitchell JB, et al: *Lung Cancer: Principles and Practice*, 2003. New York, Lippincott Williams & Wilkins, pp 1-16.
2. Langer CJ, Manola J, Bernardo P, et al: Cisplatin-based therapy for elderly patients with advanced non–small-cell lung cancer: Implications of Eastern Cooperative Oncology Group 5592: A randomized trial. *J Natl Cancer Inst* 94:173-181, 2002.
3. Kelly K, Giarritta S, Hayes S, et al: Should older patients (pts) receive combination chemotherapy for advanced stage non–small-cell lung cancer (NSCLC)? An analysis of Southwest Oncology trials 9509 and 9308. Presented at the Annual Meeting of the American Society of Clinical Oncologists, 2001.

Randomized Phase III Trial of Pemetrexed Versus Docetaxel in Patients With Non–Small-Cell Lung Cancer Previously Treated With Chemotherapy

Hanna N, Shepherd FA, Fossella FV, et al (Indiana Univ, Indianapolis; Eli Lilly and Company, Indianapolis, Ind; Univ of Texas, Houston; et al)

J Clin Oncol 22:1589-1597, 2004 7–17

Introduction.—Pemetrexed is a novel, multitargeted antifolate chemotherapy agent that is active in numerous tumor types, including non–small cell lung cancer (NSCLC). Its main mechanism of action is inhibition of the enzyme thymidylate synthase, which results in reduced thymidine needed for pyrimidine synthesis. The efficacy and toxicity of pemetrexed versus docetaxel were compared in patients with advanced NSCLC who previously underwent chemotherapy.

Methods.—Eligible participants had a performance status of 0 to 2, prior treatment with 1 chemotherapy regimen for advanced NSCLC, and adequate organ function. A total of 571 patients were randomly assigned to treatment with either pemetrexed 500 mg/m^2 IV on day 1 with vitamin B_{12}, folic acid, and dexamethasone or to docetaxel 75 mg/m^2 IV on day 1 with dexamethasone every 21 days. The major end point was overall survival.

Results.—The overall response rates for pemetrexed and docetaxel were 9.1% and 8.8% ($P = .105$), respectively, with a median progression-free sur-

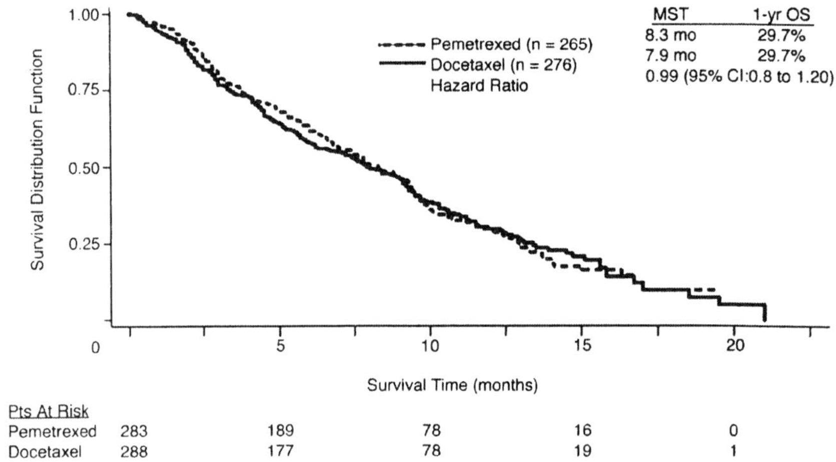

FIGURE 2.—Median survival time (*MST*). *Abbreviations: Mo*, Months; *yr*, year; *Pts*, patients. (Courtesy of Hanna N, Shepherd FA, Fossella FV, et al: Randomized phase III trial of pemetrexed versus docetaxel in patients with non–small-cell lung cancer previously treated with chemotherapy. *J Clin Oncol* 22(9):1589-1597, 2004. Reprinted with permission from the American Society of Clinical Oncology.)

vival of 2.9 months for each treatment arm (Fig 2). The 1-year survival rate for both pemetrexed and docetaxel was 29.7%. Compared with patients in the pemetrexed group, patients in the docetaxel group were more likely to have grade 3 or 4 neutropenia (40.2% vs 5.3%; $P < .001$), febrile neutropenia (12.7% vs 1.9%; $P < .001$), neutropenia with infections (3.35% vs 0.0%; $P = .004$) (Table 5), hospitalizations for neutropenic fever (13.4% vs 1.5%; $P < .001$), hospitalizations due to other drug-associated adverse events (10.5% vs 6.4%; $P = .092$), use of granulocyte colony-stimulating factor support (19.2% vs 2.6%; $P < .001$), and all grade alopecia (37.7% vs 6.4%; $P < .001$).

Conclusion.—Treatment with pemetrexed produced clinically equivalent efficacy outcomes, yet with significantly fewer side effects, compared to docetaxel in the second-line treatment of patients with advanced NSCLC.

TABLE 5.—Grade 3 and 4 Hematologic Toxicities

	% of Pemetrexed Patients (n = 265)	% of Docetaxel Patients (n = 276)	P*
Neutropenia	5.3	40.2	<.001
Febrile Neutropenia	1.9	12.7	<.001
Neutropenia with infection	0.0	3.3	.004
Anemia	4.2	4.3	.99
Thrombocytopenia	1.9	0.4	.116

Note: Toxicities are graded by the National Cancer Institute Common Toxicity Criteria version 2.
*Fisher's exact test.
(Courtesy of Hanna N, Shepherd FA, Fossella FV, et al: Randomized phase III trial of pemetrexed versus docetaxel in patients with non–small-cell lung cancer previously treated with chemotherapy. *J Clin Oncol* 22(9):1589-1597, 2004. Reprinted with permission from the American Society of Clinical Oncology.)

Pemetrexed should be considered a standard treatment option for second-line NSCLC when available.

► This multi-institutional, international phase III trial compares the standard chemotherapy agent, docetaxel, to the experimental agent, pemetrexed, in patients with advanced NSCLC previously treated with chemotherapy. Docetaxel at 75 mg/m^2 was the only Food and Drug Administration–approved chemotherapy agent in the second-line treatment of patients with NSCLC at the advent of this trial.

In this trial, pemetrexed demonstrated clinically equivalent efficacy when compared with docetaxel, but pemetrexed was associated with significantly fewer episodes of neutropenia, neutropenic fever, and infections related to neutropenia. As a result, fewer patients were hospitalized and/or required the use of granulocyte colony-stimulating factor on the pemetrexed arm. Docetaxel is frequently given by clinicians on a low-dose, weekly schedule to reduce the myelosuppression associated with the every-3-week regimen.

However, phase III trials comparing the weekly versus every-3-week docetaxel schedules have failed to justify the routine use of the more inconvenient weekly regimen.[1,2] As a result, pemetrexed, given at 500 mg/m^2 IV every 3 weeks—along with vitamin B_{12} and folate supplemenation and dexamethasone on the day before, the day of, and the day after pemetrexed—represents an attractive second-line treatment option.

N. H. Hanna, MD

References

1. Camps C, Massuti B, Jimenez A, et al: Second-line docetaxel administered every 3 weeks versus weekly in advanced non-small cell lung cancer (NSCLC): A Spanish Lung Cancer Group (SLCG) phase III trial. *Proc Am Soc Clin Oncol* 22:625 (abstract 2514), 2003.
2. Gridelli C, Illiano A, Salvagni S, et al: Effect of quality-of-life (QoL) of weekly vs 3 weekly docetaxel (D) in second-line treatment of advanced non-small cell lung cancer: The DISTAL randomized phase 3 study. *Proc Am Soc Clin Oncol* 22:625A, 2003.

Docetaxel Versus Docetaxel Plus Cisplatin as Front-line Treatment of Patients With Advanced Non–Small-Cell Lung Cancer: A Randomized, Multicenter Phase III Trial

Georgoulias V, Ardavanis A, Agelidou A, et al (Univ General Hosp of Heraklion, Crete, Greece; Agios Savas Anticancer Hosp, Greece; Sotiria Hosp, Greece; et al)

J Clin Oncol 22:2602-2609, 2004 7–18

Introduction.—Most patients with non–small cell lung cancer (NSCLC) are diagnosed with metastatic disease; without systemic chemotherapy, their median survival is 5 to 6 months, and fewer than 10% are alive at 1 year. Platinum-based regimens provide a small, yet statistically significant benefit. Cisplatin-containing regimens are significantly more toxic, compared to those without cisplatin. A prospective, multicenter, randomized, phase III trial was performed to assess the activity and toxicity of single-agent docetaxel (D) vs those of docetaxel plus cisplatin (DC) in untreated patients with advanced or metastatic NSCLC.

Methods.—Patients were selected randomly to receive either DC (n = 167; docetaxel 100 mg/m^2 on day 1, cisplatin 80 mg/m^2 on day 2, and recombinant human granulocyte colony-stimulating factor (rhG-CSF) 150 µg/m^2 on days 3 to 9) or D (n = 152; 100 mg/m^2 on day 1 without rhG-CSF every 3 weeks).

Results.—The overall response rate for DC was 36.5% (3 complete responses and 58 partial responses); for D, the rate was 21.7% (1 complete response and 32 partial responses; P = .004). The median overall survival (OS) times were 10.5 months (range, 0.5-41 months) for DC, and 8.0 months (range, 0.5-41 months) for D (P = .200). The 1- and 2-year survival rates were 44% and 19%, respectively, for DC and 43% and 15%, respectively, for D. The median time to tumor progression was 4.0 months for DC and 2.5 months for D (P = .580). Grade 2/3 anemia was significantly higher in the DC group, compared with that in the D group (33% vs 16%; P = .0001). Febrile neutropenia developed in 15 patients in the DC group and 12 in the D group (9% vs 8%). Grade 3/4 nausea/vomiting (P = .0001), diarrhea (P= .007), neurotoxicity (P= .017), and nephrotoxicity (P= .006) occurred significantly more frequently in the DC vs D group. Five treatment-associated deaths occurred in the DC group and 1 in the D group (P = .098).

Conclusion.—The DC regimen provided a higher response rate, yet there was no improvement in median time to tumor progression or OS, compared with that of D. Monotherapy with D could be a reasonable front-line chemotherapy for patients who cannot tolerate cisplatin.

▶ This article by Georgoulias et al compares D versus DC in the first-line treatment of patients with advanced NSCLC. The combination therapy resulted in a significantly higher response rate (36.5% vs 21.7%) and numerically higher median survival rates (median, 10.5 vs 8 months), although not statistically significant. Also, as expected, the combination therapy also resulted in more side effects. These study results are consistent with those of 2 other studies comparing either paclitaxel with/without carboplatin or gemcitabine with/without carboplatin.[1,2] Therefore, standard first-line treatment for good-performance-status patients with advanced NSCLC remains a platinum-based 2-drug regimen. However, single-agent therapy with either docetaxel, paclitaxel, or gemcitabine would be reasonable for some patients who cannot tolerate a platinum agent.

N. H. Hanna, MD

References

1. Lilenbaum R, Herndon J, List M, et al: Single agent (SA) versus combination chemotherapy (CC) in advanced non-small cell lung cancer (NSCLC): A CALGB randomized trial of efficacy, quality of life (QOL), and cost-effectiveness. *Proc Am Soc Clin Oncol* 21:1A, 2002.

2. Sederholm CJMF: Gemcitabine (G) compared with gemcitabine plus carboplatin (GC) in advanced non-small cell lung cancer (NSCLC): A phase III study by the Swedish Lung Cancer Study Group (SLUSG). *Proc Am Soc Clin Oncol* 21:291A, 2002.

Randomized Phase III Study of Gemcitabine and Vinorelbine Versus Gemcitabine, Vinorelbine, and Cisplatin in the Treatment of Advanced Non–Small-Cell Lung Cancer: From the German and Swiss Lung Cancer Study Group

Laack E, Dickgreber N, Müller T, et al (Univ Hosp Hamburg Eppendorf, Germany; Univ Hosp Magdeburg, Germany; Nordwest Hospital Frankfurt, Germany; et al)

J Clin Oncol 22:2348-2356, 2004 7–19

Introduction.—Cytotoxic drugs that are equally as active as cisplatin but are better tolerated are needed to optimize therapy of patients with metastatic and advanced non–small cell lung cancer (NSCLC). Three hundred patients with NSCLC stage IIIB disease with malignant pleural effusion or stage IV disease were assessed to determined whether cisplatin-based chemotherapy (gemcitabine, vinorelbine, and cisplatin [GVP]) provides better overall survival (OS) as first-line therapy, compared with that of cisplatin-free chemotherapy (gemcitabine and vinorelbine [GV]).

Methods.—Between September 1999 and June 2001, patients were selected randomly to receive GV (gemcitabine 1000 mg/m^2 plus vinorelbine 25 mg/m^2 on days 1 and 8 every 3 weeks) or GVP (gemcitabine 1000 mg/m^2 plus vinorelbine 25 mg/m^2 on days 1 and 8 plus cisplatin 75 mg/m^2 on day 2 every 3 weeks). The primary end point was OS.

Results.—Data for 287 patients (GV, 143; GVP, 144) were analyzed. At the time of analysis (April 15, 2002, 209 (73%) patients (GV, 103; GVP, 106) had died. No between-group differences were noted in OS between GV and GVP (median survival, 35.9 vs 32.4 weeks; 1-year survival rate, 33.6% vs 27.5%, P = .73). Similarly, no between-group differences were noted in event-free survival (20.4% vs 21.9%; median time-to-event, 19.3 vs 22.3 weeks; P = .35). After at least 2 treatment cycles, 214 (74.6%) patients were assessable for best response. The overall response rate for GV was 13.0%, compared with that of 28.3% for GVP (P = .004; complete responders, 0% vs 3.8%; partial responders, 13.0% vs 24.5%). Hematologic and nonhematologic toxicity was significantly less in the GV group than in the GVP group. No statistically significant differences were noted in patients' quality of life.

Conclusion.—The cisplatin-based regimen as first-line chemotherapy in advanced NSCLC provided no additional survival benefit compared with that of the cisplatin-free regimen, which was considerably better tolerated.

► This randomized trial by Laack et al compares a 2-drug non–platinum-based regimen (gemcitabine plus vinorelbine) to the same regimen with cisplatin in patients with advanced NSCLC. In this study, the addition of cisplatin increased response rates but had no impact on overall survival. Furthermore, the

3-drug regimen was associated with significantly more toxicity. These study results are consistent with many other studies that compare 3-drug regimens to 2-drug regimens in NSCLC, including the addition of a "new" chemotherapy agent to a cisplatin-regimen and the addition of a "molecularly targeted agent," such as gefitinib, erlotinib, or affinitac, to a platinum-based 2-drug regimen. Most studies comparing a platinum-based 2-drug regimen to a non–platinum-based 2-drug regimen demonstrate equivalent efficacy outcomes and toxicity profiles. Further advances in the treatment of NSCLC are unlikely to come from the empiric addition of a third agent to a standard 2-drug regimen.

N. H. Hanna, MD

Gemcitabine Plus Vinorelbine Compared With Cisplatin Plus Vinorelbine or Cisplatin Plus Gemcitabine for Advanced Non–Small-Cell Lung Cancer: A Phase III Trial of the Italian GEMVIN Investigators and the National Cancer Institute of Canada Clinical Trials Group

Gridelli C, Gallo C, Shepherd FA, et al (GEMVIN Investigators, Naples, Italy; Natl Cancer Inst of Canada, Kingston)

J Clin Oncol 21:3025-3034, 2003 7–20

Background.—Platinum-containing chemotherapy regimens are standard for treating advanced non–small cell lung cancer (NSCLC). However, toxicity is common and may significantly impair quality of life. The combination of gemcitabine plus vinorelbine was compared with the combinations of cisplatin plus gemcitabine and cisplatin plus vinorelbine to determine the effect of each regimen on patients' quality of life, without compromising survival.

Methods.—The study included 501 patients with stage IIIB or IV NSCLC who were randomly assigned to gemcitabine plus vinorelbine (group 1) or to gemcitabine plus cisplatin or vinorelbine plus cisplatin (group 2). The median patient age was 62 years; none was older than 70.

Findings.—After 2 months of treatment, the groups did not differ significantly in global quality-of-life scores. However, group 2 had significantly more worsening of appetite, vomiting, and alopecia. Group 2 patients had significantly more-frequent grade 3 or 4 myelosuppression and ototoxicity. The median survival in groups 1 and 2 were 32 weeks and 38 weeks, respectively. The median progression-free survival was 17 weeks and 23 weeks, respectively. The hazard ratio for death in group 1 was 1.15, and for progression, 1.29.

Conclusions.—The patients treated with gemcitabine plus vinorelbine did not have global improvements in quality of life compared with that of patients given cisplatin-based regimens. However, the former did have improvements in some components of quality of life. Gemcitabine plus vinorelbine was less toxic than standard cisplatin-based chemotherapy. The latter was associated with a slight, nonsignificant survival advantage.

Three-Arm Randomized Study of Two Cisplatin-Based Regimens and Paclitaxel Plus Gemcitabine in Advanced Non–Small-Cell Lung Cancer: A Phase III Trial of the European Organization for Research and Treatment of Cancer Lung Cancer Group—EORTC 08975

Smit EF, van Meerbeeck JP, Lianes P, et al (Vrije Universiteit Med Ctr, Amsterdam; Erasmus Med Centre, Rotterdam, The Netherlands; St Antonius Ziekenhuis, Nieuwegein, The Netherlands; et al)

J Clin Oncol 21:3909-3917, 2003 7–21

Background.—The cure rate for non–small cell lung cancer (NSCLC) is only approximately 15% at 5 years. This distressingly low rate is due to the high rate of unresectable diseases at presentation and the inability of systemic therapy to cure metastatic disease. The therapeutic efficacies of paclitaxel plus cisplatin (arm A), gemcitabine plus cisplatin (arm B), and paclitaxel plus gemcitabine (arm C) were compared in chemotherapy-naïve patients with advanced NSCLC.

Methods.—Four hundred eighty patients were included in the study. Treatment consisted of paclitaxel, 175 mg/m^2 in a 3-hour infusion on day 1, or gemcitabine, 1250 mg/m^2 on days 1 and 8, both combined with cisplatin, 80 mg/m^2 on day 1, or paclitaxel, 175 mg/m^2, in a 3-hour infusion on day 1, combined with gemcitabine, 1250 mg/m^2, on days 1 and 8.

Findings.—Response rates in arms A, B, and C were 31.8%, 36.6%, and 27.7%, respectively. The median survival times were 8.1 months in arm A, 8.9 months in arm B, and 6.7 months in arm C. Myelosuppression was the only secondary endpoint that differed significantly between groups, differing between arms B and A. The mean treatment costs were 25% greater in arm C than in the other 2 arms.

Conclusions.—Gemcitabine plus cisplatin and paclitaxel plus gemcitabine do not appear to increase overall survival compared with paclitaxel plus cisplatin in patients with advanced NSCLC. Most quality-of-life variables were similar among groups. The nonplatinum arm had the highest cost of the different regimens. All treatments were well tolerated.

Cisplatin Plus Gemcitabine Versus a Cisplatin-Based Triplet Versus Nonplatinum Sequential Doublets in Advanced Non–Small-Cell Lung Cancer: A Spanish Lung Cancer Group Phase III Randomized Trial

Alberola V, Camps C, Provencio M, et al (Arnau de Vilanova Hosp, Spain; Gen Univ Hosp, Valencia, Spain; Puerta de Hierro Hosp, Spain; et al)

J Clin Oncol 21:3207-3213, 2003 7–22

Background.—Several novel cytotoxic drugs have been developed for the treatment of non–small cell lung cancer (NSCLC). Research has centered on platinum-based doublets or triplets and, less often, nonplatinum-based doublets. The survival benefits of cisplatin plus gemcitabine were compared with those of a cisplatin-based triplet, and nonplatinum sequential doublets in patients with advanced NSCLC.

Methods.—The study included 557 patients with stage IIIB to IV NSCLC who were assigned randomly to (1) cisplatin 100 mg/m^2 on day 1 plus gemcitabine 1250 mg/m^2 on days 1 and 8, every 3 weeks for 6 cycles (CG group); (2) cisplatin 100 mg/m^2 on day 1 plus gemcitabine 1000 mg/m^2 plus vinorelbine 25 mg/m^2 on days 1 and 8, every 3 weeks for 6 cycles (CGV group); or (3) gemcitabine 1000 mg/m^2 plus vinorelbine 30 mg/m^2 on days 1 and 8, every 3 weeks for 3 cycles, followed by vinorelbine 30 mg/m^2 on days 1 and 8 plus ifosfamide 3 g/m^2 on day 1, every 3 weeks for 3 cycles (GV-VI group).

Findings.—Response rates were 42% in the CG group, 41% in the CGV group, and only 27% in the GV-VI group. The median survival and time to progression did not differ significantly among groups. Grade 3 to 4 neutropenia occurred in 57% for the CGV group, compared with 32% in the GC group and 27% in the GV-VI group. Neutropenic fever rates in the CGV, GC, and GV-VI groups were 19%, 4%, and 5%, respectively. The rate of grade 3 to 4 thrombocytopenia was also greatest in the GCV group, at 23%, being 19% in the CG group and only 3% in the GV-VI group. Grade 3 to 4 emesis occurred in 32% of patients in the GVC group, 22% in the GC group, and 6% in the GV-VI group.

Conclusions.—These data support the use of CG as a standard regimen for the first-line treatment of patients with advanced NSCLC. Adding vinorelbine to this combination substantially increases toxicity without improving response or survival. The benefit of noncisplatin combination has yet to be demonstrated.

► The standard treatment for advanced NSCLC has traditionally been a "platin"-based regimen, based in part upon a meta-analysis published in 1995, which showed that cisplatin-based regimens resulted in a hazard ratio of 0.73 for survival compared to best supportive care, with an absolute improvement in survival at 1 year of 10%, whereas long-term alkylating agents resulted in a hazard ratio of 1.26, and a 6%-decrease in 1-year survival. Based on these data, the American Society of Clinical Oncology treatment guidelines in 1997 for unresectable disease concluded "In Stage IV disease, chemotherapy prolongs survival and is most appropriate for individuals with good performance status.... Chemotherapy given to NSCLC patients should be a platin-based regimen."[1]

Because of the side effects associated with cisplatin, however, there has been considerable interest in nonplatin-containing doublets as a first-line treatment for NSCLC. The studies presented here (Abstracts 7–20 to 7–22) represent 2 randomized studies comparing gemcitabine plus vinorelbine (Abstract 7–20) or gemcitabine plus paclitaxel (Abstract 7–21) with cisplatin-based regimens. In the Gridelli study, the authors used as their comparator arms cisplatin/vinorelbine or cisplatin/gemcitabine, because they were the 2 most commonly used regimens in Italy and Canada at the time the study was planned. Patients were randomly assigned to the gemcitabine/vinorelbine and 2 cisplatin-based arms on a 2:1:1 ratio, and the 2 arms were combined for analysis. The hypothesis of the study was that patients receiving the noncisplatin regimen would experience similar efficacy, with quality of life as the primary endpoint. The investigators clearly demonstrated a difference in toxicity; patients receiving the cisplatin-based therapies had more myelosuppression, vomiting, renal toxicity, hair loss, ototoxicity and fatigue than patients receiving gemcitabine/vinorelbine. However, they did not achieve their major end point: despite the fact that the noncisplatin-containing arms were significantly less toxic than the gemcitabine/vinorelbine arm, it did not improve global quality of life. There was no difference in response rates (30% for the cisplatin regimens, 25% for gemcitabine/vinorelbine) or survival (38 vs 32 weeks, respectively) between the 2 regimens. However, the gemcitabine/vinorelbine had an inferior progression-free survival (32 weeks compared with 38 weeks in the cisplatin-based arms, $P = .004$), and the survival differences, although not statistically inferior, showed a trend toward inferiority for the noncisplatin-based arm ($P = .08$).

EORTC 08975, reported by Smit et al (Abstract 7–21), compared paclitaxel/cisplatin with gemcitabine/cisplatin with paclitaxel/gemcitabine. Although not statistically significant, there was a trend toward inferior median survival and 1-year survival in the paclitaxel/gemcitabine arm. Most quality-of-life parameters were similar, but costs associated with the nonplatinum arm were highest.

The Spanish Lung Cancer Group Trial, reported by Alberola et al (Abstract 7–22), compared a standard platin-doublet, cisplatin-gemcitabine, with a cisplatin triplet and a nonplatin therapy consisting of sequential doublets, gemcitabine/vinorelbine followed by vinorelbine/ifosfamide. Although response rates were higher in the cisplatin/gemcitabine arm, there was no difference in the median, 1-year, or 2-year survival. Hematologic toxicity and neutrapenic fevers were significantly higher in the triplet arm.

Other investigators have looked at nonplatin doublets with mixed results. The Hellenic Cooperative Oncology Group selected patients randomly to receive paclitaxel with either carboplatin or gemcitabine.[2] The median and 1-year survival rate were 10.4 months and 41.7% for the carboplatin/paclitaxel arm, and 9.8 months and 41.4% for the gemcitabine/paclitaxel arm, respectively. Both regimens were well tolerated. The Greek Oncology Cooperative Group compared docetaxel plus cisplatin with gemcitabine and docetaxel.[3] The median survival was 10 months in the cisplatin/docetaxel arm and 9.5 months in the gemcitabine/docetaxel arm; 1-year survival was 42% and 39%, respectively. The gemcitabine/docetaxel arm had the more favorable toxicity profile. Other studies, however, have reported a trend toward inferior survival with nonplatin-based regimens. The Greek Cooperative Group for Lung Cancer compared docetaxel plus gemcitabine with vinorelbine plus cisplatin.[4] Although not statistically significant, the median survival between the 2 groups was 9 months for docetaxel/gemcitabine and 11.5 months for vinorelbine/cisplatin. Toxicity, however, was less in the docetaxel/gemcitabine arm.

What can we conclude from all this? Taken together, these trials suggest third-generation nonplatin doublets, if not equivalent to cisplatin-containing doublets, are probably close. Toxicity appears to be somewhat improved (although quality of life does not), making these regimens particularly appropriate for frail patients who are unlikely to tolerate the toxicity of cisplatin.

The American Society of Clinical Oncology recently updated its 1997 recommendations for the treatment of advanced NSCLC[5] to read "First line chemotherapy given to patients with advanced NSCLC should be a two-drug combination. Non-platinum containing chemotherapy regimens may be used as alternatives to platinum-based regimens in the first line."

J. H. Schiller, MD

References

1. Clinical practice guidelines for the treatment of unresectable non-small-cell lung cancer. Adopted on May 16, 1997 by the American Society of Clinical Oncology. *J Clin Oncol* 15:2996-3018, 1997.
2. Kosmidis P, Mylonakis N, Nicolaides C, et al: Paclitaxel plus carboplatin versus gemcitabine plus paclitaxel in advanced non–small-cell lung cancer: A phase III randomized trial. *J Clinical Oncology* 20:3578-3585, 2002.
3. Georgoulias V, Papadakis E, Alexopoulos A, et al: Greek Oncology Cooperative Group for Lung, Platinum-based and non-platinum-based chemotherapy in advanced non–small-cell lung cancer: A randomised multicentre trial. *Lancet* 357:1478-1484, 2001.
4. Kakolyris S, Tsiafaki X, Agelidou A, et al: Preliminary results of a multicenter randomized phase III trial of docetaxel plus gemcitabine (DG) versus vinorelbine plus cisplatin (VC) in patients with advanced non–small-cell lung cancer. Presented at the Annual Meeting of the American Society of Clinical Oncology, Orlando, Fla, 2002.
5. Pfister DG, Johnson DH, Azzoli CG, et al: American Society of Clinical Oncology treatment of unresectable non–small-cell lung cancer guideline: Update 2003. *J Clin Oncol* 22:330-353, 2004.

Phase II Study of R115777, a Farnesyl Transferase Inhibitor, in Myelodysplastic Syndrome

Kurzrock R, Albitar M, Cortes JE, et al (Univ of Texas, Houston; Johnson and Johnson Pharmaceutical Research and Development, Titusville, NJ)

J Clin Oncol 22:1287-1292, 2004 7–23

Background.—RAS proteins play a critical role in many cellular functions. Farnesylation is an enzymatic step critical to the activation of RAS and other cellular proteins, and drugs that block this step (farnesyltransferase inhibitors [FTIs]) may be useful as anticancer agents. A phase I trial showed the novel FTI R115777 (Zarnestra; Johnson and Johnson Pharmaceutical Research and Development, Raritan, NJ) has some efficacy in patients with refractory leukemia. This phase II trial studied the efficacy and safety of R115777 in patients with myelodysplastic syndrome (MDS).

Methods.—The subjects were 28 patients (79% male; aged 49 to 80 years) with refractory anemia (RA; n = 5), RA with excess blasts (RAEB; n = 18), or RAEB in transformation (RAEBT; n = 5). All had intermediate or high-risk MDS. Patients were treated with oral R115777, 600 mg twice a day, for 4 weeks, followed by 2 weeks off therapy. These 6-week cycles were repeated until the patient responded (at which point he or she received maintenance therapy) or until unacceptable toxicity developed (at which point the dose was reduced to 300 mg twice daily).

Results.—One of the patients dropped out of the study because of a hip fracture during the first week of treatment. Of the 27 assessable patients, 2 had a complete response and 1 had a partial response, for an overall response rate of 11.1%. Both the patients achieving a complete response (for 4 and 11 months) had RAEB (diploid karyotype). The patient who achieved partial remission (for 2 months) had RAEB and multiple cytogenetic abnormalities. None of these 3 patients had RAS mutations. All 3 responders required dose reduction during the first month of treatment because of rash or severe cytopenia. During the induction period (first 2 cycles), 3 patients progressed to acute myelogenous leukemia; all 3 had initial International Prognostic Scoring System scores more than 2.0. During the induction period, the initial R115777 dose was associated with myelosuppression, fatigue, and nausea in >60% of patients and headache, diarrhea, rash, stomatitis, dyspnea, and chest pain or palpitations in 20% to 40% of patients. Adverse events necessitated dose reduction in 4 patients and discontinuation of therapy in 7 patients. The lower dose, however, was well tolerated.

Conclusion.—R115777 showed modest activity in these patients with MDS, but a regimen of 600 mg orally twice a day for 4 weeks is not well tolerated. Further study is warranted to determine the optimal dosing parameters for R115777 and the molecular targets in MDS most likely to respond to therapy.

► MDS is a family of disorders characterized by ineffective hematopoiesis. Farnesylation is a critical aspect of intracellular signaling in which proteins are activated and their location in the cytosol altered by the addition of farnesyl groups. A family of anticancer drugs known as FTIs have been studied in cancer and have demonstrated a moderate degree of activity in patients with acute myeloid leukemia. As a result, the investigators of this study performed a phase II trial of the FTI R115777. Patients with all forms of MDS were treated with the agent at a dose of 600 mg orally twice daily. There were 3 objective responses, including 2 complete remissions and 1 partial remission in 27 assessable patients. The responding patients all had evidence of RAEB or RABT. The major toxicity of the therapy was myelosuppression, requiring either a dose reduction or discontinuation of therapy in 41% of the patients. The authors concluded that the modest activity of this agent in the MDS population was exceeded by the more significant degree of toxicity and that a different dose and schedule need to be explored. Given the activity in patients with acute myeloid leukemia, it is reasonable to assume that once this is resolved possibly more activity and less toxicity will be seen.

M. S. Gordon, MD

Use of Gene-Expression Profiling to Identify Prognostic Subclasses in Adult Acute Myeloid Leukemia

Bullinger L, Döhner K, Bair E, et al (Stanford Univ, Calif; Univ of Ulm, Germany)
N Engl J Med 350:1605-1616, 2004 7–24

Background.—Acute myeloid leukemia (AML) is the most common form of leukemia in adults. Complete remission is induced in about 70% to 80% of younger patients (age 16 to 60 years) who undergo chemotherapy, but many of them experience a relapse and die of their disease. The presence or absence of recurrent cytogenetic aberrations has been used to identify the appropriate therapy in AML patients, but the classification system currently in use does not fully reflect the molecular heterogeneity of AML and treatment stratification is difficult, particularly in patients with intermediate-risk AML who have a normal karyotype. The molecular variation underlying the biologic and clinical heterogeneity in AML was systematically investigated. This approach has also provided insight into diffuse large B-cell lymphoma and childhood acute lymphoblastic leukemia.

Methods.—Complementary DNA microarrays were used to determine the levels of gene expression in peripheral-blood samples or bone marrow samples from 116 adults with AML (including 45 with a normal karyotype). Unsupervised hierarchical clustering analysis was used to identify molecular subgroups with distinct gene-expression signatures. A training set of samples from 59 patients was used to apply a novel supervised learning algorithm to devise a gene-expression-based clinical-outcome predictor that was then tested with an independent validation group composed of the remaining 57 patients.

Results.—New molecular subtypes of AML were identified through unsupervised analysis, including 2 prognostically relevant subgroups in AML with a normal karyotype. The supervised learning algorithm was then used to construct an optimal 133-gene clinical-outcome predictor, which accurately predicted overall survival among patients in the independent validation group, including the subgroup of patients with AML with a normal karyotype. Multivariate analysis showed that the gene-expression predictor was a strong independent prognostic factor.

Conclusions.—It would appear from these findings that the use of gene-expression profiling improves the molecular classification of AML in adults.

► The diagnosis and characterization of adult acute leukemia has classically been performed by pathologists by cytochemical or immunohistochemical stains on bone marrow aspirates and biopsies. This process fails to appreciate the novelty that is adult leukemia, and although flow cytometry has aided in the diagnosis of some cases, it has not replaced the classical FAB (French-American-British) classification system. Prognosis of AML is typically linked to the FAB class as well as the findings on cytogenetic studies. Specific cytogenetic abnormalities such as monosomy 7 are typically associated with a grim prognosis, whereas others, such as the translocation of chromosome 8 and 21, are associated with a better overall survival because of a higher complete remission rate. The investigators in this study sought to develop a gene-expression profiling system that would be especially applicable to those patients with normal cytogenetics. By using a systematic approach to developing this process, the investigators performed complementary DNA microarrays on leukemia samples from 116 patients with AML to develop a clustering analysis that would allow them to characterize leukemic samples. They then tested this on a set of 59 blinded samples and devised a predictive outcomes analysis that identified gene expression patterns that predicted survival in AML patients, including those with normal cytogenetics. In a multivariate analysis, this method of gene expression profiling was statistically significantly associated with prognosis and represents a potentially valuable tool for classifying AML, especially for those patients with normal cytogenetics for whom decisions regarding options such as bone marrow transplantation may be difficult. Subsequent prospective trials of this approach need to be performed to validate this gene expression profiling for larger scale use.

M. S. Gordon, MD

Prognostically Useful Gene-Expression Profiles in Acute Myeloid Leukemia

Valk PJ, Verhaak RG, Beijen MA, et al (Erasmus Univ, Rotterdam, The Netherlands; Leiden Univ, The Netherlands)

N Engl J Med 350:1617-1628, 2004 7–25

Background.—Clinicians must use a combination of methods to classify acute myeloid leukemia (AML), make treatment decisions, and determine prognosis. However, even this combined approach accurately provides treatment and prognostic information in only half of affected patients. Gene-expression profiles were used to identify established and novel subclasses of AML and otherwise unrecognized cases of poor-risk AML.

Methods.—Samples of peripheral blood or bone marrow were obtained from 285 patients with AML. Gene-expression profiles were determined with the use of Affymetrix U133A GeneChips (Affymetrix, Santa Clara, Calif) containing about 13,000 unique genes or expression-signature tags. Data were analyzed with Omniviz software (Omniviz, Maynard, Mass). Significance analysis of microarrays and prediction analysis of microarrays software were also performed.

Findings.—Sixteen patient groups were identified by unsupervised cluster analyses on the basis of molecular signatures. The genes defining these clusters and the minimal numbers of genes needed to identify prognostically important clusters with a high degree of accuracy were determined. The presence of chromosomal lesions, such as t(8; 21), t(15; 17), and inv(16), as well as specific genetic mutations (CEBPA) and abnormal oncogene expression (EV11) drove the clustering. Several novel clusters were also identified, some consisting of specimens with normal karyotypes. Cases of AML with poor treatment outcomes were included in a unique cluster with a distinctive gene-expression signature.

Conclusions.—A single assay can be used to identify cases of AML with known cytogenetic abnormalities as well as new clusters of AML with characteristic gene-expression signatures. Genome-wide analytic techniques will continue to advance, enabling analysis of subtle differences in gene expression and predictions of pathogenic pathways.

▶ The investigators in this study performed complementary DNA microarray on samples peripheral blood or bone marrow samples from patients with AML. From their samples, they were able to identify 16 groups of patients with distinct molecular signatures. In most cases, these distinct groups correlated with the specific cytogenetic mutations seen in the leukemic cells. In 119 of the cases, however, the karyotype was normal and these patients tended to cluster in several distinct groups that may or may not have correlated with the French-American-British (FAB) classification. Prognostically, these clusters were associated with different outcomes in terms of relapse-free and overall survival and these tended to correspond to the known prognosis of the cytogenetic abnormalities. Overall, the investigators have identified a minimum number of genes that need to be assessed to characterize the patients, and further studies to determine the validity of this analysis in contrast to cytogenetic or pathologic assessment needs to be performed. Like the study of Bullinger et al (Abstract 7–24), this process holds great promise for identifying previously unrecognized high-risk patients to allow individualization of therapy that is based on gene expression patterns.

M. S. Gordon, MD

An Innovative Phase I Clinical Study Demonstrates Inhibition of FLT3 Phosphorylation by SU11248 in Acute Myeloid Leukemia Patients

O'Farrell A-M, Foran JM, Fiedler W, et al (SUGEN Inc, South San Francisco, Calif; Univ of Alabama, Birmingham; Univ Hosp Hamburg-Eppendorf, Germany; et al)

Clin Cancer Res 9:5465-5476, 2003 7–26

Background.—Optimal clinical development of novel targeted therapies relies on direct and rapid proof of molecular activity obtained in early clinical trials. The oral multitargeted kinase inhibitor SU11248 has selectivity for fms-related tyrosine kinase 3/Flk2 (FLT3), which is a promising candidate for targeted treatment in acute myeloid leukemia (AML). A translational study was performed to demonstrate SU11248 inhibition of FLT3 phosphorylation.

Methods.—Twenty-nine patients with AML received 1 dose of SU11248 escalated from 50 to 350 mg in 50 mg increments in subgroups of 3 to 6 patients. At 7 time points during the 48 hours after SU11248 administration, FLT3 phosphorylation and plasma pharmacokinetics were assessed. In addition, FLT3 genotype was determined.

Findings.—FLT3 phosphorylation was inhibited in 50% of FLT3-wild-type (WT) patients and in all FLT3-mutant patients. Consistent with preclinical expectations, FLT3 internal tandem duplication mutations had increased sensitivity compared with FLT3-WT. Strong inhibition of FLT3 phosphorylation in more than half the patients was achieved in the groups given 200 mg and above. In addition, downstream signaling pathways were inhibited. Signal transducer and activator of transcription 5 declined mainly in internal tandem duplication patients and at later time points in FLT3-WT patients. Extracellular signal-regulated kinase activity was decreased in most patients independent of FLT3 inhibition. Adverse events related to the study drug occurred in 31% of the patients, consisting mostly of grade 1 or 2 diarrhea and nausea at higher dose levels.

Conclusions.—These data provide the first evidence of anti-FLT3 activity in patients with AML. Such proof of target inhibition is essential for developing novel oncology therapies.

▶ Among the chromosomal abnormalities that have garnered a great deal of attention in AML, those associated with the FLT3 receptor have been critically important. This receptor tyrosine kinase (RTK) is expressed and activated in the majority of AML patients. These activating mutations are thought to be viable targets for the treatment of leukemia in much the same way as the *bcr-abl* translocation has been a target for imatinib therapy in chronic myeloid leukemia. SU11248 is a small molecule tyrosine kinase inhibitor that has activity on a number of kinases, such as those associated with the c-kit receptor and the KDR VEGF-R2 receptor. SU11248 also has activity against the RTK activity of the activated FLT3 receptor and in this phase I trial, the investigators performed a phase I trial of this targeted therapy in patients with AML regardless of the pretreatment activation status of the receptor. Cohort of 3 to 6 patients were treated with a single dose of SU11248 at doses ranging from 50 to 350 mg. Serial sampling of leukemic cells allowed the assessment of FLT3 phosphorylation in response to the therapy. Because this was a single-dose study, response to treatment was not an objective. As expected, 100% of the patients with AML associated with activating mutations of FLT3 demonstrated inhibition of phosphorylation. Somewhat surprisingly, however, was the fact that 50% of the patients with FLT3-WT also had inhibition of phosphorylation suggesting that this agent is active in this setting. The question of whether inhibition of FLT3 in patients without the activating mutations is of value will need to be explored in separate clinical trials which are planned.

M. S. Gordon, MD

Results of Decitabine (5-Aza-2'Deoxycytidine) Therapy in 130 Patients With Chronic Myelogenous Leukemia

Kantarjian HM, O'Brien S, Cortes J, et al (Univ of Texas, Houston)

Cancer 98:522-528, 2003 7–27

Background.—DNA methylation silences many tumor suppressor genes, which allows tumor progression in several cancers, including chronic myelogenous leukemia (CML). Decitabine is a hypomethylating agent with activity against acute myeloid leukemia and myelodysplastic syndrome. Whether decitabine might be effective in patients with a different phase of CML was investigated.

Methods.—The subjects were 130 patients 16 to 78 years old (62% male) with CML. Of these, 123 had Philadelphia chromosome (Ph)-positive CML and 7 had Ph-negative disease. Among the patients with Ph-positive CML, 64 were in the blastic phase, 51 were in the accelerated phase, and 8 were in the chronic phase. Decitabine was administered initially in 13 patients as 100 mg/m^2 over a 6-hour period every 12 hours for 5 days every 4 to 8 weeks. Because of severe prolonged myelosuppression, however, doses were reduced to 75 mg/m^2 in the next 33 patients, then to 50 mg/m^2 in the final 84 patients. Complete hematologic response (CHR) was defined as normalization of peripheral blood counts and differentials with <5% blasts in the bone marrow for 4 weeks or more. Hematologic improvement (HI) was defined similarly to CHR, except persistent thrombocytopenia (<100 W 10^9 cells/L) and a few immature cells (<5% myelocytes or metamyelocytes, no blasts or promyelocytes) were allowed. Partial hematologic response (PHR) was defined similarly to CHR, except persistent palpable splenomegaly, thrombocytosis (>450 W 10^9 platelets/L) and a few immature cells were allowed. A return to the second chronic phase (second CP) was defined as the disappearance of blastic-phase features and a return to chronic-phase features. Additionally, patients who achieved CHR or HI were examined to determine cytogenic response.

Results.—Four patients died during the first course of decitabine, 3 from complications of myelosuppression and 1 from progressive disease. Objective responses were achieved by 18 (28%) of 64 patients in the blastic phase, including 6 with CHR, 2 with PHR, 7 with HI, and 3 who returned to the second CP. Additionally, 5 patients (8%) had a cytogenic response. Objective responses were achieved by 28 of 51 patients (55%) in the accelerated phase, including 12 with CHR, 10 with PHR, 3 with HI, and 3 who returned to the second CP. Additionally, 7 patients (14%) had a cytogenic response. Objective responses were achieved by 5 (63%) of 8 patients in the chronic phase, including 1 patient with CHR and 4 with PHR. Additionally, 1 patient (12%) had a cytogenic response. Objective responses were achieved by 4 (57%) of 7 patients with PH-negative CML, including 2 with CHR, 1 with PHR, and 1 who returned to the second CP. Results did not appear to differ according to the dose of decitabine. The median survival was 5 months for patients in the blastic phase, 13 months for patients in the accelerated phase, and 13 months for patients with Ph-negative CML. Severe, prolonged myelosuppression was the only significant adverse event, which was more severe with higher doses and often associated with febrile episodes (37% of patients) and infection (34%).

Conclusion.—Decitabine appears to have significant activity in all phases of CML. Future studies should evaluate whether lower doses of decitabine for longer periods, with or without imatinib, could reduce myelosuppression while still controlling disease.

► The treatment of CML has undergone significant transformation with the use of targeted therapies to the *BCR-ABL* translocation. As in the myelodysplastic syndromes, DNA methylation, which silences various tumor suppressor genes, is thought to be critical to the evolution of these hematologic diseases. Decitabine is a novel hypomethylating agent that has been approved for the treatment of the myelodysplastic syndromes. In this study, 130 patients with CML predominantly in the accelerated or blast crisis phases were treated with courses of decitabine. In the patients with blast crisis CML, 18 of the 64 achieved a complete hematologic response, whereas in the accelerated phase 55% had some form of a response, including complete and partial hematologic responses as well as hematologic improvement and a second CP. While the 3-year survival rate for the blast crisis patients was less than 5%, the accelerated patients had a 3-year survival rate of 27%, which was felt to be an improvement over previous studies. The major toxicity of the therapy was prolonged myelosuppression that was manageable. Since patients entering accelerated or blast crisis tend to not be optimal candidates for allogeneic bone marrow transplantation or need to have time to identify adequate matched donors, this therapy may provide an opportunity for temporary hematologic improvement before such a procedure.

M. S. Gordon, MD

Pleural Disorders

Gene Expression Profiles Predict Survival and Progression of Pleural Mesothelioma

Pass HI, Liu Z, Wali A, et al (Wayne State Univ, Detroit, Mich; Harper Univ Hosp, Detroit, Mich; Loyola Univ, Maywood, Ill; et al)

Clin Cancer Res 10:849-859, 2004 7–28

Introduction.—Clinical outcomes for patients with malignant pleural mesothelioma (MPM) are not precisely predicted by histopathology and intraoperative staging. Gene expression profiles may be able to predict time to progression and survival in surgically cytoreduced pleural mesothelioma of all stages. Gene expression data were analyzed by using 2 programs, significance analysis microarrays and dChip, to determine whether concordant genes from both analyses could correctly cluster patients into good or poor risk cohorts.

Methods.—Gene expression analyses from 21 patients with MPM with cytoreductions and identical postoperative adjuvant therapy were conducted by using the U95 Affymetrix gene chip. With both dChip and significance analysis microarrays, neural networks constructed a common 27-gene classifier that was linked with either the high-risk or low-risk group of patients. Data were verified by using real-time polymerase chain reaction and immunohistochemical staining. The 27-gene classifier was also used for validation in another set of 17 patients with MPM.

Results.—Groups predicted by the gene classifier recapitulated the actual time to progression and survival of the test set with 95.2% accuracy by 10-fold cross-validation. Clinical outcomes were independent of histology. Heterogeneity of progression and survival in early stage patients was defined by the classifier. The gene classifier had a 76% accuracy in the other validation set of MPMs.

Conclusion.—Pretherapy gene expression analysis of mesothelioma biopsies may be predictive of which patients benefit from a surgical approach.

▶ MPM is an uncommon but lethal disease. Most patients have surgically unresectable disease at diagnosis. For these patients with potentially resectable disease, surgery still results in too few cures. Gene array technologies hold the promise of being able to better predict the behavior of cancers and the effectiveness of interventions. This study evaluated gene profiles of 21 patients with MPM. When surgically staged I and II patients were grouped together, their survival was significantly different depending on their gene cluster analysis. This study describes a set of 27 genes that may have the capability of segregating good risk and poor risk patients. Further study is needed, but if validated, gene expression profiles may be used to direct clinical decision making in the future.

N. H. Hanna, MD

Prospective Randomized Trial of Intrapleural Bleomycin Versus Interferon Alfa-2b via Ultrasound-Guided Small-Bore Chest Tube in the Palliative Treatment of Malignant Pleural Effusions

Sartori S, Tassinari D, Ceccotti P, et al (St Anna Hosp, Ferrara, Italy; City Hosp, Rimini, Italy)

J Clin Oncol 22:1228-1233, 2004 7–29

Background.—Malignant pleural effusions complicate end-stage malignancy and are generally unresponsive to systemic chemotherapy. Pleurodesis is used when life expectancy is not too short. The most commonly used antineoplastic agent for pleurodesis is bleomycin. Intrapleural interferon (IFN) alfa or beta has also had some success in controlling malignant effusions. The palliative efficacy of intrapleural bleomycin was compared with that of recombinant IFN-α-2b after the effusion was completely drained with an US-guided small-bore chest catheter.

Methods.—Randomization placed 83 patients in the intrapleural bleomycin group and 77 in the IFN group. All had rapidly recurrent malignant pleural effusions. Before beginning drug treatment, an US-guided catheter was placed to completely drain the pleural effusion. A single dose of bleomycin, 0.75 mg/kg, was given, with an additional dose administered if daily fluid output did not decrease to less than 100 mL/d within 3 days. Six courses of IFN, 1 million units per 10 kg, were given at 4-day intervals. With the use of the intention-to-treat principle, outcomes were evaluated after 30 days and every 2 weeks until death or progression of disease that required thoracentesis.

Results.—Of those receiving bleomycin, 60 were given one dose and 23 a further dose. Three patients refused to continue IFN therapy after 2 or 3 courses. Three deaths occurred in each group within 30 days of chest tube removal. At 1 month, 80 bleomycin patients and 71 IFN patients had completed treatment and were still alive. The bleomycin group had a significantly higher 30-day response rate than the IFN group. The median survival with bleomycin was 96 days and that with IFN was 85 days. The bleomycin group required 96 thoracenteses and the IFN group required 235. Both groups reported mild toxic reactions, principally self-limiting fever, vomiting, and moderate chest pain. IFN patients also developed a flulike syndrome.

Conclusions.—IFN was not an effective agent for use in the palliative management of malignant pleural effusion in patients with advanced neoplastic disease. Bleomycin was more effective than IFN and provided a valid option for the management of these patients. When a second dose of bleomycin is given to patients who do not respond to the first dose, the overall outcome of treatment was markedly improved.

▶ Over the last 4 decades, a large number of agents have been introduced into the pleural space after near-complete removal of a pleural effusion, to attempt to achieve closure of the pleural space and, thus, to prevent reaccumulation of the effusion. The high order of efficacy of bleomycin as such an agent was first reported over 2 decades ago. This randomized trial compares bleomycin to IFN alfa-2b for palliative treatment of malignant pleural effusions, based on recent claims of response rates as high as 100% with the use of IFN. Bleomycin achieved a 30-day respone rate of 84%, was superior to IFN, produced fewer complications than those reported with IFN or talc, and thus represents a valid option for the treatment of pleural effusions.

J. T. Thigpen, MD

Phase II Trial of Pleural Photodynamic Therapy and Surgery for Patients With Non–Small-Cell Lung Cancer With Pleural Spread

Friedberg JS, Mick R, Stevenson JP, et al (Thomas Jefferson Univ Hosp, Philadelphia; Univ of Pennsylvania, Philadelphia)

J Clin Oncol 22:2192-2201, 2004 7–30

Introduction.—Non–small-cell lung cancer (NSCLC) with pleural spread is incurable and has been recommended to be upstaged to stage IV disease because of similar survival rates of 6 to 9 months. Surgery alone in these patients does not control local disease or extend survival beyond palliative chemotherapy. The efficacy of intrapleural porfimer sodium-mediated photodynamic therapy (PDT) at the previously established maximally tolerated dose (30 J/cm^2 of 630 light delivered 24 hours after a porfimer sodium dose of 2.0 mg/kg) was evaluated in a stratified phase II trial of patients with NSCLC with pleural dissemination.

Methods.—Twenty-two patients with NSCLC with pleural spread underwent combination surgery with intraoperative PDT. Porfimer sodium (2 mg/kg) was administered 24 hours preoperatively, at which time all gross tumor was resected and followed by illumination of the hemithorax with 630 nm light to a measured dose of 30 J/cm^2. Photosensitizer levels in tumor and surrounding normal tissue were determined.

Results.—Of 22 patients enrolled, 17 underwent complete debulking and PDT, 3 underwent partial debulking/PDT, and 2 patients were unresectable. Local control of pleural disease at 6 months was observed in 11 (73%) of 15 patients (95% confidence interval, 44.9%-92.2%). The median overall survival was 21.7 months (95% confidence interval, 17.7-25.8 months). Measured levels of porfimer sodium in tumors were greater than those observed in normal tissues; ratios ranged between 1.19 to 22.42.

Conclusion.—It appears that surgery and PDT may be performed safely and with very good local control in patients with NSCLC with pleural spread. The median survival was 21.7 months, determined from the time of surgery and PDT. Further evaluation of this encouraging therapy is warranted.

► The overall survival rates of patients with NSCLC with pleural spread are similar to those with stage IV disease. These patients are believed to be largely incurable and surgical resection is usually deferred. A major obstacle to cure is the presence of microscopic disease within the chest cavity despite apparent complete resection. PDT has anticancer activity and can spare toxicity to underlying tissues. The authors report their experience with surgical resection and PDT in patients whose tumors have pleural spread. Local control after 6 months was achieved in 73% of patients, toxicities with PDT were generally grade 1 or 2, and median survival was 21 months. These data suggest that further study of this combined modality approach is warranted.

N. H. Hanna, MD

Pleural Lavage Cytology in Non–Small Cell Lung Cancer: Lessons From 1000 Consecutive Resections

Okada M, Sakamoto T, Nishio W, et al (Hyogo Med Ctr, Japan)

J Thorac Cardiovasc Surg 126:1911-1915, 2003 7–31

Background.—When there are malignant cells in the pleural effusion of patients with lung cancer, advanced disease and poor prognosis are generally assumed to be present. However, sometimes malignant cells are in the pleural cavity but do not show up in the effusion or in macroscopic dissemination. It is not routine practice to perform cytologic examination of pleural lavage fluid before undertaking resection for lung cancer. A large prospective trial was done to analyze survival data, assess the pattern of recurrence, and identify the independent prognostic significance of the results of pleural lavage fluid cytology before resection.

Methods.—One thousand patients with non–small cell lung cancer but no pleural effusion underwent pleural lavage before tumor resection. The pleural lavage fluid was examined cytologically. Findings were linked to survival data and patterns of recurrence.

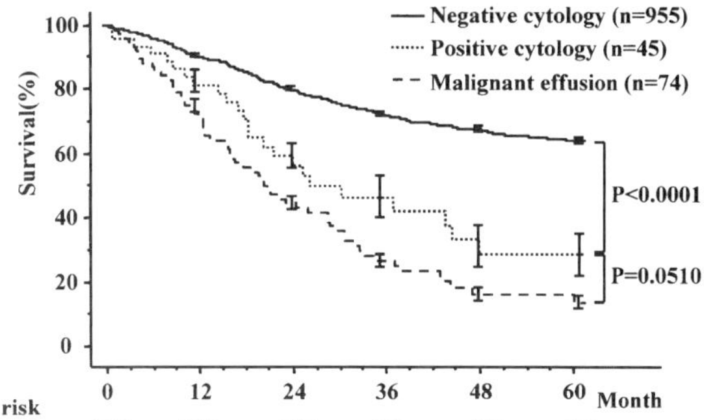

Number at risk	0	12	24	36	48	60
Negative cytology	955	809	617	454	339	237
Positive cytology	45	31	18	12	7	2
Malignant effusion	74	53	29	15	8	5

FIGURE 1.—Cumulative survival curves of patients according to cytologic status of pleural lavage fluid. There were 74 patients with malignant effusion undergoing resection of the primary tumor during the same period, but they were excluded from this study. The survival rate of patients with positive cytologic findings was significantly worse than that of patients with negative cytologic findings ($P < .0001$). In addition, patients with positive cytologic findings had a better (not significant) prognosis than those with malignant effusion ($P = .0510$). (Reprinted from Okada M, Sakamoto T, Nishio W, et al: Pleural lavage cytology in non–small cell lung cancer: Lessons from 1000 consecutive resections. *J Thorac Cardiovasc Surg* 126:1911-1915, 2003. Copyright 2003 with permission from The American Association for Thoracic Surgery.)

Results.—Positive findings were obtained in 45 patients (4.5%) and were much more common among patients with adenocarcinoma than those with squamous cell carcinoma, large cell carcinoma, or adenosquamous carcinoma. Among 587 patients with pathologic stage I disease, positive findings for malignancy were detected in 13 patients (2.2%). Six of 173 patients (3.5%) with stage II disease and 26 of 240 (10.8%) with stage III disease also had malignant cells in the pleural lavage fluid. Twenty of 658 patients without nodal involvement had malignant cells present, as did 8 of 171 patients with N1 disease and 17 of 171 patients with N2 disease. It was more common to

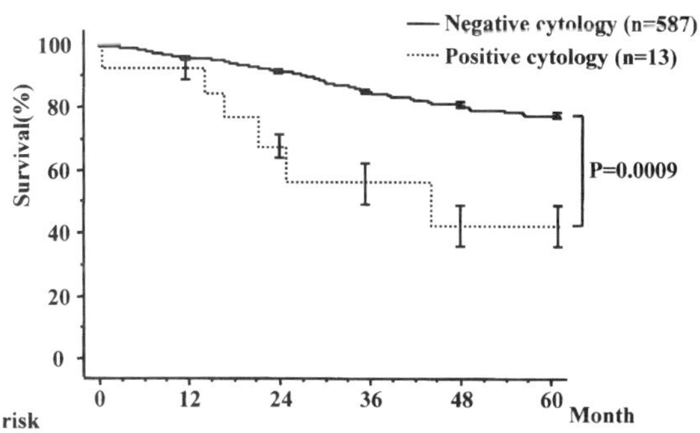

Number at risk	0	12	24	36	48	60
Negative cytology	574	524	430	324	245	173
Positive cytology	13	11	6	5	3	1

FIGURE 2.—Cumulative survival curves of patients with pathologic stage I disease according to cytologic status of pleural lavage fluid. The survival rate of patients with positive cytologic findings was significantly worse than that of patients with negative cytologic findings ($P = .0009$). (Reprinted from Okada M, Sakamoto T, Nishio W, et al: Pleural lavage cytology in non–small cell lung cancer: Lessons from 1000 consecutive resections. *J Thorac Cardiovasc Surg* 126:1911-1915, 2003. Copyright 2003 with permission from The American Association for Thoracic Surgery.)

TABLE 2.—Multivariable Analysis of Prognostic Factors (n = 1000)

Factors	Unfavorable	Favorable	Risk Ratio	95% CI	*P* Value
Sex	Male	Female	1.550	1.171-2.052	.0022
Age	≥ 65	≤ 64	1.330	1.062-1.665	.0131
CEA	Positive	Negative	1.431	1.143-1.791	.0017
Histology	Non-AD	AD	1.236	0.970-1.574	.0862
Pathologic stage	II + III	I	3.007	2.346-3.854	<.0001
Lymphatic permeation	Positive	Negative	1.377	1.079-1.759	.0101
Vascular involvement	Positive	Negative	1.307	1.171-2.052	.0237
Lavage cytology	Positive	Negative	1.634	1.051-2.539	.0290

Abbreviation: AD, Adenocarcinoma.

(Reprinted from Okada M, Sakamoto T, Nishio W, et al: Pleural lavage cytology in non–small cell lung cancer: Lessons from 1000 consecutive resections. *J Thorac Cardiovasc Surg* 126:1911-1915, 2003. Copyright 2003 with permission from The American Association for Thoracic Surgery.)

have positive results with greater lymphatic involvement. Positive cytologic findings were obtained in 16.7% of patients with pleural involvement, 10.3% of patients with lymphatic involvement, and 7.5% of patients with vascular involvement. Among patients without these findings, the rates of positive cytologic results were 1.8%, 1.8%, and 2.3%, respectively. With a higher value of preoperative serum carcinoembryonic antigen (CEA), the cytologic results were positive in 6.8% of cases; with normal CEA values, the results were positive in 3.1% of cases. The rates of positive findings were 3.6% for male and 6.6% for female patients. Significantly better survival rates were found for negative pleural fluid versus positive pleural fluid. Patients with positive findings had a 3-year survival rate of 46% and a 5-year rate of 28%. Patients with negative findings had a 3-year survival rate of 75% and a 5-year rate of 67% (Fig 1). Even in patients with stage I disease, positive cytologic findings indicated a significantly worse 5-year survival rate than negative cytologic findings (43% vs 81%) (Fig 2). The factors found to be independent and significant prognostic determinants on multivariate analysis were pleural lavage cytology, gender, age, CEA level, pathologic stage, lymphatic permeation, and vascular involvement (Table 2). Recurrences were noted in 64.4% of the 45 patients with positive findings in pleural lavage fluid (Table 3). Distant metastases were seen more often than local recurrences, affecting 65.5% versus 34.5% of patients, respectively.

TABLE 3.—Recurrence Pattern in Patients with Positive Pleural Lavage Cytologic Findings (n = 45)

	Stage I	Stage II	Stage III	Total
No. of patients	13	6	26	45
No recurrences	5	4	7	16
With recurrence	8	2	19	29
Local (pleural cavity)	2 (2)	1 (1)	7 (5)	10 (8)
Distant	6	1	12	19

(Reprinted from Okada M, Sakamoto T, Nishio W, et al: Pleural lavage cytology in non–small cell lung cancer: Lessons from 1000 consecutive resections. *J Thorac Cardiovasc Surg* 126:1911-1915, 2003. Copyright 2003 with permission from The American Association for Thoracic Surgery.)

Conclusions.—Patients with stage I disease had significantly worse prognosis and 5-year survival when their cytologic results were positive than patients whose cytologic results were negative. Pleural lavage cytologic results were found to be an independent predictor of prognosis along with gender, age, serum CEA level, pathologic stage, lymphatic permeation, and vascular involvement.

▶ This group of Japanese investigators reports on the importance of pleural lavage cytology at the time of surgery for non–small cell lung cancer. They have evaluated this prospectively in 1000 consecutive patients who went to surgery and who did not have any obvious pleural effusion. Their procedure was carried out intraoperatively with 100 mL of saline given intrapleurally immediately after the thoracotomy. Forty-five of the 1000 patients had a positive lavage, which appeared to correlate with a worse prognosis.

It would seem that this is simple enough to do and carries enough of a poor prognosis that it needs confirmation. If it is confirmed, then it probably needs to be done on a routine basis for those who are undergoing surgical resection for non–small cell lung cancer.

E. Glatstein, MD

8 Head and Neck Cancer

Molecular Marker Profiles Predict Locoregional Control of Head and Neck Squamous Cell Carcinoma in a Randomized Trial of Continuous Hyperfractionated Accelerated Radiotherapy

Buffa FM, Bentzen SM, Daley FM, et al (Mount Vernon Hosp, London; Univ College London; Barbara Ann Karmanos Cancer Inst, Detroit, Mich)

Clin Cancer Res 10:3745-3754, 2004 8–1

Introduction.—The identification of factors that assist prediction of tumor responses to radiotherapy may be helpful in refining treatment strategies and improving outcome. The possible correlation of molecular marker expression profiles with locoregional control of head and neck squamous cell carcinoma was examined in a randomized trial of conventional versus continuous hyperfractionated accelerated radiotherapy (CHART).

Methods.—Tumor material was obtained from 402 patients and underwent immunohistochemistry to evaluate Ki-67, CD31, p53, Bcl-2, and cyclin D1 expression. A hierarchical clustering algorithm with a Bayesian information criterion was used to group tumors with similar marker expression. The resulting expression profiles were comparing regarding their difference in outcome after CHART and conventionally fractionated radiotherapy.

Results.—Molecular marker profile was an independent prognostic factor for locoregional control and was verified in multivariate analysis that included these clinical variables: tumor and nodal status, primary site, histologic grade, age, and gender ($P < .001$ and $P = .006$ for local and nodal relapse, respectively). In particular, Bcl-2-positive tumors responded significantly better than average in both trial arms. Tumors negative for p53 and Bcl-2, with high and randomly patterned Ki-67 expression, responded worse than average; there was no benefit provided by CHART. Tumors with similarly negative p53 and Bcl-2, yet low Ki-67 staining and an organized pattern, benefitted significantly from the CHART schedule.

Conclusion.—It appears that molecular profiles have the potential to predict radiotherapy response of head and neck squamous cell carcinoma and to provide treatment stratification. Distinct expression profiles were associated with 3 distinct phenotypes, including good locoregional control, poor locoregional control, and an outcome strongly dependent on the fractionation schedule.

▶ The Medical Research Council conducted a randomized study comparing conventional radiation versus CHART in patients with head and neck cancer. This analysis, reported by Buffa et al, evaluated molecular marker profiles that may predict better outcome in a subset of patients treated with CHART. Tumors were stained for a variety of markers, including Bcl-2, which predicted for better outcome in both arms of the trial. Tumors that were negative for Bcl-2 and p53 but had low Ki-67 staining benefitted significantly from CHART. This study identifies the potential of molecular markers to predict response by radiation schedule in head and neck cancers. Prospective studies to correlate response to radiation with gene expression data are needed to help refine the optimal radiation schedule to be used in individual patients.

N. H. Hanna, MD

Treatment of Salivary Gland Neoplasms With Fast Neutron Radiotherapy

Douglas JG, Koh W, Austin-Seymour M, et al (Univ of Washington, Seattle)
Arch Otolaryngol Head Neck Surg 129:944-948, 2003 8–2

Background.—Salivary gland malignancies account for about 5% of all head and neck cancers. Postoperative irradiation can improve locoregional control and survival rate, especially in patients with advanced-stage disease. The efficacy of fast neutron radiotherapy in the treatment of salivary gland neoplasms was investigated in a retrospective analysis.

Methods.—The study included 279 patients who were treated with curative intent, using fast neutron radiotherapy. Of this number, 263 (94%) had evidence of gross residual disease at the time of treatment. Tumors of a major salivary gland were seen in 141 patients, and tumors of minor salivary glands were seen in 138. Patients were followed up for a median of 36 months.

Findings.—The actuarial cause-specific survival rate at 6 years was 67%. In a multivariate analysis, factors associated with a significant improvement in cause-specific survival rate were stage I to II disease, minor salivary sites, lack of skull base invasion, and primary disease. The actuarial locoregional control rate at 6 years was 59%. Factors associated with a significantly improved locoregional control rate in a multivariate analysis included tumor size of 4 cm or smaller, lack of invasion of base of skull, previous surgical resection, and no previous radiotherapy. The 6-year actuarial locoregional control rate was 100% in 16 patients with no evidence of gross residual disease. The actuarial rate of freedom from metastasis at 6 years was 64%. Variables related to decreased development of systemic metastases were negative lymph nodes at treatment and lack of skull base involvement. The 6-year actuarial rate of developing grade 3 or 4 toxicity in the long term was 10%; no patients had grade 5 effects.

Conclusions.—Neutron radiotherapy appears to be effective in patients with salivary gland neoplasms with gross residual disease. Locoregional control was excellent in patients with no evidence of gross disease.

▶ For approximately 20 years now, radiation oncologists have been told that the one tumor for which neutron therapy is indicated is a neoplasm of the salivary glands. This experience from the University of Washington reviews 279 patients who were treated with fast neutron therapy. Almost all of them had gross residual disease at the time of treatment. The median follow-up was 36 months, which is a little short for salivary gland tumors; but given the number, the follow-up is actually adequate. There is approximately an even split between major and minor salivary gland lesions among these patients. The 6-year actuarial cause specific survival rate is approximately 67%. It is unfortunate they do not give full survival curves, but rather focus on cause-specific survival. In any event, considering that these patients all have gross residual disease, this is an impressive accomplishment. The important prognostic factors associated with prolonged cause-specific survival rates relate to stage, lymph node positivity, size of lesion, base of skull involvement, prior surgery, and gross residual disease. All in all, this is a useful experience for a cancer that is uncommonly seen.

E. Glatstein, MD

Concurrent Chemotherapy and Radiotherapy for Organ Preservation in Advanced Laryngeal Cancer

Forastiere AA, Goepfert H, Maor M , et al (Johns Hopkins Univ, Baltimore, Md; Univ of Texas, Houston; Radiation Therapy Oncology Group Headquarters, Philadelphia; et al)

N Engl J Med 349:2091-2098, 2003 8–3

Background.—The use of induction chemotherapy followed by radiotherapy preserved the larynx in 64% of patients and permitted the same 68% 2-year survival rate as was achieved with the use of surgery plus adjuvant radiotherapy for patients with cancer of the larynx. The ability to preserve the larynx has led to the use of induction chemotherapy and radiotherapy as an alternative to laryngectomy for laryngeal cancer that is locally advanced. Three radiation-based treatments were evaluated for their resulting rates of laryngeal preservation in a randomized trial.

Methods.—Patients with locally advanced cancer of the larynx were randomly assigned to receive induction chemotherapy plus fluorouracil followed by radiotherapy, radiotherapy with concurrent cisplatin, or only radiotherapy. The median follow-up lasted 3.8 years. The rate of preservation of the larynx was compared among the 3 groups.

Results.—The analysis included 518 patients, all of whom had previously untreated stage III or IV laryngeal cancer. Toxic effects occurred with essentially the same severity and frequency in the group receiving induction cisplatin plus fluorouracil followed by radiotherapy as the group receiving radiotherapy alone and consisted principally of grade 3 in-field effects on the skin and mucous membranes. Patients who received radiotherapy plus cisplatin tended to have toxic effects related to the chemotherapy and increased rates of severe radiation-related effects on mucosa, the pharynx, and the esophagus. Overall, 81% of the group receiving induction cisplatin plus fluorouracil followed by radiotherapy, 82% of the group receiving radiotherapy with concurrent cisplatin, and 61% of the radiotherapy-alone group experienced severe toxic effects. Eighty-eight percent of patients receiving radiotherapy with concurrent cisplatin, 75% of those having induction chemotherapy followed by radiotherapy, and 70% of those having radiotherapy alone had an intact larynx after 2 years. Those receiving radiotherapy with concurrent cisplatin also had a significantly better local-regional control rate (78%) than the group receiving induction cisplatin plus fluorouracil followed by radiotherapy (61%) or the radiotherapy-alone group (56%). Distant metastases were less frequent among all patients receiving chemotherapy than among those having radiotherapy alone, which produced a better disease-free survival rate; however, the overall survival rates for all groups were similar.

Conclusions.—Overall survival rates among the 3 groups did not differ greatly, being approximately 75% at 2 years. Radiotherapy plus concurrent cisplatin achieved the highest rate of laryngeal preservation and had an absolute reduction in the rate of laryngectomy of 43% compared with the other groups. These findings apply only to patients with stage III or IV disease.

▶ Approximately 9500 patients in the United States each year are diagnosed with laryngeal carcinoma. Until a few years ago, the primary treatment for this disease was a total laryngectomy. More than a decade ago the Department of Veterans Affairs Laryngeal Cancer Study Group demonstrated that chemotherapy following radiation was just as effective as surgery followed by adjuvant radiotherapy.[1] The optimization of radiation and chemotherapy to minimize salvage laryngectomies was not known and is the subject of this landmark trial. The authors found that radiation therapy plus concurrent cisplatin was superior to sequential therapy with respect to laryngeal preservation and locoregional control. Toxicity is still significant and will need to be addressed in future studies. It should be noted that this study only included patients with stage III and IV laryngeal carcinoma and did not include patients with significant invasion of the tongue or gross destruction of the cartilage of the larynx. For many patients, however, this clearly seems to be the correct treatment approach.

P. J. Loehrer, Sr, MD

Reference

1. The Department of Veterans Affairs Laryngeal Cancer Study Group: Induction chemotherapy plus radiation compared with surgery plus radiation in patients with advanced laryngeal cancer. *N Engl J Med* 324:1685-1690, 1991.

Postoperative Concurrent Radiotherapy and Chemotherapy for High-Risk Squamous-Cell Carcinoma of the Head and Neck

Cooper JS, for the Radiation Therapy Oncology Group 9501/Intergroup (New York Univ; Radiation Therapy Oncology Group Headquarters, Philadelphia; Johns Hopkins Oncology Ctr, Baltimore, Md; et al)

N Engl J Med 350:1937-1944, 2004 8–4

Background.—High-risk squamous-cell carcinoma of the head and neck often recurs in the original tumor bed, despite treatment with resection and postoperative radiotherapy. Whether concurrent postoperative administration of cisplatin and radiotherapy would increase local and regional control rates was investigated.

Methods.—The study included 459 patients who were enrolled between 1995 and 2000. Total resection of all visible and palpable disease was performed in all patients. Patients were then assigned randomly to radiotherapy alone, 60 to 66 Gy in 30 to 33 fractions during 6 to 6.6 weeks; or to this treatment plus concurrent IV cisplatin, 100 mg per square meter of body-surface area on days 1, 22, and 43. The median follow-up was 45.9 months.

Findings.—Local and regional control rates were significantly greater for patients receiving combined therapy than for those given radiotherapy alone. The estimated 2-year rate of local and regional control was 82% for the combined treatment group and 72% for the radiotherapy only group. Disease-free survival was also significantly longer in the former group, though overall survival was comparable between groups. Acute adverse effects of grade 3 or worse occurred in 77% of the combined therapy group and in 34% of the radiotherapy only group. Four patients died as a direct result of combined therapy.

Conclusions.—Concurrent chemotherapy and radiotherapy after resection significantly improves local and regional control and disease-free survival rates among high-risk patients with head and neck cancer. However, this combined approach is associated with a marked increase in adverse effects, some potentially fatal.

Postoperative Irradiation With or Without Concomitant Chemotherapy for Locally Advanced Head and Neck Cancer

Bernier J, for the European Organization for Research and Treatment of Cancer Trial 22931 (Oncology Inst of Southern Switzerland, Bellinzona; Institut Gustave Roussy, Villejuif, France; Centre Hospitalier Universitaire Vaudois, Lausanne, Switzerland; et al)

N Engl J Med 350:1945-1952, 2004 8–5

Background.—Among patients with stage III or IV squamous-cell carcinoma of the head and neck, postoperative local or regional recurrences and distant metastases are common. The efficacy of concomitant cisplatin and irradiation was compared with that of radiotherapy alone as adjuvant therapy in this patient population.

Methods.—The study included 334 patients who had undergone surgery with curative intent and were assigned randomly to radiotherapy alone, 66 Gy during a 6.5-week period, or to the same radiotherapy plus cisplatin, 100 mg per square meter of body-surface area on days 1, 22, and 43. The median follow-up was 60 months.

Findings.—The combined therapy group had a significantly greater progression-free survival rate than did the radiotherapy only group. The 5-year Kaplan-Meier estimates of progression-free survival were 47% and 36%, respectively. In addition, the overall survival rate was significantly higher for patients receiving combined treatment than for those receiving radiotherapy alone, with 5-year Kaplan-Meier estimates of 53% and 40%, respectively. The cumulative incidence of local and regional recurrences in the combined treatment group was significantly less than in the radiation only group; the estimates of 5-year cumulative incidence was 31% after radiotherapy and 18% after combined treatment. Adverse effects of grade 3 or higher occurred in 41% of the patients receiving combined therapy, compared with the same adverse effects occurring in only 21% of those receiving radiotherapy alone. The types of severe mucosal adverse effects and the incidence of late adverse effects were comparable in the 2 groups.

Conclusions.—In patients with locally advanced head and neck cancer, postoperative concurrent administration of high-dose cisplatin with radiotherapy is more effective than radiotherapy alone. However, severe adverse effects were more common after combined therapy than after radiotherapy alone.

▶ Local failure rates with surgery followed by radiation therapy for patients with poor risk stage III and IV head and neck cancers remains high. A local/regional failure in the head/neck region can result in significant morbidity to the patient (pain, vascular or neurologic compromise, impingement on airway or swallowing, etc); therefore, attempts to reduce local failure after surgery is warranted. These trials reported by Cooper et al (Abstract 8–4) and Bernier et al (Abstract 8–5) evaluate the role of concomitant cisplatin given every 3 weeks for 3 treatments during postoperative radiation therapy alone compared with a control group of radiation therapy alone. Patient characteristics and numerical results for the trials differ slightly, but similar conclusions can be drawn from these studies. First, toxicity is significantly increased with the addition of cisplatin to radiation therapy compared with radiation therapy alone; however, this is mainly acute toxicity and patients can be supported through this difficulty (pain, dysphagia). Second, local failure rates are significantly reduced with the addition of cisplatin. Third, long-term survival appears slightly improved with cisplatin (statistically significant in the study by Bernier et al and numerically superior, but not statistically significant, in the study by Cooper et al). Collectively, these data provide support for the use of concurrent chemoradiation in the adjuvant setting for patients with poor-risk advanced head/neck cancers.

N. H. Hanna, MD

9 Malignant Melanoma

^{V599E}B-RAF Is an Oncogene in Melanocytes

Wellbrock C, Oglivie L, Hedley D, et al (Inst of Cancer Research, London; Inst of Cancer Research, Sutton, Surrey, England)

Cancer Res 64:2338-2342, 2004 9–1

Background.—Through the activation of various effector proteins, the RAS proteins regulate cell proliferation, survival, and differentiation. Activated RAF proteins stimulate a signaling cascade that includes both the MEK and the extracellular signal-regulated kinase (ERK) protein kinases. RAS gene mutations are found in approximately 15% to 20% of patients who have melanoma, but RAS activation in melanocytes has produced melanoma in mice only when the cell cycle progression inhibitor p16^{INK4A} was also deleted. Mutation of the RAS effector B-RAF is found in approximately 70% of cutaneous melanomas and 80% of benign melanocytic lesions (nevi). Eighty percent of the B-RAF mutations involve a glutamic acid for valine substitution at position 599, yielding a protein with elevated kinase activity in vitro and constitutive activation of ERK. Most cell lines of melanoma have elevated ERK activity. In cultures, elevated ERK signaling seems to be required for melanocyte proliferation. The conclusion is that RAS induces ERK activation with a dependence on B-RAF, then these oncogenes transform melanocytes with a common mechanism. ^{V599E}B-RAF was shown to stimulate constitutive ERK activity and transform melan a cells, making it an important melanocyte oncogene.

Methods.—Melan-a cell cultures were exposed to ^{V599E}B-RAF and wild-type B-RAF (^{WT}B-RAF). The results were then evaluated in vitro and in vivo in female CD1 nude mice.

Results.—Western blotting revealed that even with low levels of expression, all the cell lines that expressed ^{V599E}B-RAF had constitutive MEK and ERK activation. However, no increased MEK or ERK phosphorylation was found in cell lines expressing even high levels of ^{WT}B-RAF. Therefore, the overexpression of ^{WT}B-RAF was inadequate to trigger melanocytes to produce constitutive MEK/ERK signaling.

Conclusions.—B-RAF proved to be a potent oncogene during the early stages of melanoma development. In contrast, ^{WT}B-RAF was not required to produce RAS-induced pigment cell transformation. These findings are important considerations in developing therapeutic strategies for melanoma.

► Melanoma is a devastating disease that frequently arises from precursor lesions in the form of dysplastic nevi or even from the malignant transformation of previously benign nevi. B-RAF is an downstream molecule in the RAS-RAF kinase pathway and is mutated and activated in 80% of benign nevi. Initially thought to be a critical step in the development of melanoma and a valuable target for therapeutic development, inhibitors of RAF kinases have not demonstrated significant antitumor activity in this setting. The authors of this article studied the mechanisms of tumorigenicity in transformed melanocytes to determine the role of the mutated B-RAF gene. They found that while the presence of a mutated B-RAF gene is strongly associated with transformation of melanocytes to melanoma, once transformed, the melanoma cells develop redundant pathways that significantly reduce the impact of RAF kinase inhibitors as antitumor agents on their own. Hence, while this target remains attractive, it may require combinations of selective inhibitors to modulate the antitumor activity adequately enough to warrant their use as targeted therapies in melanoma treatment.

M. S. Gordon, MD

Prognostic Significance of Molecular Upstaging of Paraffin-Embedded Sentinel Lymph Nodes in Melanoma Patients

Takeuchi H, Morton DL, Kuo C, et al (John Wayne Cancer Inst, Santa Monica, Calif)

J Clin Oncol 22:2671-2680, 2004 9–2

Background.—Melanoma recurs in a significant number of patients with histopathologically negative sentinel lymph nodes (SLNs). A quantitative real-time reverse transcriptase polymerase chain reaction (qRT) assay with multiple specific mRNA markers may identify occult metastasis in paraffin-embedded (PE) SLNs to upstage and better predict disease outcomes.

Methods.—Paraffin-embedded SLNs collected from 215 clinically node-negative patients were analyzed by qRT. All patients had had lymphatic mapping and sentinel lymphadenopathy for melanoma. Follow-up was at least 8 years. A total of 308 PE SLNs were sectioned and assessed by qRT for mRNA of 4 melanoma-related genes: *MART-1*, *MAGE-A3*, *GalNAc-T*, and *Pax3*.

Findings.—Positive SLNs were identified in 25% of the patients by hematoxylin and eosin or immunohistochemistry. Thirty percent of the 162 with histopathologically negative SLNs expressed at least 1 of the 4 qRT markers. These 48 patients also had significantly increased risk of disease recurrence in a Cox proportional hazards model, with a risk ratio of 7.48. The presence of 1 or more markers in histopathologically negative SLNs was a significant, independent prognostic indicator of overall survival in a multivariate analysis (Fig 3).

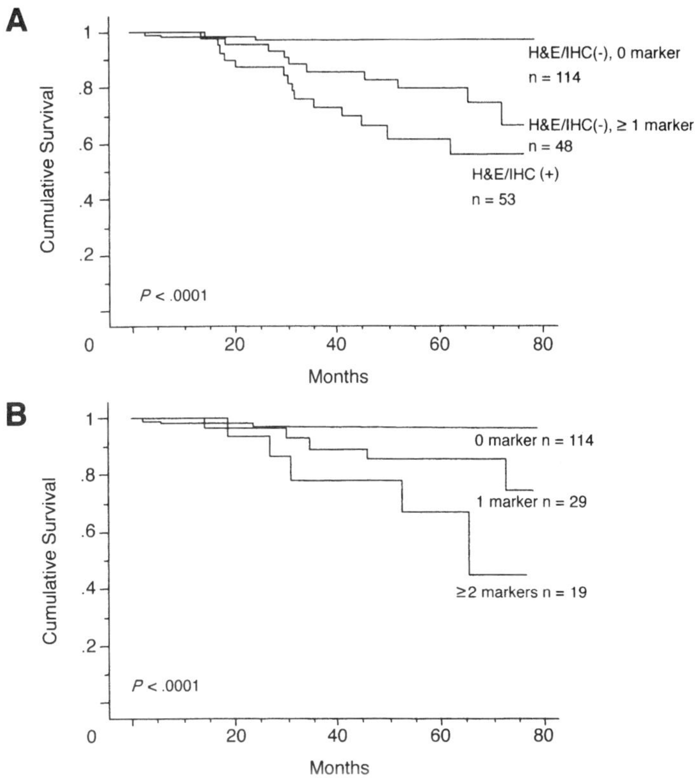

FIGURE 3.—**A**, Kaplan-Meier curve analysis of overall survival (*OS*) according to multiple marker qRT and histopathology status in 215 patients. **B**, Kaplan-Meier curve analysis of OS according to number of molecular markers in 162 SLN histopathology-negative patients. *Abbreviations: H&E*, Hematoxylin and eosin; *IHC*, immunohistochemistry. (Courtesy of Takeuchi H, Morton DL, Kuo C, et al: Prognostic significance of molecular upstaging of paraffin-embedded sentinel lymph nodes in melanoma patients. *J Clin Oncol* 22:2671-2680, 2004. Reprinted with permission from the American Society of Clinical Oncology.)

Conclusions.—This multiple-marker qRT assay can identify occult metastatic melanoma cells in PE SLN, resulting in an upstaging of early malignant melanoma. Molecular upstaging of PE histopathologically negative SLNs is a significant independent prognostic indicator for long-term disease recurrence and overall patient survival. This technique is rapid, reproducible, and quantitatively significant.

► The use of molecular markers to improve prognostic prediction for individual patients is a major area of research interest. This retrospective study suggests that the use of qRT for specific melanoma-associated markers in SLNs provides improved prediction of disease-free survival compared with standard hematoxylin and eosin or immunohistochemical examination. Although the results of this study are impressive, several caveats must be kept in mind. This is a single-institution, retrospective study. Before use in clinical practice, prospective validation is needed. In addition, the ability of multiple institutions to reproduce the technology utilized and the definition of an ideal marker panel remains uncertain. However, this is clearly an area worthy of further study to determine the implications of these findings for both local and systemic treatment.

M. Morrow, MD

Excision Margins in High-Risk Malignant Melanoma

Thomas JM, for the United Kingdom Melanoma Study Group, the British Association of Plastic Surgeons, and the Scottish Cancer Therapy Network (Royal Marsden Hosp Natl Health Service Trust, London; et al)

N Engl J Med 350:757-766, 2004 9–3

Background.—The risk of death of cutaneous melanoma is determined primarily by the tumor's thickness, the presence or absence of tumor ulcerations and microdeposits of melanoma in sentinel lymph nodes, the site of the tumor, and the sex of the patient. In the past, wide margins of excision were used to prevent lymphatic spread, but in the last 10 years these margins have become smaller because trials have suggested that narrower margins are safe. However, inadequate excision margins increase the risk of local recurrence and in-transit metastases, and unnecessarily large margins are associated with greater morbidity and increased cost. The effect of width of excision margin on the outcome of patients with high-risk malignant melanoma was investigated.

Methods.—From an enrollment of 900 patients, 453 were randomly assigned to undergo surgery with a 1-cm margin of excision, and 447 patients were assigned to surgery with a 3-cm margin of excision. The median follow-up for these patients was 60 months. The main outcome measures were local recurrence, which was defined as a recurrence within 2 cm of the scar or graft, and in-transit recurrence, which was defined as a recurrence from beyond the first 2 cm of the scar or graft to the regional nodes.

Results.—The patients who underwent surgery with a 1-cm margin of excision were at a significantly increased risk of locoregional recurrence. There were 168 cases of locoregional recurrence in the group with 1-cm margins of excision compared with 142 cases of locoregional recurrence in the group with 3-cm margins (Table 5). A total of 128 deaths attributable to melanoma were recorded in the group with 1-cm margins compared with 105 in the group with 3-cm margins. The overall survival was similar in the 2 groups.

Conclusion.—In patients with melanoma with a poor prognosis (tumor thickness 2 mm or greater), a 1-cm margin of excision is associated with a significantly greater risk of regional recurrence than is a 3-cm margin, but with a similar overall survival rate.

▶ Although the appropriate margin width for excision of melanoma has been examined in 3 randomized trials,[1-3] only 1 of these studies included patients with melanomas greater than 2 mm in thickness.[2] The randomized trial presented here demonstrates a 34% increase in locoregional events in patients

TABLE 5.—Multivariate Analysis of Locoregional Recurrence, Recurrence or Death, Death From Melanoma, and Death From Any Cause*

Factor	No. of Patients	Primary End Points				Secondary End Points			
		Locoregional Recurrence Hazard Ratio (95% CI)	*P* Value	Recurrence or Death Hazard Ratio (95% CI)	*P* Value	Death From Melanoma Hazard Ratio (95% CI)	*P* Value	Death From Any Cause Hazard Ratio (95% CI)	*P* Value
Margin of excision			0.02		0.03		0.07		0.3
3 cm†	383	1.00		1.00		1.00		1.00	
1 cm	386	1.34 (1.06-1.70)		1.25 (1.02-1.55)		1.29 (0.98-1.70)		1.14 (0.89-1.47)	
Sex			0.03		0.01		0.02		0.02
Female†	351	1.00		1.00		1.00		1.00	
Male	418	1.34 (1.03-1.74)		1.35 (1.07-1.70)		1.46 (1.07-1.98)		1.41 (1.07-1.86)	
Tumor thickness‡			<0.001		<0.001		<0.001		<0.001
2 mm	200	0.70 (0.54-0.91)		0.74 (0.59-0.94)		0.77 (0.57-1.05)		0.79 (0.59-1.04)	
3 mm†	247	1.00		1.00		1.00		1.00	
4 mm	137	1.28 (0.99-1.67)		1.24 (0.98-1.56)		1.2 (0.89-1.64)		1.19 (0.90-1.57)	
5 mm	70	1.56 (1.20-2.02)		1.46 (1.16-1.84)		1.39 (1.02-1.89)		1.35 (1.02-1.79)	
6 mm	115	1.82 (1.40-2.37)		1.67 (1.32-2.11)		1.57 (1.15-2.13)		1.51 (1.14-2.00)	
Ulceration			<0.001		<0.001		<0.001		<0.001
Absent†	472	1.00		1.00		1.00		1.00	
Present	297	1.74 (1.37-2.24)		1.71 (1.38-2.12)		2.00 (1.51-2.65)		2.04 (1.58-2.64)	
Site			0.9		0.21		0.03		0.06
Distal limb†	244	1.00		1.00		1.00		1.00	
Proximal limb	172	1.10 (0.78-1.54)		1.27 (0.94-1.71)		1.64 (1.09-2.48)		1.45 (1.00-2.09)	
Trunk	353	1.06 (0.78-1.44)		1.24 (0.95-1.63)		1.63 (1.11-2.37)		1.45 (1.04-2.02)	

*A total of 769 patients had complete data on all the factors included in the multivariate analysis. Factors that did not have independent predictive ability in the multivariate analysis were included in order to be able to make comparisons across end points (ie, the margin of excision was included in the models for melanoma-specific and overall survival, and site was included in the models for locoregional recurrence and disease-free survival).

†This group served as the reference group.

‡The tumor thickness was determined before randomization and histologic review.

(Reprinted by permission of *The New England Journal of Medicine* from Thomas JM, for the United Kingdom Melanoma Study Group, the British Association of Plastic Surgeons, and the Scottish Cancer Therapy Network: Excision margins in high-risk malignant melanoma. *N Engl J Med* 350:757-766, 2004.)

with melanomas 2 mm or greater in thickness excised to a 1 cm, rather than a 3-cm margin. Although the risk of melanoma specific death was not statistically significantly increased, a hazard ratio of 1.29 was observed in multivariate analysis. While an increased risk of death with inadequate local control seems quite feasible in a disease where systemic therapy is of limited efficacy, avoidance of the morbidity of local recurrence is a reasonable goal even in the absence of a survival benefit. This study indicates that a 1-cm margin does not provide optimal local control for melanomas 2 mm or greater in thickness, but does not provide guidance as to whether the 3-cm margin used in this study is preferable to the 2-cm margin studied in the Intergroup Melanoma Surgical Trial.[1]

M. Morrow, MD

References

1. Balch CM, Soong SJ, Smith T, et al: Long-term results of a prospective surgical trial comparing 2 cm vs. 4 cm excision margins for 740 patients with 1-4 mm melanomas. *Ann Surg Oncol* 8:101-108, 2001.
2. Cohn-Cedermark G, Rutqvist LE, Andersson R, et al: Long-term results of a randomized study by the Swedish Melanoma Study Group on 2-cm versus 5-cm resection margins for patients with cutaneous melanoma with tumor thickness of 0.8-2.0 mm. *Cancer* 89:1495-1501, 2000.
3. Veronesi U, Cascinelli N, Adamus J, et al: Thin stage I primary cutaneous malignant melanoma: Comparison of excision with margins of 1 or 3 cm. *N Eng J Med* 318:1159-1162, 1998.

► The margins for excision of melanoma have been controversial over the past several decades. Previous trials have examined tumor margins but were done largely in thin lesions.[1-3] All these previous trials (with the exception of one) included patients with thicknesses less than 2 mm and none contained patients with depth greater than 4 mm. This study demonstrates that a 3-cm margin is superior to a 1-cm margin for deeper lesions. Whether a 2-cm margin would accomplish the same as 3-cm remains to be seen.

P. J. Loehrer, Sr, MD

References

1. Balch CM, Soong SJ, Smith T, et al: Long-term results of a prospective surgical trial comparing 2 cm vs 4 cm excision margins for 740 patients with 1-4 mm melanomas. *Ann Surg Oncol* 8:101-108, 2001.
2. Cohn-Cedermark G, Rutqvist LE, Andersson R, et al: Long term results of a randomized study by the Swedish Melanoma Study Group on 2-cm versus 5-cm resection margins for patients with cutaneous melanoma with a tumor thickness of 0.8-2.0 mm. *Cancer* 89:1495-1501, 2000.
3. Veronesi U, Cascinelli N, Adamus J, et al: Thin stage I primary cutaneous malignant melanoma: Comparison of excision with margins of 1 or 3 cm. *N Engl J Med* 318:1159-1162, 1988 (erratum, *N Engl J Med* 325:292, 1991).

10 Sarcoma

Osteosarcoma Over the Age of Forty

Grimer RJ, Cannon SR, Taminiau AM, et al (Royal Orthopaedic Hosp, Birmingham, England; Royal Natl Orthopaedic Hosp, Stanmore, England; Leiden Univ Med Centre, The Netherlands; et al)
Eur J Cancer 39:157-163, 2003 10–1

Background.—Most osteosarcomas (OSs) arise in adolescence, but a second peak occurs in the seventh and eighth decades of life. Aggressive chemotherapeutic approaches are not usually used for elderly patients, who are believed to be unable to tolerate these treatments. Patients older than 40 years who had OS were retrospectively reviewed by The European Musculo Skeletal Oncology Society.

Methods.—A total of 481 patients (mean age, 55 years) with newly diagnosed OS of bone were studied. Twenty-six patients had low-grade OS, 42 had OS linked to Paget's disease, 41 had OS develop after radiation, and 270 had high-grade OS, with 48 having metastases at diagnosis. The details on treatment and outcome were analyzed.

Results.—Each year from 1955 on, more patients were added to the registry, with an average of 40 patients added each year at the end. Tumor sizes ranged from 1 to 34 cm; the average size was 11 cm. In 29% of conventional high-grade OSs, the distal femur was involved; in 14%, the proximal tibia; in 14%, the pelvis; and in 10% the humerus (Table 1). Seven of 42 patients with

TABLE 1.—Location of the Tumors Split by Main Sites/Grades

Site	Total	High Grade	Paget's	Radiation-Induced	Low Grade
Femur	189	159	12	4	14
Pelvis	72	45	12	12	3
Tibia	58	51	3	1	3
Humerus	50	33	9	6	2
Scapula	20	7	2	11	0
Rib	16	14	0	2	0
Skull	15	9	2	1	3
Jaw	11	10	0	0	1
Others	50	44	2	4	0
Total	481	372	42	41	26

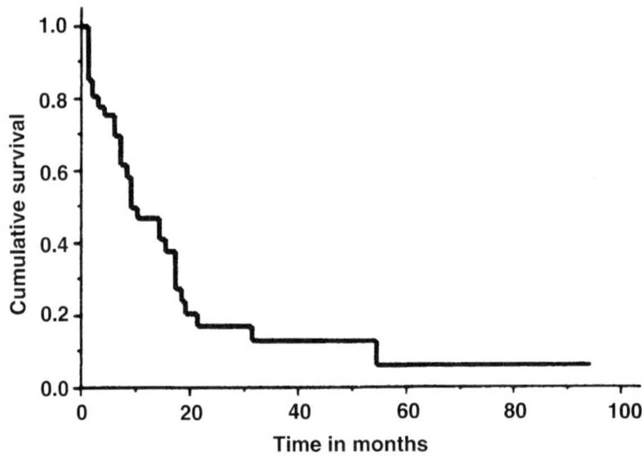

FIGURE 3.—Survivorship of patients with Paget's osteosarcoma. (Reprinted from Grimer RJ, Cannon SR, Taminiau AM, et al: Osteosarcoma over the age of forty. *Eur J Cancer* 39:157-163, 2003. Copyright 2003, with permission from Elsevier Science.)

Paget's OS had metastases at diagnosis. The femur and pelvis were most often involved. Fourteen patients had surgery, 2 had chemotherapy, and 22 had palliative radiotherapy. Local recurrence develop in 5 surgical patients. One patient survived 8 years after amputation for OS of the tibia, but the median survival was 9 months (Fig 3). Women predominated in the 41 patients with radiation-induced OS. The pelvis and scapula were the most common sites involved, reflecting sites affected by radiotherapy for ovarian/cervical cancer and breast cancer. From 6 to 23 years elapsed between radiation exposure and OS development. Chemotherapy was used for 22 patients, surgery for 29, and 15 had both. Radiotherapy was used in 3 cases. Local recurrence developed in 11 patients. Patients with metastases at diagnosis died within 15 months, but the overall median survival was 33 months, and the 5-year survival rate was 35% (Fig 4). In 26 patients with low-grade

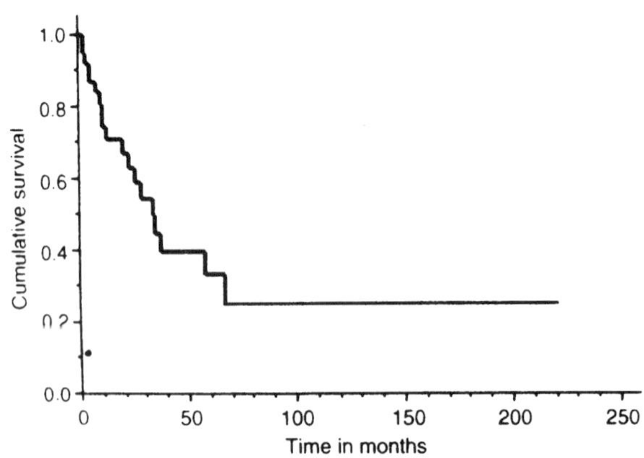

FIGURE 4.—Survivorship of patients with radiation-induced osteosarcoma. (Reprinted from Grimer RJ, Cannon SR, Taminiau AM, et al: Osteosarcoma over the age of forty. *Eur J Cancer* 39:157-163, 2003. Copyright 2003, with permission from Elsevier Science.)

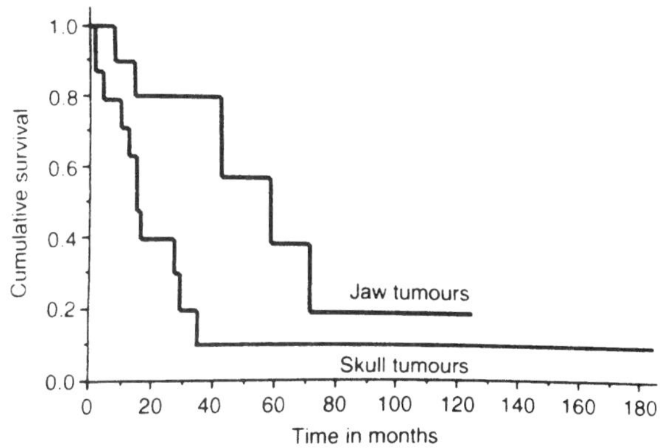

FIGURE 5.—Survival of patients with jaw and skull tumors. (Reprinted from Grimer RJ, Cannon SR, Taminiau AM, et al: Osteosarcoma over the age of forty. *Eur J Cancer* 39:157-163, 2003. Copyright 2003, with permission from Elsevier Science.)

OS, the femur, tibia, and pelvis were most often affected. Chemotherapy was used for 2 patients and surgery for 25. Local recurrence developed in 4 patients and metastatic disease in 3. The 5-year survival rate was 88%. The skull or jaw was involved in 26 patients, of whom 20 had surgery. Local recurrence developed in 6 of 11 jaw excisions and 7 of 9 skull excisions. Nine patients had radiotherapy and 9 had chemotherapy. The median survival was 57 months for jaw tumors and 15 months for skull tumors (Fig 5). Three patients had OS of the spine, and 5 had OS of the sacrum. Surgery and chemotherapy were effective in spinal OS, but all patients with sacral tumors died within 20 months of diagnosis. Pelvic OS affected 72 patients. Of 37 who had surgery, 24 also had chemotherapy; 17 had chemotherapy with or without radiation. The median survival was 14 months; only 14% survived long-term. None of the 20 patients with high-grade OS of the axial skeleton not involving the spine or pelvis survived 5 years, even with surgery and chemotherapy. The survival rate among the 41 patients with conventional OS with metastases was 12% at 5 years; all had chemotherapy and surgery. Of 238 patients with high-grade conventional OS, amputation was done in 86 patients, limb salvage surgery in 126, chemotherapy in 154, and radiotherapy in 22 cases. Local recurrence was found in 25, with most having had simple surgical excision. Five- and 10-year overall survival rates were 46% and 33%, respectively. OS of the lower limb and age younger than 60 years were significantly associated with survival at 5 years.

Conclusions.—OS among older patients is a challenging disease that requires aggressive management, including chemotherapy when possible. Cure cannot be achieved without complete surgical excision.

▶ This group of European investigators reports on patients who developed OS beyond the age of 40. They have a total of 481 patients, of whom 42 developed OS in the setting of Paget's disease. They also had 41 patients with radiation-induced sarcomas whose prognosis appeared to be similar to that of conventional OS. For those with axial tumors or metastatic tumors, the prognosis was poor. Nonetheless, of 238 patients who had nonmetastatic OS, a survival of 46% at 5 years was reported.

From time to time we see such patients, and we are hard pressed to find a lot of data on which to base our decisions. This is a useful reference in that regard. I think the thing you can take away from this is that this disease is relatively poorly studied. I know that most people would not consider radiation as part of the management because this is supposedly a "radioresistant neoplasm." Personally, I have a modest experience with unresectable osteogenic sarcomas of the torso which leads me to believe that is incorrect. I have 3 long-term survivors with unresectable OS treated with radiation alone. I have also found radiation useful as an adjuvant in resected OS of the adult in the head and neck region. It is my own belief that people have assumed that osteogenic sarcoma is "radioresistant" simply because the masses rarely shrink in size. This is true for most bony neoplasms, other than Ewing's. The fact is that most of these tumors have enough matrix and stroma associated with their malignant growth that even if all the cells are killed, the stroma and matrix persist.

E. Glatstein, MD

Neoadjuvant Chemotherapy for Ewing's Tumor of Bone: Recent Experience at the Rizzoli Orthopaedic Institute

Bacci G, Mercuri M, Longhi A, et al (Rizzoli Orthopaedic Inst, Bologna, Italy; S Orsola Hosp, Bologna, Italy)

Eur J Cancer 38:2243-2251, 2002 10–2

Background.—Standard treatment for Ewing's sarcoma of the bone at present includes neoadjuvant chemotherapy. In November 1991, a new neoadjuvant, single-arm, nonrandomized protocol (REN-3) was initiated with ifosfamide and actinomycin from the induction treatment. Results achieved between 1991 and 1997 were reported.

Methods.—One hundred fifty-seven patients with nonmetastatic Ewing's sarcoma of the bone underwent treatment according to the REN-3 protocol

TABLE 4.—Probability of Relapse According to Several Variables: Multivariate Analyses

Variable		Odds Ratio (95% CI)	*P* Value
Serum LDH	Elevated	2.484 (1.498-4.119)	$P = 0.0004$
	Normal	1	
Necrosis	Grade I and II	2.083 (1.208-3.594)	$P = 0.008$
	Grade III	1	
Fever	Present	3.460 (1.352-8.858)	$P = 0.009$
	Absent	1	
Volume	> 100 mL	2.484 (1.329-3.910)	$P = 0.002$
	> 100 mL	1	

Abbreviation: 95% CI, 95% confidence interval.

(Reprinted from Bacci G, Mercuri M, Longhi A, et al: Neoadjuvant chemotherapy for Ewing's tumor of bone: Recent experience at the Rizzoli Orthopaedic Institute. *Eur J Cancer* 38:2243-2251, 2002.

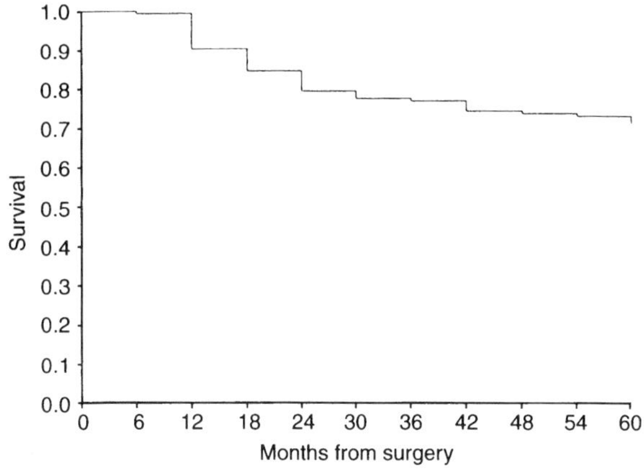

FIGURE 3.—Five-year event-free survival (71%). (Reprinted from Bacci G, Mercuri M, Longhi A, et al: Neoadjuvant chemotherapy for Ewing's tumor of bone: Recent experience at the Rizzoli Orthopaedic Institute. *Eur J Cancer* 38:2243-2251, 2002. Copyright 2002, with permission from Elsevier Science.)

at 1 center between 1991 and 1997. Induction chemotherapy consisted of 2 cycles of vincristine, doxorubicin, and cyclophosphamide (VAC) alternating with a cycle of ifosfamide and actinomycin (VIAc). After local treatment, patients were given another 3 VAC cycles; 2 VIAc cycles; 3 cycles of ifosfamide plus etoposide; and 2 cycles of vincristine, cyclophosphamide, and actinomycin. Local treatment consisted of surgery alone in 53% of the patients, surgery plus radiotherapy in 25%, and radiotherapy only in 22%.

Findings.—At a mean follow-up of 7 years, 70% of patients were continuously event-free. Forty-five patients had relapses, 33 from metastases and 12 from local recurrence associated with metastases (Table 4). Two patients died from toxicity. Event-free survival at 5 years was 71%, and overall survival at 5 years, 76.5% (Figs 3 and 4).

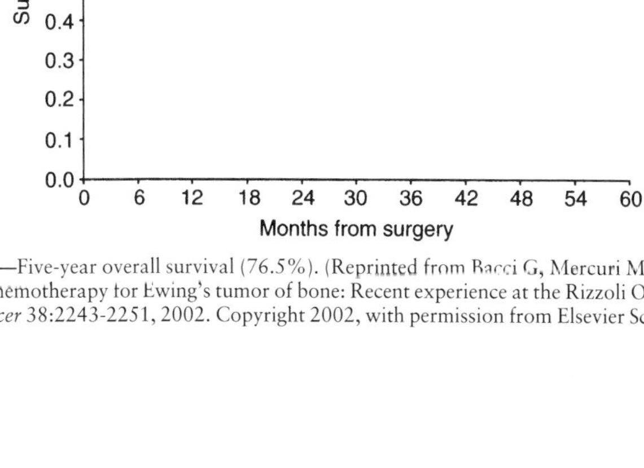

FIGURE 4.—Five-year overall survival (76.5%). (Reprinted from Bacci G, Mercuri M, Longhi A, et al: Neoadjuvant chemotherapy for Ewing's tumor of bone: Recent experience at the Rizzoli Orthopaedic Institute. *Eur J Cancer* 38:2243-2251, 2002. Copyright 2002, with permission from Elsevier Science.)

Conclusions.—Adding ifosfamide and etoposide to the classic VACAc regimen in patients with Ewing's sarcoma of the bone improves prognosis. These findings also indicate the early use of ifosfamide.

▶ This article from Italy looks at 157 patients who had Ewing's sarcoma of bone without obvious metastases. Typically, these patients have gone to surgery and then received adjuvant treatment. However, these authors are reporting on a protocol in which they started on induction chemotherapy with vincristine, Adriamycin (doxorubicin), and cyclophosphamide alternating with vincristine, ifosfamide, and actinomycin D. About a third of their patients had primary lesions that did not involve the extremities. The median follow-up was 7 years, and thus it appears to be adequate. The overall event-free survival at 5 years is about 70%, which is a good figure. The overall survival is just over 75% at 5 years. Nonetheless, the authors give no data beyond 5 years despite the median 7-year follow-up, thereby raising some question marks. The idea of giving neoadjuvant treatment as opposed to adjuvant would appear to have some real value, and one can anticipate that this will be used more commonly.

E. Glatstein, MD

Kinase Mutations and Imatinib Response in Patients With Metastatic Gastrointestinal Stromal Tumor

Heinrich MC, Corless CL, Demetri GD, et al (Oregon Univ, Portland; Portland Veterans Affairs Med Ctr, Ore; Dana-Farber Cancer Inst, Boston; et al)

J Clin Oncol 21:4342-4349, 2003 10–3

Introduction.—Most gastrointestinal stromal tumors (GISTs) express constitutively activated mutant isoforms of the receptor tyrosine kinase KIT or kinase platelet-derived growth factor receptor alpha (PDGFRA), which are potential therapeutic targets for imatinib mesylate. The association between mutations in these kinases and clinical response to imatinib was evaluated in patients with advance GIST.

Methods.—The GISTs from 127 patients enrolled in a clinical investigation of imatinib were evaluated for mutations of KIT or PDGFRA. The correlation between mutation types and clinical outcome was assessed.

Results.—Activating mutations of KIT or PDGFRA were identified in 112 (88.2%) and 6 (4.7%) GISTs, respectively. Most of the KIT mutations involved exon 9 or exon 11 (23 and 85 mutations, respectively) (Fig 1). All KIT mutant isoforms and a subset of PDGFRA mutant isoforms were sensitive to imatinib in vitro. In patients with GISTs that harbored exon 11 KIT mutations, the partial response rate was 83.5%; patients with tumors with an exon 9 KIT mutation or no detectable mutation of KIT or PDGFRA had partial response rates of 47.8% (P = .0006) and 0.0%, respectively. Patients with tumors with exon 11 KIT mutations had longer event-free and overall survival rates compared with those whose tumors expressed either exon 9 KIT mutations or had no identifiable kinase mutation (Fig 3).

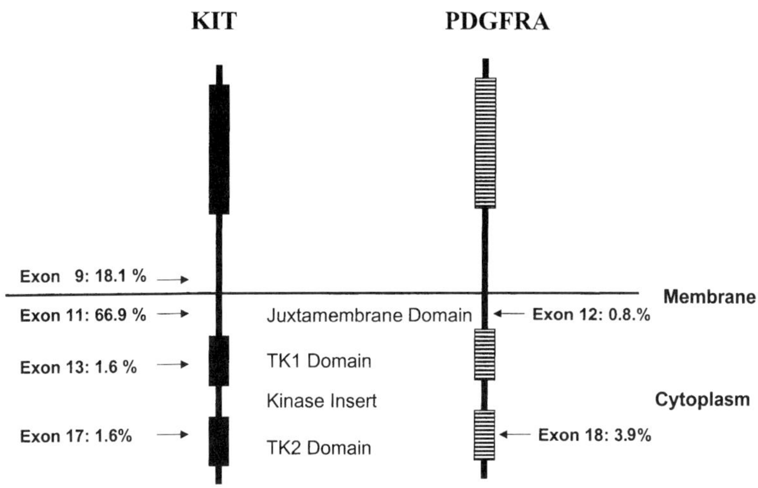

FIGURE 1.—Structure of KIT and PDGFRA. Locations of GIST-associated kinase mutations are shown in relation to the structural features of the patient. GISTs from 9 (7.1%) of 127 patients had no detectable KIT or PDGFRA mutation. (Courtesy of Heinrich MC, Corless CL, Demetri GD, et al: Kinase mutations and imatinib response in patients with metastatic gastrointestinal stromal tumor. *J Clin Oncol* 21:4342-4349, 2003. Reprinted with permission from the American Society for Clinical Oncology.)

Conclusion.—Activating mutations of KIT or PDGFRA are seen in most GISTs; the mutational status of these oncoproteins is predictive of clinical response to imatinib. The PDGFRA mutation may explain clinical response and sensitivity to imatinib in some GISTs lacking KIT mutations.

► One of the most exciting therapeutic strategies in the last few years has been that of the incorporation of imatinib for the treatment of GISTs. Like life, few things are perfect. In this case, not all patients with GIST respond favorably to imatinib. These investigators studied the impact of the activating mutations of KIT and PDGFRA with clinical outcome. One of the more interesting aspects is that some patients with GIST tumors who lack KIT mutations respond if they have gain-of-function PDGFRA mutations. Seven percent of patients will have no detectable KIT or PDGFRA mutations. This study provides further insight, bridging molecular biology and therapeutics in this unique tumor.

P. J. Loehrer, Sr, MD

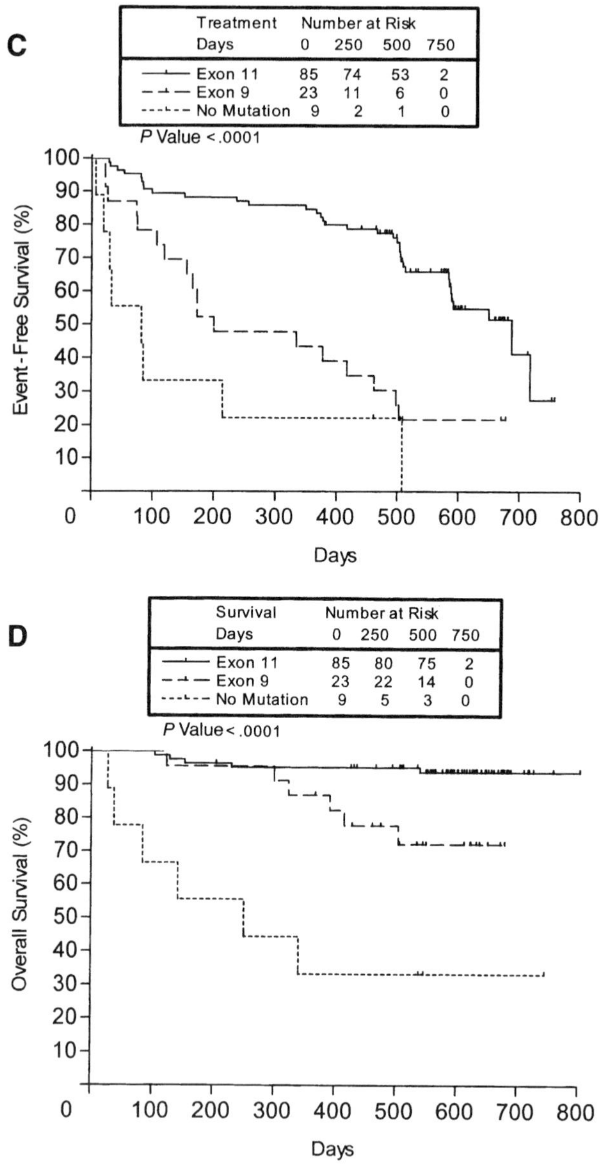

FIGURE 3.—GIST kinase genotype correlates with event-free survival and overall survival. Kaplan-Meier estimate of probability of event-free survival (**C**) and overall survival (**D**) for patients with KIT exon 11 mutation, KIT exon 9 mutation, or no mutation of KIT or PDGFRA. Log-rank *P* value is listed above each graph. (Courtesy of Heinrich MC, Corless CL, Demetri GD, et al: Kinase mutations and imatinib response in patients with metastatic gastrointestinal stromal tumor. *J Clin Oncol* 21:4342-4349, 2003. Reprinted with permission from the American Society for Clinical Oncology.)

Peritoneal Leiomyosarcomatosis Originating From Gastrointestinal Leiomyosarcomas: CT Features

Rha SE, Ha HK, Kim AY, et al (Univ of Ulsan, Seoul, Korea; Catholic Univ of Korea, Seoul)

Radiology 227:385-390, 2003 10–4

Background.—Peritoneal leiomyosarcomatosis (PL) is the peritoneal dissemination of leiomyosarcomas. Computed tomography may be useful in patients suspected of having PL, because CT can depict peritoneal nodules and determine the primary tumor site. The CT features of PL originating from gastrointestinal leiomyosarcoma were assessed. In addition, the CT features of primary gastrointestinal leiomyosarcomas in patients with and without PL were compared.

Methods.—The CT scans and medical records of 89 patients with gastrointestinal leiomyosarcoma were reviewed. The morphologic appearance of peritoneal lesions on CT scans was evaluated.

Findings.—Thirty-nine patients had metastases, and 25 had PL (Fig 2). Other metastatic sites observed were the liver in 26 patients, lymph nodes in 11, lungs in 3, and bone in 1 (Table 1). Twenty-two of the 25 patients with PL had multiple discrete peritoneal nodules on CT, and 3 had massive peritoneal lesions. In 10 patients, smudged omental infiltration was observed along with other findings. Peritoneal masses were seen in the mesentery in 18 patients, omentum in 11, paracolic gutters in 11, pelvic cavity in 8, perihepatic space in 3, and perisplenic space in 1. Ascites were present in 4 patients. Patients with and patients without PL showed significant differences in the size of the primary tumor, the mean diameter being 12.5 and 9.2 cm, respec-

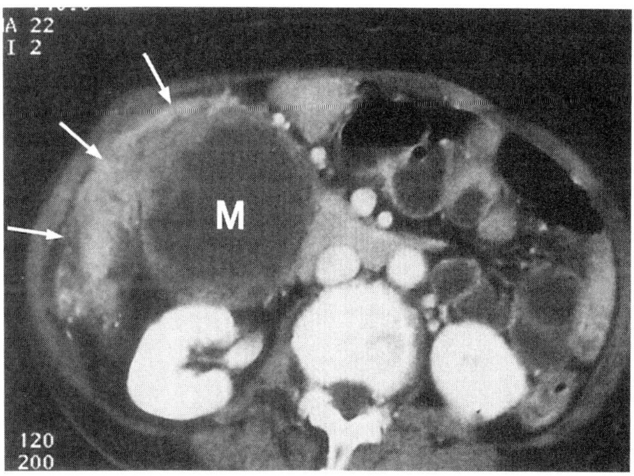

FIGURE 2.—Transverse contrast-enhanced CT scan obtained in a 69-year-old woman with PL originating from gastric leiomyosarcoma shows a large well-defined mesenteric mass (M) with extensive central necrosis combined with adjacent infiltrative omental thickening (*arrows*). (Courtesy of Rha SE, Ha HK, Kim AY, et al: Peritoneal leiomyosarcomatosis originating from gastrointestinal leiomyosarcomas: CT features. *Radiology* 227:385-390, 2003. Radiological Society of North America.)

TABLE 1.—Sites of Metastatic Leiomyosarcoma

Site	No. of Patients*
Liver	26/89 (29)
Peritoneum	25/89 (28)
Mesentery	18/25 (72)
Omentum	11/25 (44)
Paracolic gutters	11/25 (44)
Pelvic cavity	8/25 (32)
Perihepatic space	3/25 (12)
Perisplenic space	1/25 (4)
Lymph nodes	11/89 (12)
Paraaortic	6/11 (54)
Perigastric	4/11 (36)
Perirectal	1/11 (9)
Lungs	3/89 (3)
Bone	1/89 (1)

*The data on a total of 89 patients with gastrointestinal leiomyosarcoma were analyzed. Numbers in parentheses are percentages.

(Courtesy of Rha SE, Ha HK, Kim AY, et al: Peritoneal leiomyosarcomatosis originating from gastrointestinal leiomyosarcomas: CT features. *Radiology* 227:385-390, 2003.)

tively (Table 2). The prevalence of exophytic primary tumor growth also differed significantly between groups.

Conclusions.—Findings on CT scans can indicate PL in the differential diagnosis of patients with gastrointestinal leiomyosarcoma. When PL originates from large primary tumors, its prevalence appears to be greater.

► It has been my experience that CT and MR have both been relatively disappointing from the standpoint of being able to pick up peritoneal seeding. Obviously, the bigger the seed, the easier the problem is.

TABLE 2.—Comparison of CT Features of Primary Gastrointestinal Leiomyosarcoma in Patients With and Those Without PL

CT Feature	Patients With PL ($n = 25$)	Patients Without PL ($n = 64$)
Mean maximum diameter (cm)*	12.5 (4-32)	9.1 (3-18)
Most common primary site		
Small bowel	14 (56)	NA
Stomach	NA	30 (47)
Lobulated contour	23 (92)	52 (81)
Exophytic tumor growth	25 (100)	52 (81)
Necrosis	23 (92)	47 (73)
Calcification	0	7 (11)
Local tumor invasion	1 (4)	7 (11)
Lymphadenopathy	4 (16)	7 (11)
Ascites	4 (16)	3 (5)

Note: Unless otherwise noted, data are numbers of patients and numbers in parentheses are percentages.

Abbreviation: *NA*, Not applicable.

*The range of diameters is in parentheses.

(Courtesy of Rha SE, Ha HK, Kim AY, et al: Peritoneal leiomyosarcomatosis originating from gastrointestinal leiomyosarcomas: CT features. *Radiology* 227:385-390, 2003. Radiological Society of North America.)

This group of investigators from South Korea reports on 89 patients of whom somewhat less than half had intraabdominal metastases. Peritoneal seeding was actually seen in 25 patients. I think the pictures help to realize just how difficult the problem is in terms of picking up these small seeds. Once there is a mass, people are sensitive to the problem; however, in the absence of a primary mass, small peritoneal seeds remain as a major diagnostic challenge.

E. Glatstein, MD

Uterine Sarcomas Express KIT Protein but Lack Mutation(s) in Exon 11 or 17 of c-*KIT*

Rushing RS, Shajahan S, Chendil D, et al (Univ of Kentucky, Lexington)

Gynecol Oncol 91:9-14, 2003 10–5

Introduction.—Many tumors express the protein product of the proto-oncogene c-*KIT*. Some tumors respond to imatinib mesylate, a tyrosine kinase inhibitor. Tumors that respond regularly have mutation(s) in exon 11 of c-*KIT* that encodes for the regulatory juxtamembrane helix. Some tumors that express KIT protein have mutation(s) in exon 17 of c-*KIT*; these do not respond to imatinib mesylate (Fig 1). The expression of KIT protein and the mutational status of exons 11 and 17 of c-*KIT* in uterine sarcomas were evaluated.

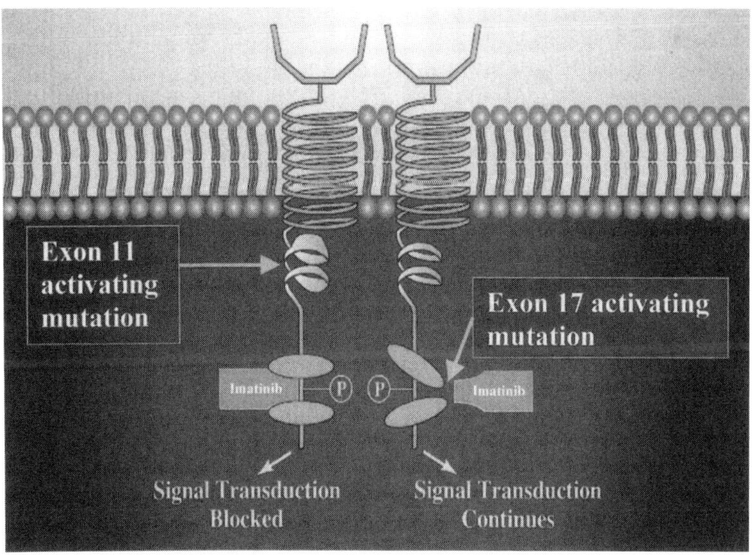

FIGURE 1.—Diagram illustrating the KIT receptor and effects of activating mutations in exon 11 and 17. Imatinib mesylate blocks signal transduction in the presence of an exon 11–activating mutation but not when the activating mutation is in exon 11 since this affects the drug-binding site. (Reprinted by permission of the publisher from Rushing RS, Shajahan S, Chendil D, et al: Uterine sarcomas express KIT protein but lack mutation(s) in exon 11 or 17 of c-*KIT*. *Gynecol Oncol* 91:9-14, 2003. Copyright 2003 by Elsevier Science Inc.)

Methods.—Twenty-five uterine sarcomas treated between 1990 and 2002 were assessed, including 14 malignant mullerian mixed tumors (MMMTs), 7 leiomyosarcomas (LMSs), 2 endometrial stromal sarcomas (ESSs), and 2 high-grade heterologous sarcomas (HGHSs). Formalin-fixed, paraffin-embedded tissue sections were immunostained with anti-KIT antibody using semiquantitative assessment. Normal myometrium, when identified in the section, was used as an internal negative control. Areas of tumors were microdissected. They underwent DNA extraction, polymerase chain reaction amplification of exons 11 and 17, single-strand conformational polymorphism, and DNA sequencing to determine the presence of mutations.

Results.—All 25 tumors expressed KIT protein at different levels, as determined by immunohistochemistry. Staining was diffuse. It was of moderate to strong intensity in 22 (88%) tumors. Staining intensity was weak in 1 each of LMSs, ESSs, and HGHSs. In MMMTs, both epithelial and sarcomatous foci stained similarly. No mutations in exons 11 or 17 of c-*KIT* were seen in 24 (96%) tumors. Deletion of both exons 11 and 17 were observed in 1 LMS.

Conclusion.—Uterine sarcomas express KIT protein, yet they lack KIT-activating mutations in exon 11 or 17 of c-*KIT*. It is not likely that these tumors will respond to treatment with imatinib mesylate.

▶ This is an interesting article from investigators from the University of Kentucky. They looked at uterine sarcomas and their expression of c-*KIT*. Obviously, the major interest in c-*KIT* is whether or not to use Gleevec. I must confess that I was unaware of the importance of the individual exon in c-*KIT* that encodes for the regulatory juxtamembrane helix. That was interesting and it was helpful for me to see that the exon 11-activating mutation seems to be the one associated with the response to Gleevec, whereas the 17 exon mutation usually does not respond to Gleevec. The reason for this distinction is that the exon 17 activating mutation actually affects the linkage of the agent itself to the c-*KIT* receptor. Thus, I actually learned something new from this article and I assume that some readers will learn from it also.

It is interesting to see the bankruptcy of thought in dealing with patients who have these sarcomas. Certainly the systemic management leaves much to be desired, and anyone who seems to express c-KIT in any way, shape, or form—regardless of mutation and of whether it is overexpressed or not—tends to be placed on Gleevec because the thinking is that it cannot hurt and just might help. Of course, the people who think this way do not have to pay for the drug, which winds up representing tens of thousands of dollars per year for a pill that is taken once a day. As Shakespeare says, "What is ought, but as tis valued?"

E. Glatstein, MD

Angiosarcoma of the Breast: A 30 Year Perspective With an Optimistic Outlook

Georgiannos SN, Sheaff M (Royal London Hosp)

Br J Plast Surg 56:129-134, 2003 10–6

Introduction.—Sarcomas of the breast are rare and account for below 1% of primary malignant mammary gland tumors. Several breast angiosarcomas have been described in single case reports. The incidence and clinicopathologic characteristics of angiosarcoma of the breast were evaluated to provide more meaningful data concerning these unusual tumors.

Methods.—A search was conducted of all cases in the pathology files of Royal London Hospital between 1970 and 2000. The search yielded 4 cases identified as primary angiosarcomas involving the breast. Medical and surgical histories, macroscopic and microscopic characteristics, and clinical outcomes with long-term follow-up were documented.

Results.—All 4 cases of angiosarcoma of the breast were in women. Two were young (aged 20 and 35 years) with no relevant medical histories; the other 2 were older (45 and 64 years) and had undergone local radiotherapy for breast carcinoma 25 and 7 years previously. Three cases were associated with "bruising" of the superficial tissues of the breast. None of the patients were smokers and all 4 had different occupations. One of the younger pa-

TABLE 1.—Clinical and Pathologic Features of 4 Cases of Angiosarcoma of the Breast

Age at Presentation (Years)	Time From Presentation to Diagnosis (Weeks)	Side	Previous Radiotherapy	Surgery	Histology	Follow-up From Initial Diagnosis (Months)
45	4	left	yes	lumpectomy followed by simple completion mastectomy	grade 1 angiosarcoma	42
64	?58	right	yes	incisional biopsy followed by completion mastectomy (segmental previously for carcinoma)	grade 3 angiosarcoma	30
20	3	left	no	initial biopsy followed by mastectomy and axillary sampling	grade 3 angiosarcoma and fibrocystic change	87
35	1 day	right	no	excision biopsy followed by simple mastectomy	grade 1 angiosarcoma with surrounding fibrocystic change	60

tients was taking oral contraceptive pills and at least 1 of the older women was receiving tamoxifen.

It appeared that diagnosis was delayed in all 4 patients. Several operative procedures were performed in all cases; all patients ultimately underwent mastectomy. Both older women shared histology features, as did both younger women (Table 1). At publication, all 4 patients were alive and free of disease.

Conclusion.—Angiosarcoma of the breast is rare, but it must be considered in the differential diagnosis, particularly with the increasing use of fine-needle aspiration and core biopsy for preoperative diagnosis. The prognosis after complete surgical excision may be better than previously believed.

▶ This article from Great Britain assesses angiosarcoma of the breast. From the Royal London Hospital, the authors evaluated records over a 30-year period and were able to come up with 4 primary angiosarcomas of the breast. This is over 10,000 breast biopsy specimens during that period. The interesting thing about this is that of their 4 cases, 2 had prior radiation (the details of which are not furnished in 1) but 2 did not. Thus, if a patient has a primary angiosarcoma of the breast, the question is: did they have radiation or not, and if they had it, was it really causative? These events are so infrequent that it is not so easy to answer those questions with confidence.

E. Glatstein, MD

11 Central Nervous System

Importance of MR Technique for Stereotactic Radiosurgery
Donahue BR, Goldberg JD, Golfinos JG, et al (New York Univ)
Neuro-Oncol 5:268-274, 2003 11–1

Background.—Triple-dose gadolinium-enhanced MR with 1 mm-thick magnetization-prepared rapid gradient echo (MPRAGE) images (SRS3×Gado) is currently used at the authors' center just before radiosurgery. The authors investigated how frequently this imaging procedure identifies previously unrecognized cerebral metastases in patients imaged initially using conventional MR with single-dose gadolinium (1×Gado).

Methods.—Forty-seven patients underwent radiosurgical procedures for cerebral metastases between July 1998 and July 2000. The diagnoses for these patients were based initially on the 1×Gado protocol. In July 1998, the use of SRS3×Gado was initiated as the routine imaging procedure to prepare for targeting lesions for radiosurgery. The procedure involved triple-

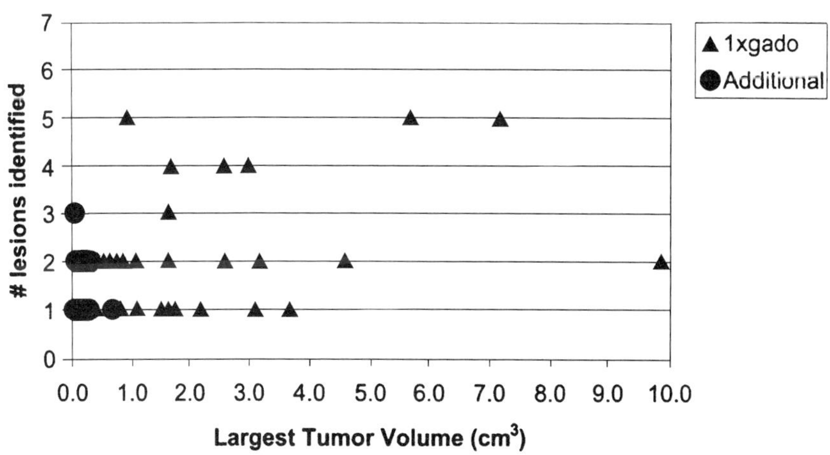

FIGURE 3.—Largest tumor volume versus the number of lesions identified, classified by whether they were identified on 1×Gado or as additional lesions on 3×Gado. (Courtesy of Donahue BR, Goldberg JD, Golfinos JG, et al: Importance of MR technique for stereotactic radiosurgery. *Neuro-Oncol* 5:268-274, 2003.)

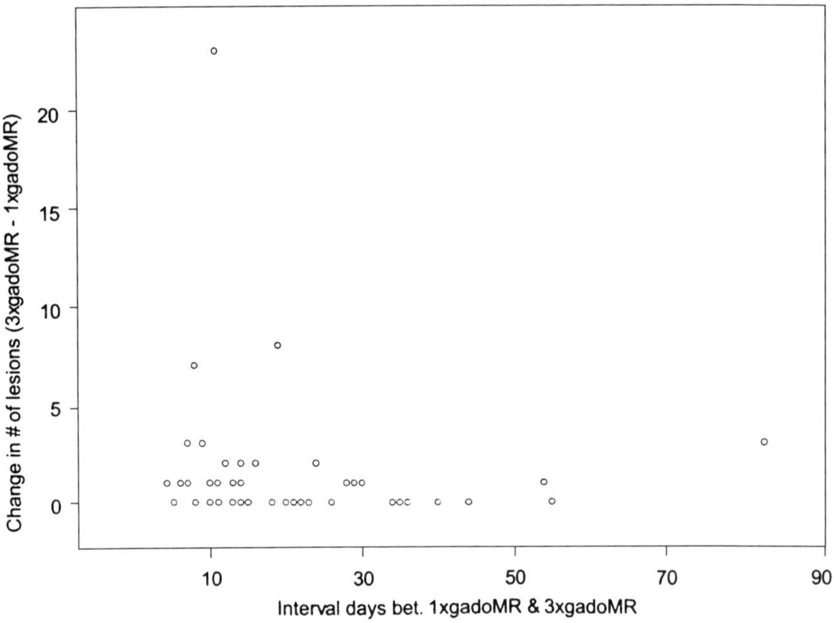

FIGURE 4.—Change in number of lesions between 1×Gado and SRS3×Gado MR by time interval between 1Gado and SRS3Gado MR (days). (Courtesy of Donahue BR, Goldberg JD, Golfinos JG, et al: Importance of MR technique for stereotactic radiosurgery. *Neuro-Oncol* 5:268-274, 2003.)

dose gadolinium and acquisition of contiguous 1-mm T1-weighted axial images. The number of brain lesions identified on the 2 protocols was compared.

Findings.—In 49% of the patients, an additional 1-23 lesions per patient were found on SRS3×Gado scans (Figs 3 and 4). More than half of these patients had only 1 additional lesion identified. The average interval between the 1×Gado and the SRS3×Gado scans was 20.6 days. The number of additional lesions found and interval between the 2 scans were negatively correlated. The number of lesions found on SRS3×Gado correlated only with the number of lesions on the 1×Gado. There were no associations with any other patient or tumor pretreatment characteristics, such as age, gender, greatest tumor volume on the 1×Gado, or number of days between 1×Gado and SRS3×Gado or previous surgery.

Conclusions.—Identifying additional lesions with SRS3×Gado MR may have implications for patients treated with stereotactic radiosurgery alone with single-dose gadolinium imaging. The use of SRS3×Gado scans for radiosurgery is advocated.

► This is a provocative article from investigators at NYU on 47 patients undergoing radiosurgery for cerebral metastases. Typically patients undergoing radiosurgery have had a diagnostic MR study using gadolinium. In preparation for radiosurgery and the localization process, these investigators required and actually used a triple dose of gadolinium and discovered that additional metastases were seen in almost half the patients compared with what was recognized after the conventional dose of gadolinium. These additional metastases ranging from 1 to 23 lesions were almost one half of the patients. Of those patients in whom additional lesions were seen, 13 patients had only 1 additional lesion identified. Nonetheless, this is a crucial finding in patients who were planned for stereotactic radiosurgery without associated whole brain irradiation. These findings appear to be important and make one wonder why we do not do more triple dose gadolinium scanning on a routine basis.

E. Glatstein, MD

Focal Lesion in the Splenium of the Corpus Callosum on FLAIR MR Images: A Common Finding With Aging and After Brain Radiation Therapy

Pekala JS, Mamourian AC, Wishart HA (Dartmouth-Hitchcock Med Ctr, Lebanon, NH; Finley Hosp, Dubuque, Iowa)

AJNR Am J Neuroradiol 24:855-861, 2003 11–2

Background.—In general, focal high signal intensity in the splenium of the corpus callosum on fluid-attenuated inversion-recovery (FLAIR) images is considered abnormal. High signal intensity has been observed in the splenium on FLAIR images in elderly patients with otherwise normal images and in patients who have undergone radiation therapy to the brain. The frequency of this finding in these patient populations was further investigated.

Methods.—The study included 67 patients imaged for suspicion of CNS disease (group 1) and 18 consecutive patients with a history of brain radiation therapy (group 2). Medical records and FLAIR images were reviewed. Autopsy specimens from an additional 2 patients with a history of chest and neck radiation therapy were also examined.

Findings.—In group 1, focal high signal intensity in the splenium correlated with aging, radiation therapy, and white matter changes. In group 2, focal high signal intensity in the splenium was apparent on the FLAIR images of 16 patients (Fig 2). Histologic evaluation of the autopsy specimens showed isomorphic gliosis.

Conclusions.—High signal intensity in the splenium of the corpus callosum on FLAIR images is commonly seen in patients with a history of radiation therapy to the brain. This finding also appears to be associated with aging.

▶ This is an article on a radiologic finding of which I was unaware, but I think it has some importance in following up patients who have had radiation therapy to the brain. Apparently, following radiation treatment, the splenium may be a focus of high signal intensity on MRI. The pictures are certainly impressive, and this is worth knowing about in the follow-up. Apparently, there is no functional correlate that is described, so this is a radiologic finding that needs to be factored into the interpretation.

E. Glatstein, MD

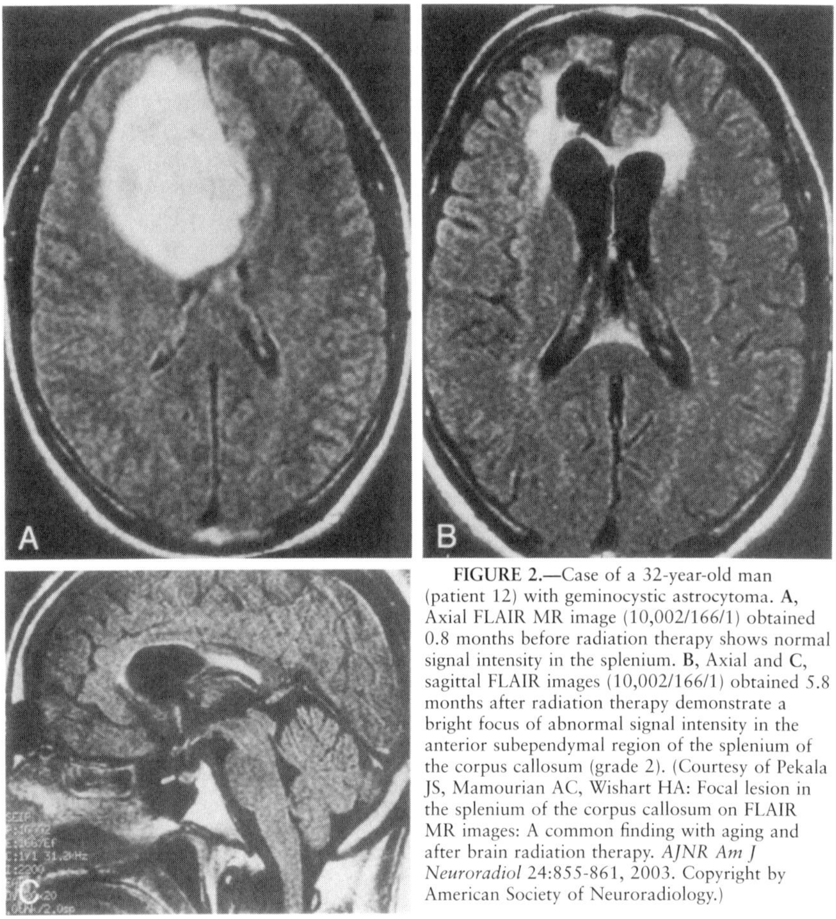

FIGURE 2.—Case of a 32-year-old man (patient 12) with geminocystic astrocytoma. **A**, Axial FLAIR MR image (10,002/166/1) obtained 0.8 months before radiation therapy shows normal signal intensity in the splenium. **B**, Axial and **C**, sagittal FLAIR images (10,002/166/1) obtained 5.8 months after radiation therapy demonstrate a bright focus of abnormal signal intensity in the anterior subependymal region of the splenium of the corpus callosum (grade 2). (Courtesy of Pekala JS, Mamourian AC, Wishart HA: Focal lesion in the splenium of the corpus callosum on FLAIR MR images: A common finding with aging and after brain radiation therapy. *AJNR Am J Neuroradiol* 24:855-861, 2003. Copyright by American Society of Neuroradiology.)

Clear Cell Ependymoma: A Clinicopathologic and Radiographic Analysis of Patients

Fouladi M, Helton K, Dalton J, et al (St Jude Children's Research Hosp, Memphis, Tenn; Henry Ford Hosp, Detroit, Mich; Johns Hopkins Univ, Baltimore, Md)

Cancer 98:2232-2244, 2003 11–3

Background.—Clear cell ependymoma (CCE), an uncommon CNS tumor, may histologically mimic oligodendroglioma, central neurocytoma, hemangioblastoma, and renal cell carcinoma. This tumor has a predilection for the supratentorial region in children. The clinical, radiographic, and pathologic characteristics and treatment outcomes were reviewed in a group of children with CCE.

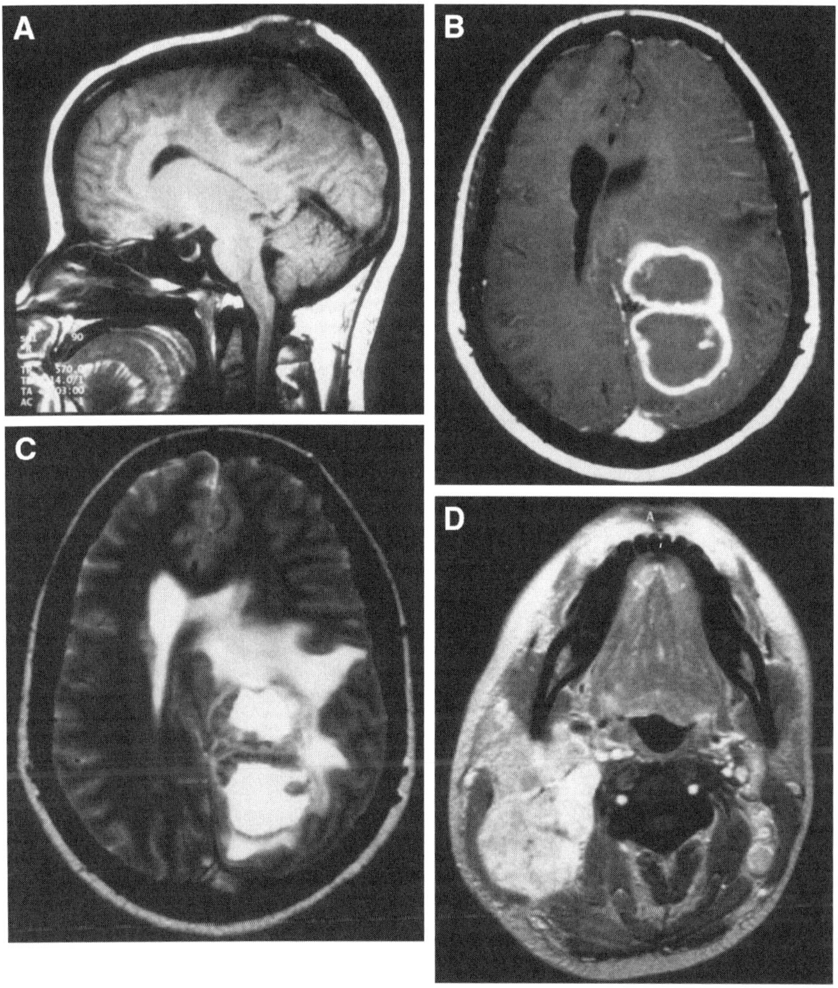

FIGURE 1.—Imaging studies from Patient 4. A sagittal, T1-weighted (T1W), precontrast image (**A**) demonstrates transcalvarial and subgaleal extension of a large parietal tumor approximately 4 years after the initial diagnosis. Postcontrast (**B**) and T2W (**C**) images demonstrate a hypercellular, multicystic mass with enhancing tumor thrombus in the superior sagittal sinus 4 years after diagnosis. (**D**) An axial, T1W, postcontrast image demonstrates bilateral anterior cervical lymph node masses (right > left) 4 years and 10 months after the initial diagnosis, respectively. (Courtesy of Fouladi M, Helton K, Dalton J, et al: Clear cell ependymoma: A clinicopathologic and radiographic analysis of patients. *Cancer* 98:2232-2244, 2003. Copyright 2003 American Cancer Society. Reprinted by permission of Wiley-Liss, Inc, a subsidiary of John Wiley & Sons, Inc.)

Methods and Findings.—The study included 10 children, 1 to 19 years old at the time of diagnosis, who were treated at one center between 1984 and 2003. Tumors were supratentorial in 9 patients. Fluorescence in situ hybridization (FISH) was done in all patients. All tumors were found to have rounded nuclei, with surrounding, clear halos, with at least focal perivascular pseudorosettes. Anaplastic features wee observed in 7 tumors. No deletions involving 1p, 19q, chromosomes or gene *NF2* (22q12) were seen. Tumors from 5 of 7 children with anaplasia showed losses of chromosome CEP18 and gene *DAL-1*. All tumors enhanced radiographically. Nine tumors had associated cysts with enhancing walls (Fig 1). Gross total resection was performed in 7 patients. In 5 patients, local radiotherapy was delivered immediately after surgery. The other 3 children, who were initially diagnosed as having pilocytic astrocytoma or oligodendroglioma, were observed only. Progression-free and overall survival rates were 34% and 75%, respectively, at 5 years. Follow-up ranged from 5 to 239 months. Local recurrence developed within a median of 9 months after diagnosis in 5 children. In another 2, extracranial soft tissue and lymph node metastases developed.

Conclusions.—CCEs had a predilection for extraneural metastases and early recurrence. Characteristic radiographic findings, anaplastic histologic features, and chromosome 18 losses were observed. Resection followed by local radiotherapy is the preferred treatment for affected children.

▶ This report represents an uncommon tumor with 10 patients treated at St Jude for this type of ependymoma. This particular entity of the CCE tends to be supratentorial and often seems to have a chromosome 18 deletion. These tumors appear to enhance and often have associated cysts. The most interesting feature of this group of patients is what appears to be a relatively high risk for extraneural metastases. This appears to be a discrete entity largely recognized only in the last 15 years.

E. Glatstein, MD

12 Gastrointestinal

Esophagus, Stomach

Early Gastric Cancer in Young, Asymptomatic Carriers of Germ-line E-Cadherin Mutations

Huntsman DG, Carneiro F, Lewis FR, et al (British Columbia Cancer Agency, Vancouver, Canada; Univ of British Columbia, Vancouver; Victoria Gen Hosp, British Columbia; et al)

N Engl J Med 344:1904-1909, 2001 12–1

Background.—Families with inherited diffuse gastric cancer have been found to have germline truncating mutations in the E-cadherin (*CDH1*) gene. Because gastric cancer has developed in 3 of every 4 carriers of this mutant gene, predictive genetic testing should be performed in members of these families. Genetic screening, surgical management, and pathologic findings were noted in young individuals with the mutant gene from 2 unrelated families.

Methods.—Testing was carried out using the polymerase chain reaction amplification method; then restriction-enzyme digestion and DNA sequencing were used in the first family. The second family underwent heteroduplex analysis. In 5 carriers of the mutation (age range, 22-40 years), prophylactic total gastrectomy was performed. The stomach's entire mucosa was extensively sampled for microscopic analysis.

Results.—All 5 patients who underwent the gastrectomy had superficial infiltrates of malignant signet-ring cells in the samples taken. Three cases were multifocal, and 1 revealed infiltrates of malignant signet-ring cells in 65 of the 140 tissue blocks evaluated (aggregate less than 2% of gastric mucosa).

Conclusion.—The neoplastic lesions found were not apparent on gross examination, and extensive pathologic study was required. The prophylactic gastrectomy in these cases was presumably curative. Both genetic counseling and consideration of prophylactic gastrectomy should be applied to young carriers of germline truncating mutations of the *CDH1* gene who belong to families with a history of diffuse gastric cancer.

▶ Classic genetic syndromes are important to know (even after one takes the board examinations). Such identified patients point to other high-risk family members in whom increased screening and/or prophylactic surgery should be considered. The familial gastric cancer syndrome is associated with diffuse gastric cancer appearing at a young age. The *CDH1* gene is highly predictive for gastric cancer, as 3 of 4 carriers of mutant *CDH1* will have malignancy develop. As gastrectomy is a procedure with potentially significant morbidity and even mortality rates, this mutation guides clinicians to advising surgery only for high-risk patients.

P. J. Loehrer, Sr, MD

Gene-Expression Profile Changes Correlated With Tumor Progression and Lymph Node Metastasis in Esophageal Cancer

Tamoto E, Tada M, Murakawa K, et al (Hokkaido Univ, Sapporo, Japan)
Clin Cancer Res 10:3629-3638, 2004 12–2

Introduction.—Several molecular markers for tumor progression and prognosis of esophageal cancer have been identified. This information is too limited to clarify the carcinogenesis, tumor progression, and invasiveness of esophageal cancer. Expression profiling that collectively examines expression of many genes by using a cDNA array may be promising for identifying molecular mechanisms independently of previous knowledge. Molecular clues to tumor progression and lymph node metastasis in esophageal cancer were examined, along with their value as predictive markers.

Methods.—The gene expression profiles in cDNA array data of a 35-tissue training set of esophageal squamous cell carcinoma (ESCC) were evaluated by using generalized linear regression analysis and a feature subset selection algorithm. The application of the identified optimal feature sets (predictive gene sets) made it possible to train and develop ensemble classifiers consisting of multiple probabilistic neural networks combined with AdaBoosting to predict tumor stages and lymph node metastasis. The classifier abilities were validated in 18 independent cases of ESCC.

Results.—A total of 71 genes of 1289 cancer-associated genes of which the expression correlated with tumor stages were identified. Forty-seven of 71 genes differed significantly between the tumor-node-metastasis pT1/2 and pT3/4 stages. Cell cycle regulators and transcription factors possibly promoting the growth of tumor cells were highly expressed in the early stages of ESCC; adhesion molecules and extracellular matrix–related molecules possibly promoted invasiveness increased in later stages. Forty-four genes with predictive values for lymph node metastasis were identified, including cell adhesion molecules and cell membrane receptors showing higher expression in node-positive cases and cell cycle regulators and intracellular signaling molecules demonstrating higher expression in node-negative cases. The ensemble classifiers trained with the selected features predicted tumor stage and lymph node metastasis in the validation cases; accuracy was 94.4% and 88.9%, respectively, illustrating the predictive value and reproducibility of these features.

Conclusion.—These characteristic genes may provide useful data for understanding the malignant nature of ESCC and for individualizing treatments.

▶ Esophageal cancer, especially when discovered beyond pathologic stage I, carries a poor prognosis. Optimal therapy for stage II and III disease is not well defined. Results from clinical trials evaluating the role of combined modality therapy vary significantly. This may, in part, be due to the heterogeneity of the disease. In an effort to better understand the clinical behavior of esophageal cancer, Tamoto et al analyzed the gene expression profiles from tumors in 54 patients. The analysis detected 47 genes that were upregulated and 24 that were downregulated according to pT stage. Expression of 87 genes showed a difference in lymph node metastasis. There were 14 common genes that distinguished both pT stage and lymph node status. These selected genes may be used to predict the clinical behavior, including tumor progression and invasiveness of esophageal cancer. However, given the complex gene networks, more study of gene and protein profiles is required to better understand the malignant nature of esophageal cancer.

N. H. Hanna, MD

Helicobacter pylori Infection and Gastric Atrophy: Risk of Adenocarcinoma and Squamous-Cell Carcinoma of the Esophagus and Adenocarcinoma of the Gastric Cardia

Ye W, Held M, Lagergren J, et al (Karolinska Institutet, Stockholm, Sweden; Internatl Epidemiology Inst, Rockville, Md; Karolinska Hosp, Stockholm, Sweden; et al)

J Natl Cancer Inst 96:388-396, 2004 12–3

Introduction.—An inverse correlation between *Helicobacter pylori* infection and esophageal adenocarcinoma has been reported that may be caused by diminished acidity from inducing atrophic gastritis from producing ammonia. The link between *H pylori* infection, gastric atrophy, and the risk of esophageal adenocarcinoma, esophageal squamous cell carcinoma, and gastric cardia adenocarcinoma was examined in a large population-based case-control investigation.

Methods.—Self-reported data were collected during interviews. Serum was obtained from 97 patients with incident esophageal adenocarcinoma, 85 patients with incident esophageal squamous cell carcinoma, 133 patients with incident cardia adenocarcinoma, and 499 randomly chosen control subjects. Serum antibodies against whole *H pylori* cell-surface antigens (HP-CSAs) and cytotoxin-related gene A (CagA) antigens were evaluated by using an immunoglobulin G enzyme-linked immunosorbent assay and immunoblotting, respectively. Gastric atrophy was evaluated by serum levels of pepsinogen I. Multivariate logistic regression with adjustment for potential confounding factors was used to investigate associations.

Results.—*H pylori* infection, assayed by HP-CSA or CagA antibodies, was statistically significantly linked with a decreased risk of esophageal adenocarcinoma (for HP-CSA antibodies, odds ratio [OR], 0.3; 95% confidence interval [CI], 0.2-0.6; for CagA antibodies, OR, 0.5; 95% CI, 0.3-0.8; for both, OR, 0.2; 95% CI, 0.1-0.5). Gastric atrophy was not linked with the risk for esophageal adenocarcinoma (OR, 1.1; 95% CI, 0.5-2.5). Serum CagA antibodies and gastric atrophy were linked with increased risk for esophageal squamous cell carcinoma (OR, 2.1; 95% CI, 1.1-4.0 and OR, 4.3; 95% CI, 1.9-9.6, respectively). The risk of gastric cardia adenocarcinoma was not linked with *H pylori* infection. Gastric atrophy was correlated with increased risk for gastric cardia adenocarcinoma (OR, 4.5; 95% CI, 2.5-7.8).

Conclusion.—Infection with *H pylori* may diminish the risk of esophageal adenocarcinoma; it is not likely to do so by atrophy-reduced acidity. Gastric atrophy and infection with CagA-positive strains of *H pylori* may escalate the risk for esophageal squamous-cell carcinoma.

▶ This study clarifies the association of *H pylori* infection associated with squamous cell carcinoma of the esophagus and a negative association with adenocarcinoma. This is a well-researched study that brings science to the epidemiologic observations of this unique syndrome.

P. J. Loehrer, Sr, MD

---

p53 and VEGF Expression Are Independent Predictors of Tumour Recurrence and Survival Following Curative Resection of Gastric Cancer

Fondevila C, Metges JP, Fuster J, et al (Univ of Barcelona; Centre Hospitalier Universitaire Cavale Blanche and Morvan, Brest, France)

Br J Cancer 90:206-215, 2004 12–4

Background.—Gastric cancer was, until the 1980s, one of the most commonly occurring tumors in the world and a leading cause of cancer death. In the past 2 decades, the incidence of gastric cancer has declined, but the prognosis for this disease in Western countries has not improved; the 5-year survival is reported to range from 20% to 30%. Surgical resection is the most effective treatment for improving prognosis, and the factor that most adversely affects prognosis is delayed diagnosis, which results in advanced disease. In patients who undergo curative resection, the biologic nature of the tumor is the determining factor in survival because nearly half of these patients will die of recurrent cancer. The value of tumor microvessel density (MVD), expression of p53, and expression of vascular endothelial growth factor (VEGF) as prognostic markers for recurrence in patients with gastric cancer who undergo surgery with curative intent was determined.

Methods.—A total of 156 patients with curatively resected gastric cancer were enrolled in this blinded retrospective evaluation. The patients were treated with either surgery alone (n = 53) or surgery plus chemotherapy (n =

103). The main outcome measures—tumor MVD, p53 expression, and VEGF expression—were assayed with immunohistochemical techniques.

Results.—After a mean follow-up of 43 months, 41% of patients had died and 35% developed recurrence of tumor. Positive correlations were found between MVD and both p53 and VEGF expression. Both MVD of 100 or greater and positive VEGF expression were associated with shorter disease-free survival, and positive VEGF expression was also associated with shorter duration of overall survival. Multivariate analysis showed that, in addition to the pathologic tumor stage, lymph node ratio, and the extent of lymphadenectomy and perineural invasion, p53 expression and VEGF expression were independently associated with both disease-free survival and overall survival. In addition, patients whose tumors did not show p53 expression were found to be at a survival benefit compared with patients who expressed p53 when treated with adjuvant chemotherapy.

Conclusions.—The expression of p53 and VEGF are independent prognostic factors for both disease-free and overall survival in patients with curatively resected gastric cancer, and p53 status may also influence the response to chemotherapy.

▶ These Spanish investigators looked at the value of tumor MVD, the expression of p53, and the expression of VEGF as prognostic markers in patients with gastric cancer who were operated on with curative intent. There are 156 such patients in this series, but two thirds of them received adjuvant chemotherapy, and there is not a real analysis of the chemotherapy efficacy per se. The survival and the disease-free survival curves (see Fig 4 in original article) look amazingly similar, and their Table 7 (see original article) suggests to me that the chemotherapy may have been (at least in part) responsible for the correlations of p53 and VEGF with outcome.

In summary, the conclusions derived in this article do not seem justified by the data themselves.

E. Glatstein, MD

Pancreatic

Main-Duct Intraductal Papillary Mucinous Neoplasms of the Pancreas: Clinical Predictors of Malignancy and Long-term Survival Following Resection

Salvia R, Castillo CF, Bassi C, et al (Univ of Verona, Italy; Massachusetts Gen Hosp, Boston)

Ann Surg 239:678-687, 2004 12–5

Background.—Intraductal papillary mucinous neoplasms (IPMNs) are being increasingly diagnosed. However, diagnosing this malignancy preoperatively is problematic, and studies of long-term survival after resection for IPMNs have yielded conflicting findings. The clinical characteristics and outcomes of 1 large cohort with IPMNs of the pancreas affecting the main pancreatic duct were reported.

Methods and Findings.—One hundred forty consecutive patients undergoing resection between 1990 and 2002 were included in the study. The mean patient age was 65 years. Forty-two percent of the patients had invasive carcinoma, 28% had borderline tumors, 18% had carcinoma in situ, and 12% had adenomas. Patients with benign IPMN were a median 6.4 years younger than those with malignant tumors. The most common symptoms were abdominal pain in 65%, weight loss in 44%, acute pancreatitis in 23%, jaundice in 17%, and onset or worsening of diabetes in 12%. Twenty-seven percent of the patients had no symptoms. Jaundice and diabetes correlated significantly with malignancy. Patients with noninvasive tumors had a cancer-specific survival of 100% at 5 and 10 years. The 58 patients with invasive carcinoma had 5- and 10-year cancer-specific survival rates of 60% and 50%, respectively.

Conclusions.—In this cohort, 60% of patients with main-duct IPMNs have cancer. Patients with malignancy tend to be older than those with benign disease and are more likely to have jaundice or new-onset diabetes. These data are consistent with the notion of benign IPMN progression to invasive cancer as well as an aggressive policy of resection at diagnosis.

Cystic Pancreatic Neoplasms: Observe or Operate

Spinelli KS, Fromwiller TE, Daniel RA, et al (Med College of Wisconsin, Milwaukee)

Ann Surg 239:651-659, 2004 12–6

Background.—Pancreatic cystic lesions are being identified with increased frequency. The incidence, natural history, and predictors of neoplasia in pancreatic cysts were investigated to determine which patients can be managed by observation and which require surgery.

Methods.—All radiologic, surgical, and pathologic records of patients seen between 1995 and 2002 were reviewed for the presence of pancreatic cysts. For the analysis of natural history, only patients with 2 scans more than 1 month apart were included. Serous cystadenomas, solid and cystic papillary tumors, lymphoepithelial cysts, and simple cysts were classified as benign. Mucinous cystic neoplasms, intraductal papillary mucinous neoplasm, cystic neuroendocrine tumors, and cystadenocarcinomas were classified as premalignant or malignant.

Findings.—From a review of 24,039 CT or MR scans, 290 patients were identified as having pancreatic cysts, for an incidence of 1.2%. Of these patients, 168 (0.7%) had no documentation of pancreatitis. Seventy-nine of these patients, with a total of 103 cysts, had more than 1 scan at a mean 16-month interval. The size of these cysts increased in 19%, were unchanged in 59%, and decreased in 22%. Forty-nine patients had surgery for 14 benign, 25 premalignant, or 10 malignant lesions. Neoplasia could not be predicted by cyst size or patient sex. However, the presence of symptoms predicted a premalignant or malignant pathology in 60%. Age older than 70 years also correlated with malignancy.

Conclusions.—Cystic pancreatic neoplasms occurred in 0.7% of this large cohort. These cysts increased in size in 19% of patients during 16 months. In patients older than 70 years, these cysts are likely to be malignant. Surgical excision is recommended for pancreatic cysts that increase under observation, are symptomatic, or are found radiologically in healthy elderly persons.

► The term *pancreatic neoplasms* encompasses a broad range of lesions, both benign and malignant, with a wide variation in outcomes. The increasing use of abdominal imaging studies, such as CT scanning and MRI, has resulted in more frequent detection of small, asymptomatic pancreatic lesions and earlier tumors more amenable to surgical resection. Appropriate management of these lesions would be enhanced by improved knowledge of their natural history, predictors of malignancy, and outcome of surgical therapy. The ability to provide this information has been limited by the relative rarity of these lesions and, in some cases, lack of agreement on diagnostic criteria. The report by Spinelli et al (Abstract 12–6) confirms that clinical and imaging criteria cannot reliably distinguish benign from malignant and premalignant cystic lesions. Salvia et al (Abstract 12–5) draw the same conclusion in a study of a well-defined group of IPMNs, a specific tumor subtype sometimes grouped with cysts. In both studies surgical resection was accomplished with low rates of morbidity and mortality. In IPMNs with invasive cancer, the 5-year survival was 60%, substantially better than survival rates observed for resectable pancreatic adenocarcinomas. These articles emphasize that even elderly patients with pancreatic lesions should be evaluated by surgeons familiar with the spectrum of pancreatic neoplasia to assess the risk/benefit ratio of surgical exploration, rather than be observed until obvious signs of malignancy occur.

M. Morrow, MD

A Randomized Trial of Chemoradiotherapy and Chemotherapy After Resection of Pancreatic Cancer

Neoptolemos JP, for the European Study Group for Pancreatic Cancer (Liverpool Univ, England; et al)

N Engl J Med 350:1200-1210, 2004 12–7

Background.—Pancreatic cancer has a very poor prognosis. Surgical resection improves prognosis, but only a minority of patients are eligible. Adjuvant therapy could improve survival. The European Study group for Pancreatic Cancer initiated a large multicenter trial (ESGPC-1) to examine the possible benefits of adjuvant therapy for patients with resectable pancreatic cancer.

Study Design.—Patients with resectable pancreatic cancer were randomly assigned to treatment with chemoradiotherapy (73 patients), chemotherapy (75), chemoradiotherapy followed by chemotherapy (72) and observation (69). Patients were followed up at 3 month intervals until death or the end of the study (up to 62 months). The primary outcome measure was 2-year survival. Secondary outcomes included adverse effects, recurrence, and quality of life. Analysis was by intention-to-treat.

Findings.—At a median follow-up of 47 months, there were 237 deaths among the 289 patients with resectable pancreatic cancer. The estimated 5-year survival rate was 10% among those who were randomly assigned to receive chemoradiotherapy and 20% among those who did not receive chemoradiotherapy. The 5-year survival rate was 21% among those who received chemotherapy and 8% among those who did not receive chemotherapy. The benefit of chemotherapy persisted after adjustment for prognostic factors.

Conclusion.—There was a significant survival benefit associated with adjuvant chemotherapy. Adjuvant chemoradiotherapy did not show a significant survival benefit. Standard care for patients with resectable pancreatic cancer should include adjuvant chemotherapy.

▶ Much of what we do in medicine is based on dogma as much as data. Pancreatic cancer is a disease in which we have made only minor progress in therapy. Therapy for stage IV disease has definitely improved with the use of gemcitabine. Therapy for resected stage II and III disease has been largely based on a trial done several decades ago by the GI Tumor Study Group, which reported an improvement in overall survival with 5-fluorouracil and radiation therapy compared with no additional therapy. This trial had fewer than 50 total patients entered.

This trial by Neoptolemos et al was presented previously[1] and undercuts the notion that radiation therapy has a positive benefit for patients with resected pancreatic cancer. This is a complicated article to read. The original study published in *The Lancet* included patients who were not randomized; in this subgroup of patients who included only randomized patients. It appears that radiation therapy may not benefit patients. Several reasons may explain this: (1) selection bias, (2) increased morbidity of postoperative versus preoperative radiation therapy, (3) poor synergy with radiation and fluorouracil, and (4) inadequate fields or dosages of radiation therapy.

This study lays down the gauntlet—all treatments (surgery, radiation, and chemotherapy) need to be subjected to well-designed prospective clinical trials. An ongoing intergroup trial is under way that evaluates gemcitabine alone versus gemcitabine and radiation therapy in patients with locally advanced disease. This will prospectively test the synergy of radiation therapy with a more active drug, gemcitabine, as well as prospectively evaluate quality of life.

P. J. Loehrer, Sr, MD

Reference

1. Neoptolemos JP, Dunn JA, Stocken DD, et al: Adjuvant chemoradiotherapy and chemotherapy in resectable pancreatic cancer: A randomized controlled trial. *Lancet* 358:1576-1585, 2001.

Hepatobiliary

Role of Vitamin K_2 in the Development of Hepatocellular Carcinoma in Women With Viral Cirrhosis of the Liver

Habu D, Shiomi S, Tamori A, et al (Osaka City Univ, Japan)
JAMA 292:358-361, 2004 12–8

Introduction.—Vitamin K_2 (menaquinone) has been shown to help prevent bone loss in women with viral cirrhosis of the liver. There is some evidence that vitamin K_2 may have a role in reducing the risk of hepatocellular carcinoma. Women with viral liver diagnosis were evaluated to determine whether vitamin K_2 has preventive effects on the development of hepatocellular carcinoma in this population.

Methods.—Forty women with viral liver cirrhosis admitted to a university hospital between 1996 and 1998 were randomly assigned to treatment with 45 mg/d of vitamin K_2 or placebo. The original goal was to evaluate the long-term effects of vitamin K_2 on bone loss in women with viral liver cirrhosis. Participants also satisfied criteria for examination of the effects of such treatment on development of hepatocellular carcinoma. Participants in both groups received symptomatic treatment of ascites, if needed, and dietary advice. The primary outcome measure was cumulative proportion of patients with hepatocellular carcinoma.

Results.—Two of 21 women randomly assigned to treatment with vitamin K_2 and 9 of 19 control subjects had hepatocellular carcinoma. The cumulative proportion of patients witch hepatocellular carcinoma was smaller in the treatment group (log-rank test, $P = .02$). Univariate analysis showed that the risk ratio for development of hepatocellular carcinoma in the treatment group versus control group was 0.20 (95% confidence interval, 0.04-0.91; $P = .04$). Multivariate analysis with adjustment for age, alanine aminotransferase activity, serum albumin, total albumin, platelet count, α-fetoprotein, and history of treatment with interferon alfa showed a risk ratio of 0.13 (95% confidence interval, 0.02-0.99; $P = .05$) for development of hepatocellular cancer among women treated with vitamin K_2.

Conclusion.—Vitamin K_2 may have a role in the prevention of hepatocellular carcinoma in women with viral cirrhosis.

► This trial was originally designed to prove a salutorious impact of Vitamin K_2 on bone loss in women with viral-induced hepatic cirrhosis. The findings of this study, however, provided a more provocative observation: a decrease in incidence of hepatocellular carcinoma. There are numerous reasons why Vitamin K_2 may benefit patients with cirrhosis. This observation needs to be studied further in a larger prospective trial.

P. J. Loehrer, Sr, MD

Colon and Anus

Do Young Colon Cancer Patients Have Worse Outcomes?

O'Connell JB, Maggard MA, Liu JH, et al (Univ of California, Los Angeles; Veterans Administration Greater Los Angeles Healthcare System; Univ of Texas, Dallas)

World J Surg 28:558-562, 2004 12–9

Background.—Previous research on colon cancer has shown increasing incidence rates among young persons and suggests that such patients may have more aggressive disease with worse 5-year survival rates than older patients with colon cancer. A nationwide population-based cancer registry was used to investigate colon cancer presentations and outcomes in younger and older populations.

Methods.—Patient records were obtained from the Surveillance, Epidemiology, and End Results (SEER) national cancer database from the years 1991 through 1999. Two cohorts were formed on the basis of age at diagnosis: 1334 patients comprised the 20- to 40-year-old group, and 46,457 comprised the 60- to 80-year-old group. The groups were compared for patient and tumor characteristics, treatment, and 5-year cancer-specific survival rates. Predictors of survival were identified in a multivariate Cox regression model.

Findings.—The younger cohort included a higher proportion of black and Latino patients compared with the older cohort. The younger group also had fewer cases of stage I or II disease, more cases of stage III or IV disease, and worse tumor grade. Stage-specific survival at 5 years was similar for pa-

TABLE 4.—Cox Multivariate Regression Analysis

Variable	Hazard Ratio	*P*	95% Confidence Interval
Young[a]	0.630	< 0.0001	0.574,0.691
AJCC II[b]	1.087	0.002	1.041,1.136
AJCC III[b]	1.935	< 0.0001	1.855,2.017
AJCC IV[b]	6.821	< 0.0001	6.550,7.103
Black[c]	1.195	< 0.0001	1.142,1.250
Hispanic[c]	0.951	0.2346	0.876,1.033
Asian[c]	0.830	< 0.0001	0.777,0.885
Other race[c]	0.771	0.0005	0.666,0.892
Male[d]	1.095	< 0.0001	1.065,1.126
Low-grade[e]	0.741	< 0.0001	0.719,0.763
Underwent irradiation[f]	1.016	0.6582	0.946,1.092
Underwent surgery[g]	0.302	< 0.0001	0.289,0.316

[a] Reference group is older.
[b] Reference group is American Joint Committee on Cancer stage I.
[c] Reference group is white.
[d] Reference group is female.
[e] Reference group is high grade.
[f] Reference group did not undergo irradiation.
[g] Reference group did not undergo surgery.

tients with stage I and III disease; however, it was significantly better for the younger patients with stage II and IV disease (Table 4).

Conclusions.—This analysis of data from a nationally representative cancer registry indicates that younger patients with colon cancer have later stage and higher grade disease that do older patients with colon cancer. However, 5-year cancer-specific survival rates among younger patients are comparable to or better than the rates among older patients. The findings from this population-based study are not consistent with previous reports from single centers.

► Assessing the impact of age as an independent prognostic factor is often difficult due to the need to control for multiple other factors known to influence cancer prognosis and the infrequent occurrence of many cancers in younger individuals. This report examines a population-based dataset of 47,791 patients, including 1334 aged 40 years or younger. Although age was a predictor of survival in univariate analysis, after controlling for factors such as stage, grade, and race, survival was found to be equal or better in younger patients than in their older counterparts. This study does not support modification of the intensity of treatment solely on the basis of age in the absence of other unfavorable prognostic features.

M. Morrow, MD

Effect of Calcium Supplementation on the Risk of Large Bowel Polyps

Wallace K, Baron JA, Cole BF, et al (Dartmouth-Hitchcock Med Ctr, Lebanon, NH; Univ of North Carolina, Chapel Hill; Univ of Southern California, Los Angeles; et al)

J Natl Cancer Inst 96:921-925, 2004 12–10

Background.—There is extensive experimental animal evidence that high calcium intake has an antineoplastic effect in the large bowel; however, epidemiologic studies have produced inconsistent results. There is stronger evidence that calcium is protective against colorectal adenomas, but few studies have examined the effect of calcium on the risk of different types of colorectal lesions or dietary determinants of this effect. The chemopreventive effect of calcium supplements was explored, specifically the effect of calcium treatment on the risk of hyperplastic polyps, tubular adenomas, and adenomas with advanced histology or large size.

Methods.—This analysis was conducted with patients from the Calcium Polyp Prevention Study, a randomized, double-blind, placebo-controlled chemoprevention trial among patients with a recent colorectal adenoma. A total of 930 patients were randomly assigned to calcium carbonate (1200 mg/d) or placebo. Follow-up colonoscopies were conducted approximately 1 and 4 years after the qualifying examination. General estimating equation and generalized linear regression analyses were used to compute risk ratios and 95% confidence intervals to assess the effect of calcium treatment versus placebo on the risk of hyperplastic polyps, tubular adenomas, and more advanced lesions. General estimating equation analyses were also used to compare the calcium treatment effects for various types of polyps with that for tubular adenomas. The interaction between calcium treatment and baseline intake of dietary calcium, fat, and fiber was also examined.

Results.—The calcium risk ratio for hyperplastic polyps was 0.82; the ratio for tubular adenomas was 0.89. The ratio for histologically advanced neoplasms was 0.65 compared with patients assigned to placebo. No statistically significant differences were observed between the risk ratio for tubular adenomas and that for other types of polyps. The effect of calcium supplementation on adenoma risk was most evident on among patients with high dietary intakes of calcium and fiber and with low intake of fat; however, the interactions were not statistically significant.

Conclusion.—Calcium supplementation may have a more significant antineoplastic effect on advanced colorectal lesions than on other types of polyps.

▶ This is a potentially important trial that confirms the role of high calcium intake in the prevention of all types of colonic polyps. This study clarifies that not all polyps are the same. The greatest benefit seems to be in histologically advanced neoplasms when compared with placebo. It should be noted that these include patients taking more than 1200 mg/d for 4 years. The additional impact of increased fiber is not well characterized at this time but also requires further studies. This is a provocative study worthy of further investigation.

P. J. Loehrer, Sr, MD

Estrogen Plus Progestin and Colorectal Cancer in Postmenopausal Women

Chlebowski RT, for the Women's Health Initiative Investigators (Harbor-UCLA, Torrance, Calif; et al)
N Engl J Med 350:991-1004, 2004 12–11

Introduction.—Observational studies report a reduced incidence of colorectal cancer and a lowered risk of death from the disease in women taking postmenopausal hormone therapy. As reported in 2002 by the Women's Health Initiative (WHI), a randomized trial identified more risks than benefits with hormone use, but found the combination of estrogen plus progestin to be associated with a significant decrease in the incidence of colorectal cancer. The features of the colorectal cancer that did develop were analyzed, together with their relation to patient characteristics.

Methods.—The WHI trial randomly assigned 16,608 postmenopausal women aged 50 to 79 years to a combination of conjugated equine estrogens (0.625 mg/d) plus medroxyprogesterone acetate (2.5 mg/d) or placebo. All women included in the study had an intact uterus, and none had a history of breast cancer or a medical condition likely to result in death within 3 years. The trial was stopped after a mean follow-up of 5.2 years because of the overall risk of adverse outcomes. Instances of colorectal cancer were confirmed by blinded adjudication.

Results.—A total of 115 invasive colorectal cancers occurred during follow-up, 43 in the hormone group and 72 in the placebo group. Compared with cancers in the placebo group, those in the hormone group had similar histologic features and grade. The number of positive lymph nodes was greater, however, in the hormone therapy group, and the cancers were more advanced. Regional or metastatic disease was present in 76.2% of women who received hormone therapy versus 48.5% of women given placebo. Colorectal cancer caused 9 deaths in the hormone group and 8 in the placebo group.

Conclusion.—The risk of colorectal cancer was decreased in women with relatively short-term use of estrogen plus progestin, but the colorectal cancers than did develop in women randomly assigned to hormone therapy were more advanced than those in women randomly assigned to placebo. Hormone therapy cannot be used to reduce the risk of colorectal cancer, and postmenopausal women who receive hormone therapy should undergo regular bowel screening.

▶ Although advantages and disadvantages to hormone replacement therapy have been noted, this report suggests a decreased risk of colon cancer in this population. It should be noted, however, that patients who were ultimately diagnosed with colon cancer presented in more advanced stages. Whether this is of significant biologic importance is uncertain. This may be somewhat reminiscent of finasteride in treatment with prostate cancer in which the overall incidence of prostate cancer is reduced but higher-grade lesions are found in the finasteride-treated population. Ultimately the impact of hormonal therapy in colorectal cancer should be more clearly defined.

P. J. Loehrer, Sr, MD

A Founder Mutation of the *MSH2* Gene and Hereditary Nonpolyposis Colorectal Cancer in the United States

Lynch HT, Coronel SM, Okimoto R, et al (Creighton Univ, Omaha, Neb; Ohio State Univ, Columbus; Leiden Univ, The Netherlands; et al)

JAMA 291:718-724, 2004 12–12

Introduction.—Hereditary nonpolyposis colorectal cancer (HNPCC; also known as Lynch syndrome) is caused by mutations in the mismatch repair genes, which carry an extraordinarily high risk of colorectal, endometrial, and other cancers. Carriers of these mutations should be identified, counseled, and offered clinical surveillance; these mutations are presently not tested for in mutation analyses. The prevalence of a large genomic deletion encompassing exons 1 to 6 of the *MSH2* gene that is widespread in the U.S. population as a result of founder effect was evaluated.

Methods.—An ongoing genealogic and historic investigation was performed to evaluate the origin and spread of an *MSH2* mutation previously identified in 9 apparently unrelated families with putative HNPCC who lived in widely different geographic locations in the United States. The primary outcome measures were classification of family members as carriers versus noncarriers of the *MSH2* mutation and spread of the *MSH2* mutation across the continental United States.

Results.—A total of 566 family members of the 9 known probands were identified as being at risk and were counseled; 137 were tested and 61 carry the founder mutation. Three families were determined genealogically to have descended from a German immigrant family that settled in Pennsylvania in the early 1700s. Movements of branches of this family have been documented from Pennsylvania through North Carolina, Alabama, Kentucky, Missouri, Iowa, Nebraska, Utah, Texas, and California. Carriers of the mutation have been diagnosed in 14 states. The deletion was not identified among 407 European and Australian families with HNPCC.

Conclusion.—The postulated high incidence and continent-wide geographic distribution of a cancer-predisposing founder mutation of the *MSH2* gene in a large outbred (vs genetically isolated) population and the ease with which the mutation can be identified indicate that routine testing of persons at risk for HNPCC in the United States should include an assay for this mutation until more is understood regarding its presence.

▶ Dr Lynch has been one of the pioneers in clinical epidemiology in cancer. He was the first to describe HNPCC. This article is a wonderfully written case study that provides insight into this unique disease. The search for a founder mutation of the *MSH2* gene is a wonderful story. The discussion portion of the report is an excellent primer for those not immersed in cancer genetics.

P. J. Loehrer, Sr, MD

Cancer Risk in Hereditary Nonpolyposis Colorectal Cancer Due to *MSH6* Mutations: Impact on Counseling and Surveillance

Hendriks YM, Wagner A, Morreau H, et al (Leiden Univ, The Netherlands; Erasmus Univ Med Ctr, Rotterdam, The Netherlands; VU Univ Med Ctr, Amsterdam; et al)

Gastroenterology 127:17-25, 2004 12–13

Introduction.—A mutated mismatch repair (MMR) gene causes hereditary nonpolyposis colorectal carcinoma (HNPCC), which accounts for 1% to 6% of all cases of colorectal carcinoma. The cumulative risk of developing cancer in a large series of *MSH6* mutation carriers was determined.

Methods.—Mutation analysis was conducted in 20 families with a germline mutation in *MSH6*. The cancer risks between *MSH6* and *MLH1/MSH2* mutation carriers were compared. Microsatellite instability (MSI) analysis and immunohistochemistry were conducted in the available tumors.

Results.—A total of 146 *MSH6* mutation carriers were seen. The cumulative risk for colorectal carcinoma was 69% for men, 30% for women, and

TABLE 2.—Mean Percentage Cancer Risks at Age 30, 50, and 70 Years for Carriers of a Mutation in *MLH1, MSH2,* or *MSH6*

Gene	Age (Yr) (95% Confidence Intervals) 30	50	70
All HNPCC-related tumours			
MLH1	4.2 (1.6-6.8)	34 (27-41)	76 (62-85)
MSH2	1.1 (0-2.3)	50 (42-57)	80 (70-86)
MSH6	0.7 (0-2.1)	22 (13-29)	73 (60-82)
Colorectal carcinoma in men			
MLH1	4.1 (0.1-7.9)	31 (19-41)	65 (39-80)
MSH2	2.0 (0-4.4)	39 (28-48)	63 (49-73)
MSH6	1.7 (0-5.0)	17 (4.4-28)	69 (42-83)
Colorectal carcinoma in women			
MLH1	4.3 (0.9-7.7)	26 (17-34)	53 (33-66)
MSH2	0	30 (18-40)	68 (43-82)
MSH6	0	10 (2.4-17)	30 (12-44)
Endometrial carcinoma			
MLH1	0	7.2 (1.4-13)	27 (14-38)
MSH2	0	23 (12-32)	40 (21-54)
MSH6	0	13 (5.3-22)	71 (50-83)

(Reprinted from Hendriks YM, Wagner A, Morreau H, et al: Cancer risk in hereditary nonpolyposis colorectal cancer due to *MSH6* mutations: Impact on counseling and surveillance. *Gastroenterology* 127:17-25, 2004. Copyright 2004, with permission from American Gastroenterology Association.)

71% for endometrial carcinoma at 70 years of age in these carriers (Table 2). The risk for all HNPCC-associated tumors was significantly lower in *MSH6* compared with *MLH1* or *MSH2* mutation carriers ($P = .002$). In female *MSH6* mutation carriers, the risk for colorectal cancer was significantly lower ($P = .0049$) and the risk for endometrial cancer significantly higher ($P = .02$) than *MLH1* and *MSH2* mutation carriers. In male carriers, the risk for colorectal cancer was lower in *MSH6* mutation carriers; the difference was not significant ($P = .0854$). Sensitivity of the MSI analysis in colorectal tumors was 86% for predicting a MMR defect. Sensitivity of immunohistochemistry for predicting a mutation in *MSH6* was 90%.

Conclusion.—Colonoscopic surveillance is recommended beginning at age 30 years in women with *MSH6* mutations. Prophylactic hysterectomy may be efficacious in carriers older than 50 years. Both MSI and immunohistochemistry analysis are sensitive tools for identifying families eligible for *MSH6* mutation analysis.

▶ The identification of genetic mutations predisposing to cancer revolutionized the field of risk assessment and management. Subsequent work is now focusing on factors responsible for variable penetrance of these mutations and differences in both level of risk and type of cancer associated with different sites of mutation on the same gene. This information has practical relevance for the development of appropriate screening strategies. This article focuses on differences in the risk of colon and endometrial carcinoma and differences in the ages of onset in patients with hereditary nonpolyposis colorectal carcinoma based on which mismatch repair gene is mutated. The 71% cumulative incidence of endometrial carcinoma in women with *MSH6* mutations supports the discussion of prophylactic hysterectomy in this subpopulation in particular.

M. Morrow, MD

Computed Tomographic Virtual Colonoscopy to Screen for Colorectal Neoplasia in Asymptomatic Adults

Pickhardt PJ, Choi JR, Hwang I, et al (Natl Naval Med Ctr, Bethesda, Md; Uniformed Services Univ of the Health Sciences, Bethesda, Md; Natl Cancer Inst, Bethesda, Md)

N Engl J Med 349:2191-2200, 2003 12–14

Introduction.—Colonoscopy has important drawbacks as a screening test, including the need to insert an IV catheter to administer sedatives, recovery time of 30 to 60 minutes, and need for someone to drive the patient home. Virtual colonoscopy requires the same bowel-cleansing preparation as conventional colonoscopy, along with the insertion of a rectal tube and insufflation of air or carbon dioxide for colon distension. Sedation is not needed and time required for the procedure is approximately 10 to 15 minutes, with an additional 30 minutes for interpretation, compared with 2 hours for colonoscopy. Described is the largest prospective evaluation to date of virtual colonoscopy as a colorectal screening test.

Methods.—Same-day virtual and optical colonoscopy were performed in 1233 asymptomatic adults (mean age, 57.8 years). The 3-dimensional endoluminal display was used for the initial detection of polyps on CT virtual colonoscopy. For the initial evaluation of each colonic segment, the colonoscopists were blinded to the findings on virtual colonoscopy, which were available to them before any subsequent reexamination. Sensitivity and specificity of virtual colonoscopy and sensitivity of optical colonoscopy were determined by using findings of the final, unblinded optical colonoscopy as the reference standard.

Results.—Sensitivity of virtual colonoscopy for adenomatous polyps was 93.8% for polyps a minimum of 10 mm in diameter, 93.9% for polyps a minimum of 8 mm in diameter, and 88.7% for polyps at least 6 mm in diameter. Sensitivity of optical colonoscopy for adenomatous polyps was 87.5%, 91.5%, and 92.3%, respectively, for the 3 polyp sizes. Specificity of virtual colonoscopy for adenomatous polyps was 96.0% for polyps a minimum of 10 mm in diameter, 92.2% for polyps a minimum of 8 mm in diameter, and 79.6% for polyps a minimum of 6 mm in diameter. Both of the malignant polyps were identified on virtual colonoscopy; 1 was missed on optical colonoscopy before results of virtual colonoscopy were divulged.

Conclusion.—Virtual colonoscopy in this large, asymptomatic screening population yielded detection rates for adenomas similar to those achieved by using conventional colonoscopy.

► This year, words that I expressed to my patients over the years took on a more personal meaning: "The prep is worse than the procedure." The question this study asks is whether virtual colonoscopy replaces standard endoscopic procedures. Unfortunately for the consumer of either procedure, the prep is the same for both. This trial was slanted toward virtual colonoscopy in that it would appear that sedation was not used for colonoscopy. A result of the side effect profile was worse. The clear advantage of colonoscopy is that it allows for a tissue diagnosis to be obtained at the same time as identifying a lesion. Ultimately the decision to utilize either of these screening procedures in a routine population is likely to be determined by economic factors. New technology may also help drive toward noninvasive procedures. There is clearly more to come on this topic.

P. J. Loehrer, Sr, MD

Histologic Analysis of the Irradiated Anal Sphincter

da Silva GM, Berho M, Wexner SD (Cleveland Clinic Florida, Weston; Cleveland Clinic Foundation, Ohio)

Dis Colon Rectum 46:1492-1497, 2003 12–15

Background.—Increasing evidence suggests that pelvic irradiation adversely affects anorectal function. However, no published histologic evidence of sphincter injury has been reported. Histologic examinations of collagen deposition and nerve fiber changes in the internal anal sphincters of patients with rectal cancer undergoing abdominoperineal resection after adjuvant chemoradiation treatment were discussed. In addition, the degree of histologic changes was correlated with the interval between chemoradiotherapy and abdominoperineal resection.

Methods.—Anal canal specimens were obtained prospectively from patients undergoing abdominoperineal resection. One pathologist unaware of patients' treatment evaluated collagen deposition and nerve fiber densities in the internal anal sphincter.

Methods.—The study included 12 patients who underwent radiation for rectal cancer (chemoradiotherapy group). Another 6 were treated by surgery alone, including 4 patients with rectal cancer and 2 with Crohn's disease. The chemoradiotherapy group showed a trend toward increased fibrosis and nerve density compared with that of the control group. As the interval from chemoradiotherapy to abdominoperineal resection increased, nerve density significantly increased.

Conclusions.—These data demonstrate that pelvic irradiation damages the myenteric plexus or the internal anal sphincter of patients with rectal cancer. These changes seem to be time-dependent. In addition, a trend toward increased collagen deposition was noted. These findings provide a morphologic basis to previously reported physiologic and clinical changes in the anal sphincter of patients undergoing radiation therapy for rectal cancer.

▶ These investigators from the Cleveland Clinic report in a small series of the histopathologic changes resulting from chemoradiation therapy for rectal cancer. There were only 12 patients who received chemoradiation, and the role of the chemotherapy seems entirely neglected in the analysis. All the changes are attributed to radiation, which may or may not be the case. There were 6 patients who were treated with surgery alone. This small number of patients appears to show an increase in fibrosis over time as well as some nerve changes. The essential point is what these changes mean functionally. That is entirely neglected in this article, which surprisingly has no radiation oncologist involved. The authors note the lack of statistical significance in their analysis but believe "that the trend for increased fibrous tissue in the internal sphincter of irradiated patients may lead to reduced sphincter elasticity, influencing muscle tone and responsiveness in the sphincter and resulting in increased fecal leakage." Unfortunately, the authors show no evidence of that at all in this analysis. There is a disconnect between their observations and their conclusion.

E. Glatstein, MD

Pooled Analysis of Fluorouracil-Based Adjuvant Therapy for Stage II and III Colon Cancer: Who Benefits and by How Much?

Gill S, Loprinzi CL, Sargent DJ, et al (Mayo Clinic, Rochester, Minn; British Columbia Cancer Agency, Vancouver, Canada; Queens Univ, Kingston, Ont, Canada; et al)

J Clin Oncol 22:1797-1806, 2004 12–16

Introduction.—Decisions concerning adjuvant chemotherapy need to be based on accurate estimates of baseline prognosis and magnitude of incremental benefit that can be achieved. In the absence of such information, patients may have misperceptions regarding the risks of their disease and an incomplete understanding of the rationale for adjuvant treatment. A pooled analysis was performed to improve the understanding of the magnitude of adjuvant therapy benefit seen in specific patient subgroups.

Methods.—A total of 3302 patients with stage II and III colon cancer from 7 randomized trials comparing fluorouracil (FU) + leucovorin or FU + levamisole to surgery alone were evaluated. Treatment, age, gender, tumor location, T stage, nodal status, and grade were examined for both prognostic and predictive significance. Model derived estimates of 5-year disease-free survival and overall survival for surgery alone and surgery plus FU-based therapy were determined for a range of patient subsets.

Results.—Nodal status, T stage, and grade were the only prognostic factors independently significant for both disease-free survival and overall survival; age was significant only for overall survival. Multivariate analysis revealed that adjuvant therapy provided a beneficial treatment effect across all subsets. The treatment benefits were consistent across gender, location, age, T stage, and grade. A significant stage by treatment interaction was present, with treatment benefiting stage III patients to a greater extent than stage II patients.

Conclusion.—Patients with high-risk resected colon cancer receive benefit from FU-based therapy across subsets of age, gender, location, T stage, nodal status, and grade. Model estimates of survival stratified by T stage, nodal status, grade, and age may be found at http://www.mayoclinic.com/calcs. These data may be used to enhance patient and physician understanding regarding potential benefits of adjuvant therapy.

▶ How patients process clinical information is extremely variable; so are the communications skill sets of physicians. The authors pooled analysis of randomized trials to clarify the impact of adjuvant therapy for prognostic and predictive characteristics. These investigators at the Mayo Clinic then created a novel Web site (http://www.mayoclinic.com/calcs) that helps patients identify their individual risk analysis profile. The result is a unique way to communicate risk and benefits to patients with colorectal cancer.

P. J. Loehrer, Sr, MD

Oxaliplatin, Fluorouracil, and Leucovorin as Adjuvant Treatment for Colon Cancer

André T, for the Multicenter International Study of Oxaliplatin/5-Fluorouracil/Leucovorin in the Adjuvant Treatment of Colon Cancer (MOSAIC) Investigators (Hôpital Tenon, Paris; et al)

N Engl J Med 350:2343-2351, 2004 12–17

Introduction.—Fluorouracil plus leucovorin (FL) is the standard adjuvant treatment for patients with colon cancer. Oxaliplatin enhances the efficacy of this combination in patients who have metastatic colon cancer. The efficacy of treatment with FL plus oxaliplatin was evaluated in the postoperative adjuvant setting to determine whether oxaliplatin can also be beneficial at an earlier disease stage.

Methods.—A total of 2246 patients who had undergone curative resection for stage II or III colon cancer were randomly assigned to 6 months of adjuvant treatment with either FL plus oxaliplatin or FL alone. The major end point was disease-free survival.

Results.—At a median follow-up of 37.9 months, 237 patients in the FL plus oxaliplatin group had a cancer-associated event compared with 293 patients in the FL group (21.1% vs 26.1%; hazard ratio for recurrence, 0.77; $P = .002$). The incidence of disease-free survival at 3 years was 78.2% (95% confidence interval, 75.6-80.7%) in the combination group versus 72.9% (95% confidence interval, 70.2-75.7%) in the FL group ($P = .002$) (Fig 1). In the combination group, the rate of febrile neutropenia was 1.8%, gastrointestinal adverse effects were low, and the incidence of grade 3 neuropathy was 12.4% during treatment, dropping to 1.1% at 1-year follow-up. Six patients from each treatment assignment died during treatment (death rate, 0.5%).

Conclusion.—The addition of oxaliplatin to a treatment regimen of FL improves the adjuvant treatment of colon cancer. The primary safety concern with oxaliplatin is peripheral neuropathy. The incidence of grade 3 pe

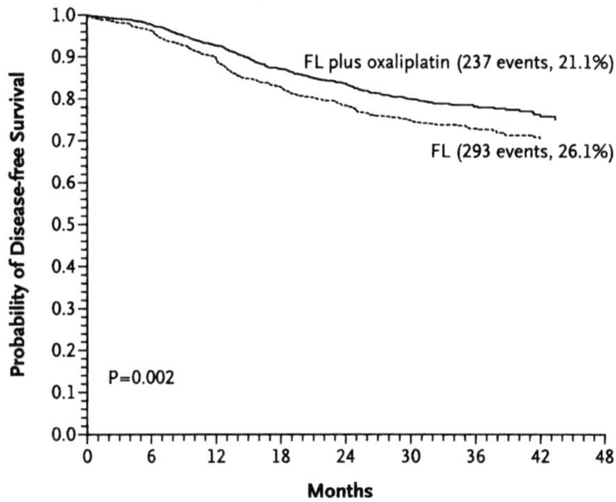

No. at Risk

FL+oxaliplatin	1123	1086	1023	959	888	663	395
FL	1123	1066	981	903	817	619	356

FIGURE 1.—Kaplan-Meier estimates of disease-free survival in the group given FL and the group given FL plus oxaliplatin, according to the intention to treat. Hazard ratio for recurrence in the group given FL plus oxaliplatin, compared with the FL group, was 0.77 (95% confidence interval, 0.65 to 0.91; $P = .002$). (Reprinted by permission of *The New England Journal of Medicine* from André T: for the Multicenter International Study of Oxaliplatin/5-Fluorouracil/Leucovorin in the Treatment of Colon Cancer (MOSAIC) Investigators: Oxaliplatin, fluorouracil, and leucovorin as adjuvant treatment for colon cancer. *N Engl J of Med* 350:2343-2351, 2004. Copyright 2004, Massachusetts Medical Society. All rights reserved.)

ripheral neuropathy dropped from 12.4% to 1.1% at 1 year in the combination group.

► Logic would lead one to think that the best adjuvant therapy is also the best therapy for metastatic disease. Three-drug regimens with FL and either CPT-11 or oxaliplatin (see Abstract 12–28) are now clearly considered standards for stage IV colorectal cancer.

This trial by André et al demonstrates an improvement in the 3-year disease-free survival with FOLFOX chemotherapy, which they feel will translate to an improved overall survival at 5 years. Of note, with a median follow-up of 3 years, the survival of FOLFOX versus 5-fluorouracil therapy was 87.7% and 86.6%, respectively ($P =$ NS). Interestingly, when one looks at various prognostic factors that predict response (age >65 years, stage II disease, presence of perforation, and postoperative elevated carcinoembryonic antigen), they did not help distinguish whether chemotherapy would be helpful. This trial clearly suggests a therapeutic advantage. Further follow-up with overall survival clearly needs to be seen. This 3-drug regimen should be part of a treatment discussion with patients with resected stage III disease.

P. J. Loehrer, Sr, MD

Randomized Trial of Intraportal and/or Systemic Adjuvant Chemotherapy in Patients With Colon Carcinoma

Labianca R, for the ACOI/GIVIO/GISCAD Investigators (Ospedali Riuniti, Bergamo, Italy; et al)

J Natl Cancer Inst 96:750-758, 2004 12–18

Introduction.—5-Fluorouracil-based adjuvant chemotherapy is standard treatment for patients who have undergone surgical resection of colon cancer. The choice of the optimal delivery route for systemic (IV vs oral) or regional (intraportal [IP], intraperitoneal, or hepatic arterial infusion) is controversial. The benefits of chemotherapy delivered by these routes individually or in combination were examined in a prospective, randomized, controlled trial.

Methods.—Between April 2, 1992, and April 30, 1998, 1084 eligible patients with Dukes stage B or C colon carcinoma were randomly assigned to treatment assignments: 369 patients to the IP regimen of continuous portal vein infusion of 5-fluorouracil at 500 mg/m^2 body surface daily and heparin 5000 IU daily for 7 consecutive days, starting on the day of surgery; 358 patients to the systemic regimen of six 28-day courses of systemic leucovorin at 100 mg/m^2 daily on days 1 through 5, then systemic bolus 5-fluorouracil at 370 mg/m^2 daily on days 1 through 5, with treatment started 15 to 35 days postoperatively; and 357 to the IP + systemic regimen (the IP regimen, followed by the systemic regimen, with the same scheduling). Survival rates were determined by using the log-rank statistic and a Cox multivariable regression model; all statistical tests were 2 sided.

Results.—At a median follow-up of 99 months, there were 389 events, including recurrences, second malignancies, or deaths; 261 patients died. Sites of first recurrences were similar among the 3 treatment arms. At 5 years, overall and event-free survival were similar among patients in the IP (74% and 68%, respectively), systemic (78% and 71%), and IP + systemic (73% and 67%) treatment arms. Compared with the systemic group, the risk for death associated with IP (hazard ratio [HR]) was 1.05 (95% confidence interval [CI], 0.82-1.36) and was similar to the IP + systemic group (HR, 1.12; 95% CI, 0.78-1.45; $P = .69$), as were risks for first event (HR, 1.07; 95% CI, 0.84-1.37 and HR, 1.10; 95% CI, 0.86-1.41, respectively).

Conclusion.—The overall and event-free survival rates were similar for all 3 treatment arms. The combined regimen yielded no better outcomes than either single regimen alone.

▶ The concept of IP therapy for the treatment of colorectal cancer has been advocated for nearly 50 years and supported by a pivotal trial by Dr Taylor and his colleagues.[1,2] This is the largest prospective trial to test this concept. I would hope that it would finally put this concept to rest.

P. J. Loehrer, Sr, MD

References

1. Morales F, Bell M, McDonald GD, et al: The prophylactic treatment of cancer at time of operation. *Ann Surg* 146:588-593, 1957.
2. Taylor I, Machin D, Mullee ME, et al: A randomized controlled trial of adjuvant portal vein cytotoxic perfusion in colorectal cancer. *Br J Surg* 72:359-363, 1985.

Phase III Study of Adjuvant Chemotherapy and Radiation Therapy Compared With Chemotherapy Alone in the Surgical Adjuvant Treatment of Colon Cancer: Results of Intergroup Protocol 0130

Martenson JA Jr, Willett CG, Sargent DJ, et al (Mayo Clinic, Rochester, Minn; Radiation Therapy Oncology Group, Philadelphia; Missouri Valley Cancer Consortium, Omaha, Neb; et al)

J Clin Oncol 22:3277-3283, 2004 12–19

Background.—In some patients with colon cancer, the risk of local recurrence after surgery is high. Whether radiation therapy added to an adjuvant chemotherapy regimen improves outcomes in these high-risk patients was investigated.

Methods.—Two hundred twenty-two patients with resected colon cancer and tumor adherence or invasion of surrounding structures or with T3N1 or T3N2 tumors of the ascending or descending colon were enrolled in the study. By random assignment, the patients received fluorouracil and levamisole treatment with or without radiation therapy. Patients receiving chemotherapy and radiation therapy were given 45 to 50.4 Gy in 25 to 28 fractions, beginning 28 days after the start of chemotherapy. One hundred eighty-seven patients were evaluable.

Findings.—Overall, the 5-year survival rates were 62% in the chemotherapy group and 58% in the chemotherapy plus radiation therapy group. Disease-free survival at 5 years was 51% in both groups. Toxicity of grade 4 or worse was documented in 42% of those receiving chemotherapy only and 54% of those receiving combination therapy. Leukopenia of grade 3 or worse occurred in 10% and 22%, respectively. The 2 groups did not differ significantly in nonhematologic toxicity, those rates being 35% and 44%, respectively.

Conclusions.—Overall and disease-free survival were similar in patients receiving chemotherapy only or in combination with radiation therapy. Toxicity was higher in the latter group.

► Periodically, the topic arises which suggests that if radiation therapy is useful in rectal cancer, then should it not be also useful in high-risk colon cancer patients. This may have particular importance for these high-risk patients in terms of reducing local-regional occurrences. This is indeed an important study that attempts to address this issue. Unfortunately, only 222 patients of the original goal of 700 patients were accrued, and despite this, if anything, the chemotherapy arm was superior to the chemotherapy plus radiation therapy with respect to overall survival (62% vs 58%), though this did not reach statistical significance. It would seem that the burden of proof still remains with those who wish to use radiation therapy for colon cancer. This trial outlines some of the numerous difficulties in accruing patients to important studies such as these. Nonetheless, these have important physiologic and economic issues that need to be defined.

P. J. Loehrer, Sr, MD

A Comparison of Laparoscopically Assisted and Open Colectomy for Colon Cancer: The Clinical Outcomes of Surgical Therapy Study Group

Nelson H, for the Clinical Outcomes of Surgical Therapy Study Group (Mayo Clinic, Rochester, Minn; et al)

N Engl J Med 350:2050-2059, 2004 12–20

Introduction.—Minimally invasive laparoscopically assisted surgery was initially considered in 1990 for patients undergoing colectomy for cancer. There was concern that this approach would compromise survival by not being able to achieve a proper oncologic resection or adequate staging or by modifying patterns of recurrence, based on frequent reports regarding tumor recurrences within surgical wounds. In 1994, a prospective randomized trial was started that compared laparoscopically assisted and open surgery for curable colon cancer in multiple, diverse surgical practices.

Methods.—A noninferiority trial was performed at 48 institutions. A total of 872 patients with adenocarcinoma of the colon were randomly assigned to undergo open or laparoscopically assisted colectomy performed by credentialed surgeons. The median follow-up was 4.4 years. The major end point was the time to tumor recurrence.

Results.—At 3-year follow-up, the incidence of recurrent disease was similar for both groups: 16% for the laparoscopic group and 18% for the open group (2-sided $P = .32$; hazard ratio for recurrence, 0.86; 95% confidence interval, 0.63-1.17). Recurrence rates in surgical wounds were less than 1% for both groups ($P = .50$). Overall survivals at 3 years were similar (86%, laparoscopic group; 85%, open colectomy group; $P = .51$; hazard ratio for death in the laparoscopic group, 0.91; 95% confidence interval, 0.68-1.21). There were no between-group differences in time to recurrence or overall survival among patients with any stage of cancer (Fig 2). Perioperative recovery was quicker in the laparoscopic group than in the open group, as demonstrated by a shorter median hospital stay (5 vs 6 days; $P < .001$) and shorter use of parenteral narcotics (3 vs 4 days; $P < .001$) and oral analgesics (1 vs 2 days; $P = .02$). The incidence of intraoperative complications, 30-day postoperative mortality, complications at discharge and 60 days, hospital readmission, and reoperation were similar between groups.

Conclusion.—The incidence of cancer recurrence was similar after laparoscopically assisted colectomy and open colectomy, indicating that the laparoscopic approach is acceptable as an alternative to open surgery for colon cancer.

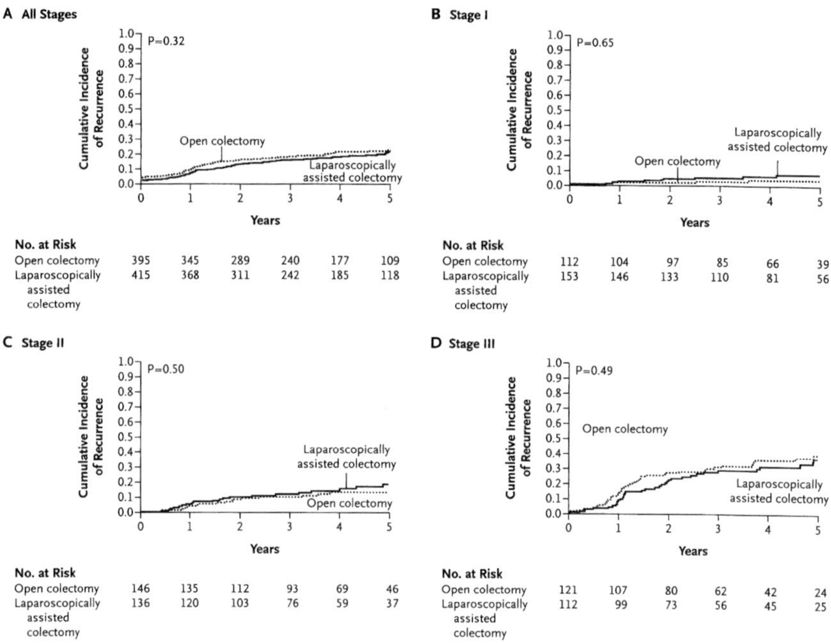

A All Stages

No. at Risk	0	1	2	3	4	5
Open colectomy	395	345	289	240	177	109
Laparoscopically assisted colectomy	415	368	311	242	185	118

B Stage I

No. at Risk	0	1	2	3	4	5
Open colectomy	112	104	97	85	66	39
Laparoscopically assisted colectomy	153	146	133	110	81	56

C Stage II

No. at Risk	0	1	2	3	4	5
Open colectomy	146	135	112	93	69	46
Laparoscopically assisted colectomy	136	120	103	76	59	37

D Stage III

No. at Risk	0	1	2	3	4	5
Open colectomy	121	107	80	62	42	24
Laparoscopically assisted colectomy	112	99	73	56	45	25

FIGURE 2.—A, Cumulative incidence of recurrence among patients with colon cancer at any stage. The tumor-node-metastasis stage was used. Patients with benign pathologic conditions were excluded from this analysis. (Reprinted by permission of *The New England Journal of Medicine* from Nelson H, for the Clinical Outcomes of Surgical Therapy Study Group. *N Engl J Med* 350:2050-2059, 2004. Copyright 2004, Massachusetts Medical Society. All rights reserved.)

► Although laparoscopic surgery is an established technique for the management of benign intraabdominal problems, concerns that the procedure might not be appropriate for patients with malignancy have been expressed. This important study documents that in the hands of experienced surgeons, recurrence rates and survival do not differ after open and laparoscopically assisted colon resection for early stage colon cancer. Several facets of this study are worthy of note. First, concerns that laparoscopic surgery would understage patients are not supported by the equal incidence of metastases in both arms of the study, as well as the lack of survival difference between stages. Surgeons were required to have performed 20 laparoscopic colon resections before trial participation, and oncologic technique was assessed by videotape. In spite of this, 21% of laparoscopic patients were converted to open colectomy, and operating time in the laparoscopic group (150 minutes) was significantly longer than that in the open group (90 minutes; $P < .001$). Although significant differences in median hospital stay and use of parenteral narcotics were observed that favored the laparoscopic group, the absolute magnitude of the differences was small.

This study clearly demonstrates that laparoscopically assisted colon resection is safe, but surgeons in practice should ensure that adequate experience with laparoscopic procedures is obtained before utilizing this approach for colon cancer. In addition, careful selection of patients with early stage disease and conversion to open resection should be carried out if the laparoscopic approach appears to compromise oncologic principles.

M. Morrow, MD

Colon Cancer Survival Is Associated With Increasing Number of Lymph Nodes Analyzed: A Secondary Survey of Intergroup Trial INT-0089

Le Voyer TE, Sigurdson ER, Hanlon AL, et al (Fox Chase Cancer Ctr, Philadelphia; Cancer and Leukemia Group B, Chicago; Southwest Oncology Group, San Antonio, Tex; et al)

J Clin Oncol 21:2912-2919, 2003 12–21

Introduction.—The most significant determinant of prognosis in patients with carcinoma of the colon is lymph node involvement. Yet the number of lymph nodes reported in colon cancer surgery varies greatly, and the effect of the number of nodes removed and examined continues to be unknown. The largest prospective database for stage II and stage III colon cancer was reviewed to determine the relationship between the number of lymph nodes recovered and survival.

Methods.—The Intergroup Trial INT-0089 was a mature trial of adjuvant chemotherapy for high-risk patients with stage II or stage III colon cancer. A secondary analysis of this group was performed. The primary end point was overall survival and the secondary end points were cause-specific survival and disease-free survival.

Results.—The median number of lymph nodes removed at the time of colectomy was 11 (range, 1-87). Of 3411 assessable patients, 648 had no evidence of lymph node metastasis. Multivariate analyses were performed separately on the node-positive and node-negative groups to determine the effect of lymph node removal. Survival dropped with increasing lymph node involvement ($P = .0001$ for all 3 survival end points). After controlling for the number of nodes involved, survival increased as more nodes were evaluated ($P = .0001$ for all 3 end points). Even when no nodes were involved, overall survival and cause-specific survival improved as more lymph nodes were examined ($P = .0005$ and $P = .007$, respectively).

Conclusion.—The number of lymph nodes examined for staging colon cancers is a prognostic outcome variable. This variable may be important to include in assessing future trials.

▶ An increasing body of data indicates that locoregional control improves survival in a variety of cancers. This study examines the impact of the number of lymph nodes removed in a colon resection on survival and finds a strong association with improved survival in both node-positive and node-negative patients. These findings are somewhat puzzling. One benefit of more extensive nodal sampling is the greater likelihood of identifying nodal metastases, allowing properly staged patients to receive adjuvant therapy. However, all patients in the Intergroup Trial analyzed by Le Voyer et al received adjuvant therapy, so this does not explain the observed survival benefit.

In patients with nodal metastases, tumor-bearing nodes that are not removed have the potential to act as sites for reseeding and contribute to mortality. It is more difficult to explain why the removal of larger numbers of uninvolved nodes contributes to survival. In those with nodal involvement, the highest survival rates were seen after removal of 35 to 40 nodes. In the node-negative group, this occurred after the removal of more than 20 nodes. It is possible that the number of nodes removed is a surrogate for other technical aspects of the operative procedure which influence survival. Alternatively, examination of more than 20 nodes may be required to reliably stage a patient as node-negative. Regardless of the explanation, review of the number of nodes removed during colon resection appears to be a low-cost method of quality assessment which can be easily undertaken in any practice setting

M. Morrow, MD

New Tumor-Node-Metastasis Staging Strategy for Node-Positive (Stage III) Rectal Cancer: An Analysis

Greene FL, Stewart AK, Norton HJ (Carolinas Med Ctr, Charlotte, NC; American College of Surgeons, Chicago)
J Clin Oncol 22:1778-1784, 2004 12–22

Background.—Traditional strategies of tumor-node-metastasis (TNM) system staging of rectal cancer have grouped patients with mesenteric nodal involvement into the stage III category despite variations in the depth of tumor penetration of the rectal wall. A recent study has suggested that stage III colorectal cancer is heterogeneous in survival patterns when differences in T and N categories are considered. An analysis of a large dataset of patients reported to the National Cancer Data Base (NCDB) has demonstrated the value of stratification of patients with stage III colon cancer.

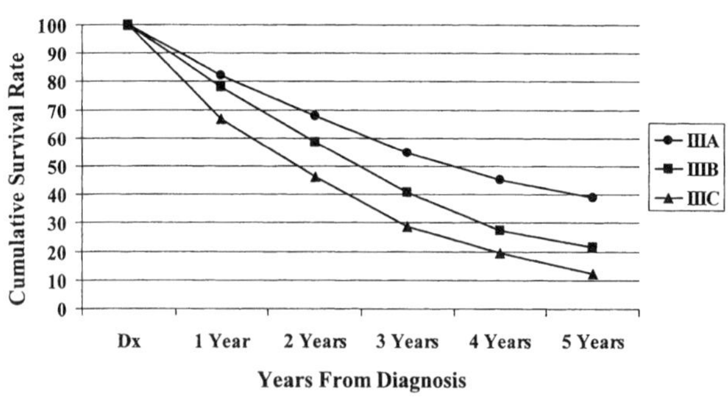

FIGURE 6.—Five-year observed survival rates: stage III rectal cancers treated by surgery alone by American Joint Committee on Cancer (Sixth Edition) subgroup. Cases diagnosed 1991 to 1993. *Abbreviation: Dx*, Diagnosis. (Courtesy of Greene FL, Stewart AK, Norton HJ: New tumor-node-metastasis staging strategy for node-positive (stage III) rectal cancer: An analysis. *J Clin Oncol* 22:1778-1784, 2004. Reprinted with permission from the American Society of Clinical Oncology.)

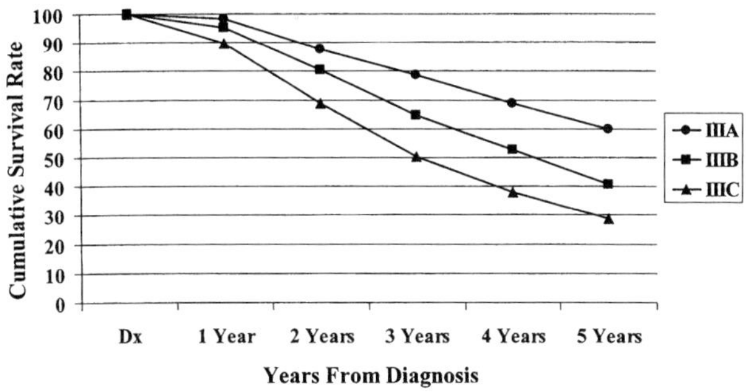

FIGURE 7.—Five-year observed survival rates: stage III rectal cancers treated with surgery, radiation, and chemotherapy by American Joint Committee on Cancer (Sixth Edition) subgroup. Cases diagnosed 1991 to 1993. *Abbreviation: Dx*, Diagnosis. (Courtesy of Greene FL, Stewart AK, Norton HJ: New tumor-node-metastasis staging strategy for node-positive (stage III) rectal cancer: An analysis. *J Clin Oncol* 22:1778-1784, 2004. Reprinted with permission from the American Society of Clinical Oncology.)

Overall survival when node-positive patients were stratified into 3 new subsets was analyzed.

Methods.—Data entered into the NCDB database for 5987 stage III patients with rectal cancer between 1991 and 1993 were analyzed. Survival was calculated with 3 new subgroups (IIIA: T 1/2, N1; IIIB: T3/4, N1; IIIC: any T, N2). Survival after surgery and adjuvant therapy was assessed. The observed survival rates were calculated and compared by the log-rank method. The Cox regression model was used to assess subgroup differences.

Results.—The 5-year observed survival rates for stage III subcategories were 55.1% in IIIA, 35.3% in IIIB, and 24.5% in IIIC (Fig 6). Stratifying for treatment outcome, stage IIIA patients having surgery alone (278 patients) had poorer observed 5-year survival (39%) than the 765 patients treated with surgery and adjuvant chemotherapy or radiation (chemo/XRT) therapy (60%) (Fig 7). Outcomes were similar in IIIB (surgery alone, 21.7% vs chemo/XRT, 40.9%) and in IIIC (surgery alone, 12.2% vs chemo/XRT, 28.9%). The differences were significant in all stages (Table 4).

Conclusions.—The traditional stage III designation of rectal cancer does not account for invasion (T1-4) and number of involved nodes (N1, N2). The stratification of stage III patients into 3 subsets is recommended for use

TABLE 4.—Observed and Relative Survival of Stage III Subsets Relating to Treatment

	Observed Survival (%)		Relative Survival (%)	
Stage	Surgery	Surgery + Chemo/XRT	Surgery	Surgery + Chemo/XRT
IIIA	39.0 (n = 278)	60.0 (n = 765)	53.2	69.7
IIIB	21.7 (n = 726)	40.9 (n = 2,130)	30.0	48.1
IIIC	12.2 (n = 467)	28.9 (n = 1,621)	17.3	33.6

(Courtesy of Greene FL, Stewart AK, Norton HJ: New tumor-node-metastasis staging strategy for node-positive (stage III) rectal cancer: An analysis. *J Clin Oncol* 22:1778-1784, 2004. Reprinted with permission from the American Society of Clinical Oncology.)

in future analyses of rectal cancer. The effect of postoperative adjuvant therapy was found to be beneficial in all subsets.

▶ There are many conflicting prognostic factors in rectal cancer, including stage, age, and grade of tumor. This study examines the current staging system and segregates stage III patients into 3 subgroups (IIIA, IIIB, IIIC) with differing outcomes depending on whether patients receive adjuvant therapy. Other factors such as age, grade, and first cancer treatment are still independent factors. This staging system improves predictability.

P. J. Loehrer, Sr, MD

Morphologic Predictors of Lymph Node Status in Rectal Cancer With Use of High-Spatial-Resolution MR Imaging With Histopathologic Comparison

Brown G, Richards CJ, Bourne MW, et al (Univ of Wales College of Medicine, Cardiff, England)
Radiology 227:371-377, 2003 12–23

Background.—The preoperative assessment of lymph node status in patients with rectal cancer is important because the patient's prognosis is affected by the number of involved nodes and because the risk of recurrence is increased with the presence of tumor-containing lymph nodes near the mesorectal fascia, unless the standard excision plane is altered. Extended lymphadenectomy may be required for nodes lying outside the mesorectal fascia to achieve clearance of the tumor. Signal intensity and border characteristics of lymph nodes at high-spatial-resolution MRI in patients with rectal cancer were evaluated, and these findings were compared with the size in prediction of nodal status.

Methods.—The study group comprised 42 patients who underwent total mesorectal excision of the rectum to determine whether they had rectal carcinoma were studied with preoperative thin-section MRI. Lymph nodes were harvested from 42 transversely sectioned surgical specimens, and the slice of each lymph node was carefully matched with its location on the corresponding MR images. Nodal size, border contour, and signal intensity on MR images were characterized and correlated with histologic involvement with metastases. Method 10 by Newcombe was performed to calculate differences in sensitivity and specificity with border or signal intensity. Method 10 of Newcombe was used to calculate differences in sensitivity and specificity with border or signal intensity.

Results.—Of the 437 nodes harvested, 102 were less than 3 mm in diameter and thus too small to be depicted on MR images (Fig 1); only 2 of these contained metastases. In 15 of 22 patients with nodal metastases (68%), the size of normal or reactive nodes was equal to or greater than that of positive nodes in the same specimen. Fifty-one nodes were above the area imaged, and 7 of these nodes contained metastases. The diameter of benign nodes was similar to that of malignant nodes, so size was not a good predictor of

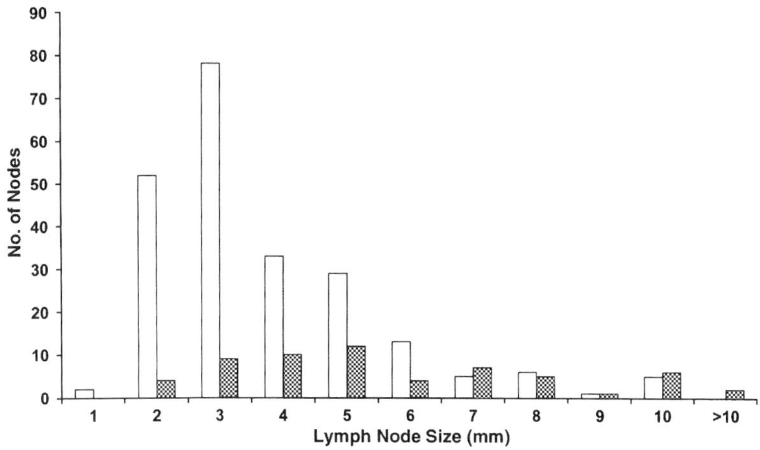

FIGURE 1.—Histogram shows the number of normal (white bars) and malignant (gray bars) nodes seen on MR images, according to diameter (which is measured in millimeters). (Courtesy of Brown G, Richards CJ, Bourne MW, et al: Morphologic predictors of lymph node status in rectal cancer with use of high-spatial-resolution MR imaging with histopathologic comparison. *Radiology* 227:371-377, 2003. Radiology Society of North America.)

nodal status (Figs 3 and 5). In nodes defined as suspicious because of an irregular border or mixed signal intensity, superior accuracy was obtained and resulted in a sensitivity of 85% and specificity of 97%.

Conclusion.—The value of MRI in prediction of nodal involvement in patients with rectal cancer is increased by the use of the border contour and signal intensity characteristics of lymph nodes rather than size criteria.

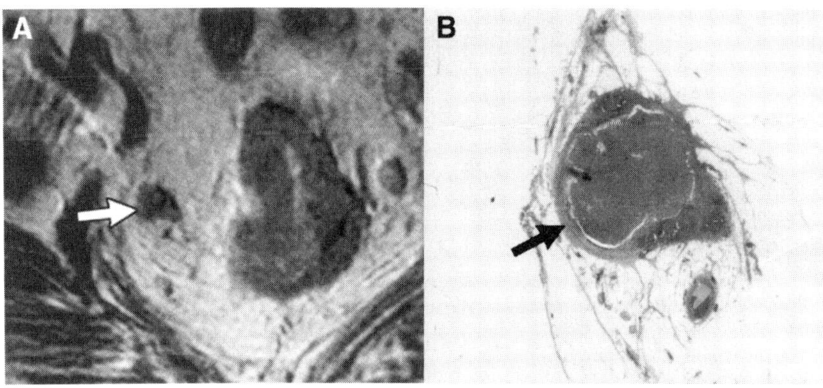

FIGURE 3.—**A**, T2-weighted fast spin-echo transverse MR image (2,500/100) through the upper portion of the rectum. A node with an irregular border (*arrow*) located close to the right lateral mesorectal margin contains mixed signal intensity. **B**, Photomicrograph shows corresponding node (*arrow*) harvested from the right lateral mesorectal margin of the specimen contains proteinaceous extracellular mucin. (Hematoxylin-eosin stain; original magnification, ×6.) (Courtesy of Brown G, Richards CJ, Bourne MW, et al: Morphologic predictors of lymph node status in rectal cancer with use of high-spatial-resolution MR imaging with histopathologic comparison. *Radiology* 227:371-377, 2003. Radiology Society of North America.)

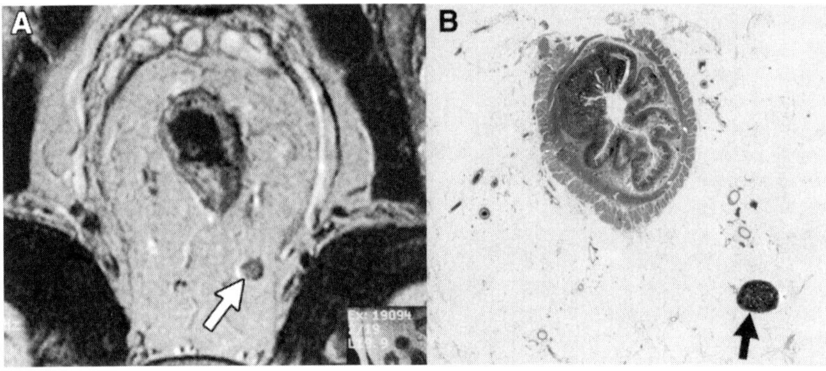

FIGURE 5.—A, T2-weighted fast spin-echo transverse MR image (>2,500/100) through the middle portion of the rectum. A high-signal-intensity node with smooth borders (*arrow*) of homogeneous signal intensity is demonstrated close to the right posterolateral border of the mesorectum. B, Corresponding histologic wholemount slice from total mesorectal excision revealed benign node (*arrow*). (Hematoxylin-eosin stain; original magnification, ×1.) (Courtesy of Brown G, Richards CJ, Bourne MW, et al: Morphologic predictors of lymph node status in rectal cancer with use of high-spatial-resolution MR imaging with histopathologic comparison. *Radiology* 227:371-377, 2003. Radiology Society of North America.)

► I really like this article because it illustrates what I think is a very important point in interpreting diagnostic images of cancer. In today's world of CT and MR, usually the only criterion for abnormality of the lymph node is size. The problem is that the cutoff is actually quite arbitrary. And anyone who thinks a millimeter one side or the other of some arbitrary threshold is important is fooling himself. These investigators from Wales determined that the diameter of benign and malignant nodes was similar and that size was not a good predictor of nodal involvement. They found that a node was defined as suspicious because of either an irregular border or some sort of mixed signal intensity. The sensitivity was about 85% although the specificity was over 90%. In any event, I think that the points made are good ones and the illustrations are excellent.

E. Glatstein, MD

Preoperative Radiotherapy Combined With Intraoperative Radiotherapy Improve Results of Total Mesorectal Excision in Patients With T_3 Rectal Cancer

Pacelli F, Di Giorgio A, Papa V, et al (Catholic Univ, Rome)
Dis Colon Rectum 47:170-179, 2004 12–24

Background.—A number of trials have suggested the value of preoperative adjuvant radiotherapy, alone or in combination with chemotherapy, in the surgical treatment of T_3 rectal cancer, with or without positive lymph nodes. However, there is much controversy regarding whether preoperative treatments offer additional survival to rectal tumor resection performed with total mesorectal excision (TME). One prospective, randomized study has reported a significant reduction in local recurrence after preoperative ra-

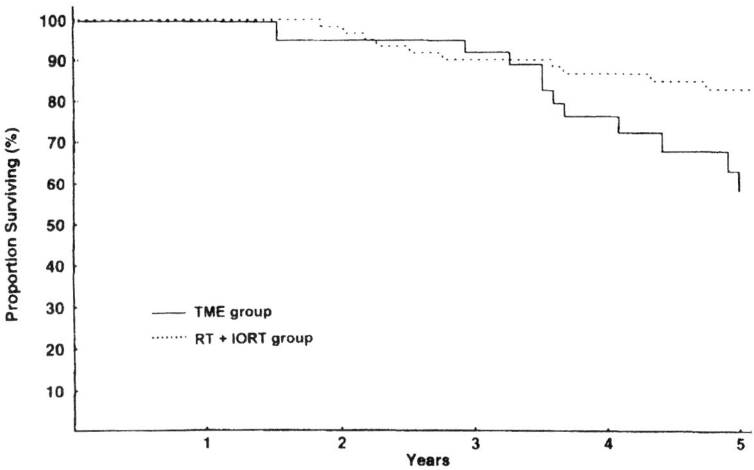

FIGURE 1.—Disease-specific survival curves according to type of treatment. *Abbreviations: TME,* Total mesorectal excision; *RT,* radiotherapy; *IORT,* intraoperative radiotherapy. (Courtesy of Pacelli F, Di Giorgio A, Papa V, et al: Preoperative radiotherapy combined with intraoperative radiotherapy improve results of total mesorectal excision in patients with T_3 rectal cancer. *Dis Colon Rectum* 47[2]:170-179, 2004. Copyright Springer-Verlag.)

diotherapy (RT), but the follow-up was too short to evaluate the long-term survival. Early and long-term results of preoperative RT plus intraoperative RT (IORT) were evaluated in a homogeneous population of T_3 middle and lower rectal cancer patients submitted to TME at a single institution.

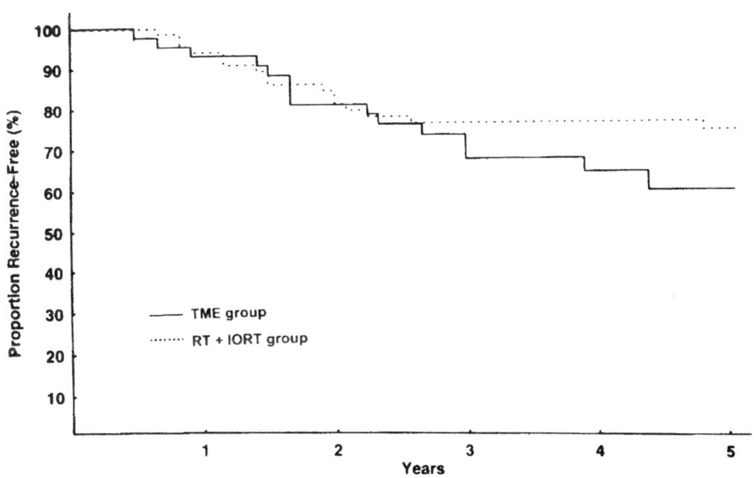

FIGURE 2.—Disease-free survival curves according to type of treatment. *Abbreviations: TME,* Total mesorectal excision; *RT,* radiotherapy; *IORT,* intraoperative radiotherapy. (Courtesy of Pacelli F, Di Giorgio A, Papa V, et al: Preoperative radiotherapy combined with intraoperative radiotherapy improve results of total mesorectal excision in patients with T_3 rectal cancer. *Dis Colon Rectum* 47[2]:170-179, 2004. Copyright Springer-Verlag.)

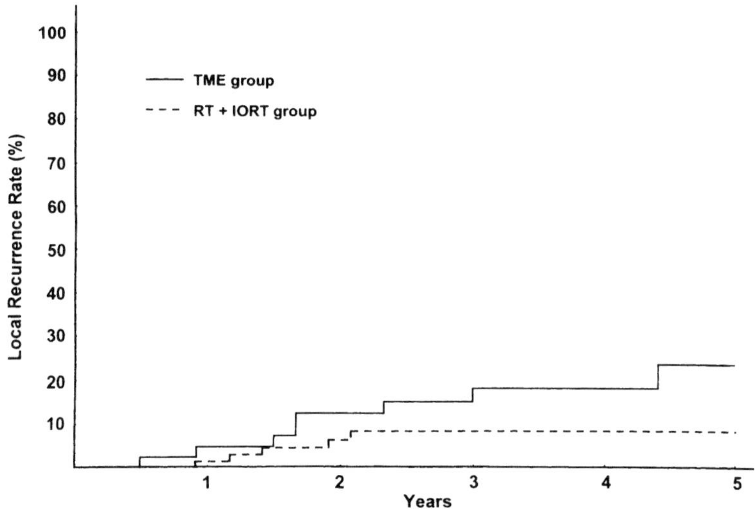

FIGURE 3.—Local recurrence rates according to type of treatment. *Abbreviations: TME,* Total mesorectal excision; *RT,* radiotherapy; *IORT,* intraoperative radiotherapy. (Courtesy of Pacelli F, Di Giorgio A, Papa V, et al: Preoperative radiotherapy combined with intraoperative radiotherapy improve results of total mesorectal excision in patients with T_3 rectal cancer. *Dis Colon Rectum* 47[2]:170-179, 2004. Copyright Springer-Verlag.)

Methods.—A series of 113 patients with middle and lower T_3 rectal cancer who underwent TME at a single surgical unit from 1991 to 1997 were divided into 2 groups on the basis of neoadjuvant treatment: preoperative RT plus IORT (n = 69) and no preoperative treatment (TME, n = 44). Standard statistical analyses were used to evaluate early results (downstaging, intraoperative factors, hospital morbidity, and mortality rates) and long-term outcomes (recurrence and survival).

Results.—Overall, 68.2% of patients were downstaged by the preoperative regimens (T_0 specimens in 3 cases). Postoperative complications were comparable in the 2 groups. The 5-year disease-specific survival was 81.4% in the preoperative RT plus IORT group and 58.1% in the TME group (Fig 1). The figures for disease-free survival were 73.1% and 57.2%, respectively (Fig 2), and the rates of local recurrence at 5 years were 6.6% and 23.2%, respectively (Fig 3).

Conclusions.—Preoperative RT plus IORT in association with TME was shown to reduce the local recurrence rate of T_3 rectal cancer and improve survival when compared with TME alone.

► These investigators from Rome have a series of 113 patients with T_3 rectal cancer treated with TME. Sixty-nine of those patients were treated with neoadjuvant treatment including preoperative RT as well as 1000 cGy of IORT. The remaining 44 had no preoperative or intraoperative treatment. The authors conclude that preoperative RT with IORT improves survival in these T_3 patients.

I certainly cannot agree with that conclusion. As perhaps one of the few radiation oncologists who has ever studied IORT in a prospective randomized way, we were able to see very little benefit, and certainly nothing statistically important, with IORT in the management of retroperitoneal sarcomas, gastric carcinomas, and pancreatic carcinomas. Perhaps it is different with advanced rectal cancer, but it is hard to see why. The main problem from the standpoint of the prospective studies to which I allude was that about 70% of those patients disseminated with intraperitoneal disease and carcinomatosis. It is not clear from this article that patients were not given postoperative RT or chemotherapy on an ad hoc basis. The "survival curve" is actually disease-specific survival; the absence of a survival curve that accounts for death from all causes represents a major flaw. That in itself makes this article dubious in terms of conclusions.

Having had considerable interest in IORT in the past, I think it takes not only a prospective study, but also one in which the surgeon decides that he really has *no really good* surgical procedure to offer at the time the patient is explored. By that I mean that if the patient really has a good surgical option in the eyes of the surgeon, then IORT is probably not going to accomplish a great deal. It is really the patient whose tumor when finally seen by the surgeon causes the surgeon to gulp, who may be a patient in whom IORT may have a true role to play. It is this difficult group with only a marginal procedure to carry out that may benefit from IORT. These are the ones in which one wonders whether IORT could be helpful. Until someone is willing to do that kind of study, I think it is premature to make any conclusion about the importance of IORT in the management of locally advanced disease in any location.

The final point to make is with only 113 total patients, even assuming that they are comparable, the curves really do not look different enough for me to assume that they are really statistically significant. With larger numbers, perhaps they might be.

E. Glatstein, MD

Impact of Preoperative Staging and Chemoradiation Versus Postoperative Chemoradiation on Outcome in Patients With Rectal Cancer: A Decision Analysis

Telford JJ, Saltzman JR, Kuntz KM, et al (Brigham and Women's Hosp, Boston; Dana-Farber Cancer Inst, Boston; Harvard Univ, Boston; et al)
J Natl Cancer Inst 96:191-201, 2004 12–25

Background.—Radical resection and postoperative chemoradiation have been the standard therapy for patients with rectal cancer, but preoperative staging by local imaging and chemoradiation are widely used. However, several centers have reported excellent results from uncontrolled prospective studies evaluating the preoperative chemoradiation for patients with locally advanced rectal cancer. These 2 approaches to rectal cancer management were compared by decision analysis.

Methods.—A decision model was developed to compare survival outcomes after postoperative chemoradiation versus preoperative staging and chemoradiation in patients aged 70 years with resectable rectal cancer. The cohorts of patients treated with each strategy were entered into a Markov model that incorporated age-adjusted and disease-specific mortality. Outcomes were evaluated by modeling 5-year disease-specific survival for preoperative chemoradiation as less than, equal to, or greater than that of postoperative chemoradiation. Base-case probabilities were derived from published data. The primary outcome measures were life expectancy and quality-adjusted life expectancy.

Results.—Life expectancy and quality-adjusted life expectancy were 9.72 and 8.72 years, respectively, in the postoperative chemoradiation strategy. In the preoperative staging and chemoradiation strategy, life expectancy was 8.71, 9.04, and 9.37 years when 5-year disease-specific survival was less than, equal to, or greater than that of postoperative chemoradiation, respectively. The decision model was sensitive to differences in the long-term toxicity of preoperative and postoperative chemoradiation. When the 5-year disease-specific survival for patients after preoperative or postoperative chemoradiation was equal, the decision model was sensitive to surgical mortality and to the probability of residual lymph node disease after local excision.

Conclusions.—Preoperative staging for selection of patients for treatment with preoperative chemoradiation of locally advanced rectal cancer is beneficial if efficacy and toxicity after preoperative chemoradiation are equal to or better than that after postoperative chemoradiation.

▶ Preoperative chemoradiotherapy has become the standard of care for many patients with rectal cancer, in part because it may allow for less morbid surgical procedures (eg, colostomy) in some patients. However, it may also overtreat patients in whom surgical excision of disease is all that is needed for cure. This integrated approach, which uses a Markov model, supports the positive impact of preoperative therapy. These results have recently been confirmed by prospective randomized trials conducted in Europe.

P. J. Loehrer, Sr, MD

Relationship of Baseline Serum Bilirubin to Efficacy and Toxicity of Single-Agent Irinotecan in Patients With Metastatic Colorectal Cancer

Meyerhardt JA, Kwok A, Ratain MJ, et al (Dana-Farber Cancer Inst, Boston; Pfizer Oncology, New York; Univ of Chicago)

J Clin Oncol 22:1439-1446, 2004 12–26

Background.—Irinotecan is active against a variety of malignancies, such as colorectal, lung, gastric, esophageal, ovarian, and head and neck carcinomas, yet this agent can also cause significant adverse effects. The predictive value of baseline serum bilirubin measures for chemotherapy-related toxicity or efficacy among patients with metastatic colorectal cancer treated by irinotecan was determined.

Methods.—Data were obtained on 287 patients enrolled in a multicenter phase III study with single-agent irinotecan given weekly or once every 3 weeks. For this secondary analysis, patients were classified on the basis of baseline bilirubin values (0-0.4, 0.5-0.9, and 1.0-1.5 mg/dL). The median follow-up was 15.8 months.

Findings.—Baseline serum bilirubin levels did not predict 1-year survival, those rates being 42.4% in the 1 to 0.4 group, 42.3% in the 0.5 to 0.9 group, and 48.1% in the 1 to 1.5 group. Baseline levels also did not predict median overall survival (10.1, 9.7, and 15.6 months, respectively) or median time to progression (2.8, 3, and 4.1 months, respectively). The risk of grade 3 to 4 neutropenia was significantly increased in patients with elevated bilirubin levels. However, this was noted only in the group treated weekly. Other toxicities did not differ significantly among bilirubin level groups.

Conclusions.—Modest increases in bilirubin appear to correlate with a greater risk of grade 3 and 4 neutropenia in patients treated weekly with irinotecan for metastatic colorectal cancer. However, baseline serum bilirubin measures do not reliably predict overall irinotecan-related toxicity or efficacy.

▶ There are far too few articles that address the usage of common chemotherapeutic agents in patients with organ dysfunction. This article is helpful, as many patients with colorectal cancer do have liver metastases with mild liver dysfunction. The scheduling of irinotecan every 3 weeks as opposed to weekly seems to abrogate the potential toxicity in these patients.

P. J. Loehrer, Sr, MD

Efficacy of 5-Fluorouracil-Based Chemotherapy in Elderly Patients With Metastatic Colorectal Cancer: A Pooled Analysis of Clinical Trials

Folprecht G, Cunningham D, Ross P, et al (Univ Hosp, Dresden, Germany; Royal-Marsden Hosp, Sutton, England; Univ of Uppsala, Sweden; et al)

Ann Oncol 15:1330-1338, 2004 12–27

Background.—Recent research has shown that elderly patients are underrepresented in clinical trials and are less often given standard therapies. To date, no large series has reported the influence of age on efficacy of chemotherapy in patients with metastatic colorectal cancer.

Methods.—Data on 3825 patients receiving 5-fluorouracil (5-FU)-containing treatment in 22 European trials were reviewed. Six hundred twenty-nine patients were aged 70 years or older.

Findings.—These elderly patients had an overall survival of 10.8 months, compared with 11.3 months in the younger patients (Fig 1). Response rates in the 2 age groups were 23.9% and 21.1%, respectively, a nonsignificant difference. Elderly patients had a marginally prolonged progression-free survival—5.5 compared with 5.3 months. In both age groups, infusional 5-FU significantly increased response rates, overall survival, and progression-free survival compared with bolus FU.

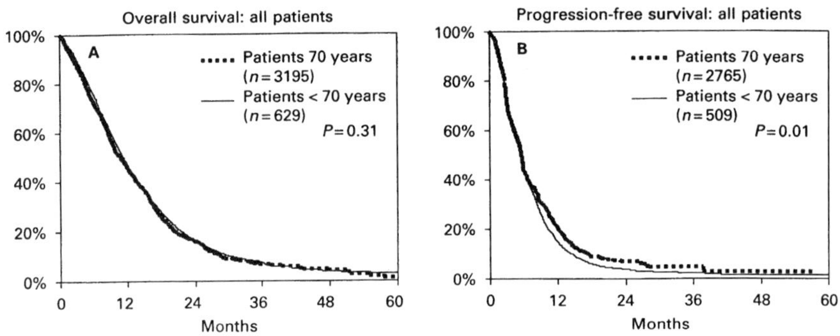

FIGURE 1.—A, Overall survival of younger patients is not different from that of elderly patients (log-rank test: $P = .31$). B, Progression-free survival was significantly prolonged in patients ≥ 70 years of age compared with younger patients (log rank test: $P = .01$). (Courtesy of Folprecht G, Cunningham D, Ross P, et al: Efficacy of 5-fluorouracil-based chemotherapy in elderly patients with metastatic colorectal cancer: A pooled analysis of clinical trials. *Ann Oncol* 15:1330-1338, 2004. Reprinted by permission of Oxford University Press.)

Conclusions.—Fit elderly patients with metastatic colorectal cancer benefit as much as younger patients from palliative chemotherapy with 5-FU. Infusional 5-FU is more effective than bolus 5-FU in patients of any age. Standard palliative chemotherapy should be offered to elderly patients. Furthermore, elderly persons should not be excluded from clinical studies.

▶ This article addresses one issue: Does adjuvant chemotherapy benefit the elderly to the same degree as younger patients? The simple answer is yes. This article also suggests the benefit of infusional 5-FU over the bolus administration of the same drug.

The field of geriatric oncology is still in its "infancy." The efforts of the Hartford Foundation and other organizations are to enhance training, develop new clinicians, and encourage evidence-based medicine for the older population. As this has a huge economic impact, this should be a high priority.

P. J. Loehrer, Sr, MD

FOLFIRI Followed by FOLFOX6 or the Reverse Sequence in Advanced Colorectal Cancer: A Randomized GERCOR Study

Tournigand C, André T, Achille E, et al (GERCOR, France; Hôpital Saint-Antoine, France; Hôpital Tenon, France; et al)

J Clin Oncol 22:229-237, 2004 12–28

Introduction.—Phase III trials have demonstrated the superiority of fluorouracil (FU) with leucovorin (LV) in combination with irinotecan or oxaliplatin versus FU + LV alone in patients with metastatic colorectal cancer. Two sequences were examined in a phase III trial: folinic acid, FU, and irinotecan (FOLFIRI) followed by folinic acid, FU, and oxaliplatin (FOLFOX6) (arm A), and FOLFOX6 followed by FOLFIRI (arm B).

Methods.—Previously treated patients with assessable disease were randomly assigned to receive either a 2-hour infusion of I-LV 200 mg/m^2 followed by a FU bolus 400 mg/m^2 and a 46-hour infusion of 2400 to 3000 mg/m^2 every 46 hours every 2 weeks, either with irinotecan 180 mg/m^2 or with oxaliplatin 100 mg/m^2 as a 2-hour infusion on day 1. At progression, irinotecan was replaced with oxaliplatin in arm A; in arm B, oxaliplatin was replaced by irinotecan.

Results.—The median survival was 21.5 months for 109 patients in arm A and 20.6 months for 111 patients in arm B (P = .99). The median second progression-free survival (PFS) was 14.2 for arm A and 10.9 for arm B (P = .64). For first-line therapy, FOLFIRI achieved a response rate (RR) of 56% and a median PFS of 8.5 months; FOLFOX6 achieved an RR of 54% and a median PFS of 8.0 months (P = .26). Second-line FOLFIRI achieved a 4% RR and 2.5-month median PFS; FOLFOX6 achieved 15% RR and a 4.2-month PFS (Fig 2). For first-line therapy, National Cancer Institute Common Toxicity Criteria grade 3/4 mucositis, nausea/vomiting, and grade 2 alopecia were more common with FOLFIRI treatment; grade 3/4 neutropenia

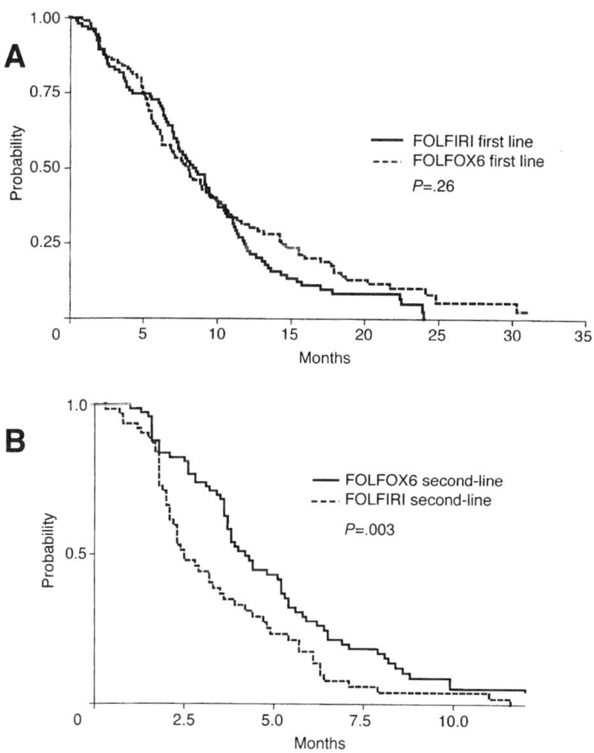

FIGURE 2.—PFS in first-line therapy (**A**) and second-line therapy (**B**). (Courtesy of Tournigand C, André T, Achille E, et al: FOLFIRI followed by FOLFOX6 or the reverse sequence in advanced colorectal cancer: A randomized GERCOR Study. *J Clin Oncol* 22:229-237, 2004. Reprinted with permission from the American Society of Clinical Oncology.)

TABLE 3.—Frequency of Common Toxicities (Percentage)

	First-Line									Second-Line								
	Arm A: FOLFIRI (n = 110)†				Arm B: FOLFOX6 (n = 110)†					Arm A: FOLFOX6 (n = 82)				Arm B: FOLFIRI (n = 68)				
Toxicity	Grade 1	Grade 2	Grade 3	Grade 4	Grade 1	Grade 2	Grade 3	Grade 4	*P* (Grade 3/4)	Grade 1	Grade 2	Grade 3	Grade 4	Grade 1	Grade 2	Grade 3	Grade 4	*P* (Grade 3/4)
Neutropenia	19	33	15	9	18	20	31	13	.003	17	24	15	2	21	18	21	0	NS
Thrombocytopenia	15	1	0	0	57	21	5	0	.01	59	9	0	1	34	4	0	0	NS
Anemia	27	12	2	1	39	12	3	0	NS	35	9	2	1	49	13	3	0	NS
Febrile neutropenia	—	0	4	3	—	1	0	0	.007	0	0	0	0	0	0	1	0	NS
Nausea	29	30	13	0	39	25	3	0	.005	37	21	6	0	26	21	0	0	.03
Vomiting	17	23	8	2	22	17	3	0	.027	17	17	4	1	16	16	3	0	NS
Diarrhea	26	23	9	5	28	13	9	2	NS	22	7	4	1	29	16	7	1	NS
Mucositis	26	15	10	0	35	10	1	0	.003	24	10	4	0	15	7	3	0	NS
Cutaneous	18	5	2	0	17	5	2	0	NS	21	2	1	0	12	1	0	0	NS
Alopecia	36	24	NA	NA	19	9	NA	NA	.003‡	13	9	NA	NA	26	13	NA	NA	NS
Neurological	10	0	0	NA	26	37	34	NA	<.001	45	29	20	0	1	0	1	0	<.001
Fatigue	15	27	4	0	17	15	3	0	.028§	9	22	5	0	12	21	1	0	NS

*Maximum toxicity per patient.
†One patient randomized in arm B received FOLFIRI as first-line treatment.
‡Comparison grade 2.
§Comparison grade 2-3.
(Courtesy of Tournigand C, André T, Achille E, et al: FOLFIRI followed by FOLFOX6 or the reverse sequence in advanced colorectal cancer: A randomized GERCOR Study. *J Clin Oncol* 22:229-237, 2004. Reprinted with permission from the American Society of Clinical Oncology.)

and neurosensory toxicity were more common with FOLFOX6 treatment (Table 3).

Conclusion.—The A and B treatment arms achieved prolonged survival and similar efficacy; they had different toxicity profiles.

▶ As was seen with the Grothey et al article (see Abstract 12–29), the introduction of oxaliplatin and irinotecan into systemic therapy has had a major impact in metastatic colorectal cancer. In this country, FOLFOX was compared with the IFL regimen (as described by Saltz et al[1]) in the intergroup trial N9741. The authors of this trial have purported superiority of FOLFOX to the IFL regimen. However, there were several different variables in that study that included the use of infusional 5-FU therapy in the FOLFOX regimen compared with bolus 5-FU in the IFL regimen. In addition, patients were crossed over to receive irinotecan before obvious progression on oxaliplatin. This artificially improved PFS. Finally, in the trial by Goldberg et al,[2] not all patients received oxaliplatin as salvage therapy in the IFL group.

This article by Tournigand et al underscores the use of 3 drugs as optimal therapy. The choice of oxaliplatin or irinotecan as front-line therapy can be largely felt by the investigator and the patient. The side effects of oxaliplatin, particularly that of cold-induced dysesthesias and neuropathy, often lead to early discontinuation (particularly when administered in cold weather). Irinotecan has a greater propensity for developing diarrhea (though not found in this study). In my mind both are useful treatment options as the basis of front-line therapy for patients with metastatic disease.

P. J. Loehrer, Sr, MD

References

1. Saltz LB, Cox JV, Blanke C, et al: Irinotecan plus fluorouracil and leucovorin for metastatic colorectal cancer. Irinotecan Study Group. *N Engl J Med* 343:905-914, 2000.
2. Goldberg RM, Morton RF, Sargent DJ, et al: N9741: Oxaliplatin or CPT-11 plus 5-fluorouracil/leucovorin or oxaliplatin plus CPT-11 in advanced colorectal cancer. Updated efficacy and quality of life data from an intergroup study. *Proc Am Soc Clin Oncol* 22:252, 2003 (abstr. 1009).

Survival of Patients With Advanced Colorectal Cancer Improves With the Availability of Fluorouracil-Leucovorin, Irinotecan, and Oxaliplatin in the Course of Treatment

Grothey A, Sargent D, Goldberg RM, et al (Mayo Clinic, Rochester, Minn; Univ of North Carolina, Chapel Hill; Univ of Halle, Germany)

J Clin Oncol 22:1209-1214, 2004 12–29

Introduction.—Fluorouracil (FU)-leucovorin (LV), irinotecan, and oxaliplatin administered alone or in combination are effective as treatment of advanced colorectal cancer (CRC). Combination protocols that use FU-LV with either irinotecan or oxaliplatin are considered standard first-line

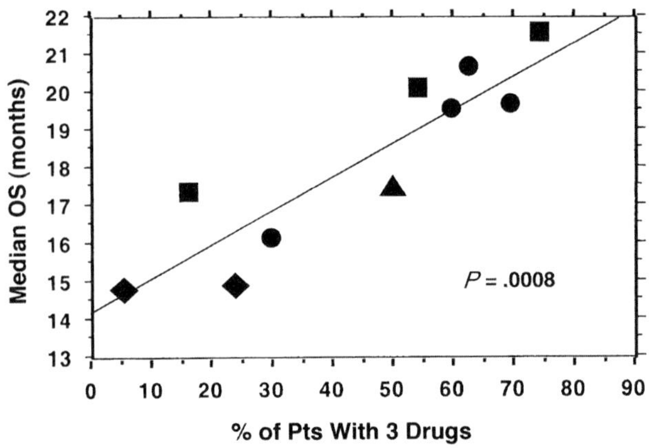

FIGURE 1.—Regression plot and relation between percentage of patients (*pts*) receiving FU-LV, irinotecan, and oxaliplatin (3 drugs) in the course of their disease and reported median OS. Mathematical equitation of regression (based on a weighted model [*solid line*]): median OS (months) = 14.09 + 0.09 × (% patients with drugs). First-line therapies: *circles*, infusional FU-LV + oxaliplatin; *squares*, infusional FU-LV + irinotecan; *diamonds*, bolus FU-LV + irinotecan; *triangle*, irinotecan + oxaliplatin. (Courtesy of Grothey A, Sargent D, Goldberg RM, et al: Survival of patients with advanced colorectal cancer improves with the availability of fluorouracil-leucovorin, irinotecan, and oxaliplatin in the course of treatment. *J Clin Oncol* 22:1209-1214, 2004. Reprinted with permission from the American Society of Clinical Oncology.)

therapies for treatment of CRC. The importance of the availability of all 3 active cytotoxic agents, FU-LV, irinotecan, and oxaliplatin, on overall survival (OS) has not been evaluated and was therefore investigated by reviewing existing data from 7 recently published or presented phase III trials in patients with advanced CRC.

Methods.—Data from the 7 trials were analyzed to correlate the percentage of patients receiving second-line therapy and the percentage of patients receiving all 3 agents. The median OS was reported by using a weighted analysis.

Results.—The reported median OS from the 7 phase III trials was significantly correlated with the percentage of patients receiving all 3 drugs during their disease course (P = .0008) (Fig 1); it was not correlated with the percentage of patients who received a second-line therapy (P = .19). The use of combination protocols as first-line therapy was linked with significant improvement in median survival of 3.5 months (95% confidence interval, 1.27-5.73 months; P = .0083).

Conclusion.—These data support the strategy of making these 3 active drugs available to all patients with advanced CRC who are candidates for such therapy to maximize OS. With the availability of salvage options, OS should no longer be considered the most appropriate end point by which to evaluate the efficacy of a palliative first-line treatment in patients with CRC.

► In a stealthlike manner, the progress of metastatic CRC has steadily improved over the last few decades. Skeptics would say the progress is based on improved technology and stage migration, but a number of prospective randomized trials during this period have clearly demonstrated improvement in progression-free survival and OS with novel regimens. This report by Grothey et al confirms these data and underlines the importance of newer antineoplastic agents such as irinotecan and oxaliplatin. Patients with stage IV colorectal cancer can now expect a 3- to 4-fold increase in survival compared with similar patients diagnosed a few decades ago.

P. J. Loehrer, Sr, MD

Longterm Results After Resection of Simultaneous and Sequential Lung and Liver Metastases From Colorectal Carcinoma

Mineo TC, Ambrogi V, Tonini G, et al (Tor Vergata Univ, Rome; La Sapienza Univ, Rome)

J Am Coll Surg 197:386-391, 2003 12–30

Background.—Simple lung or liver metastasectomy because of colorectal cancer has become an accepted therapy worldwide with a curative intent in a select group of patients. However, significant controversy has persisted regarding the value of simultaneous bi-organ metastasectomy and the selection of patients for this aggressive multiorgan surgery. An experience with a series of patients who underwent both pulmonary and hepatic metastasectomy because of colorectal cancer was reviewed.

Methods.—From a total of 155 patients who underwent surgery for lung or liver colorectal metastases from March 1987 to December 1998, 29 patients were seen with simultaneous (12 patients) or sequential (10 patients) liver-to-lung or lung-to-liver metastases (7 patients) and were selected for retrospective evaluation. All metastases were successfully resected in a total of 56 separate procedures. In 35 thoracic procedures, 45 metastases were removed by wedge resection (36 patients) or lobectomy (9 patients). In addition, 47 liver metastases were resected with the wedge procedure (24), a segmentectomy (13), or a lobectomy (10). No perioperative deaths occurred, and the morbidity rate was just 10.7%. All patients were followed up for a minimum of 3 years. Univariate and multivariate analyses were used to determine factors possibly influencing survival.

Results.—The median survival from the second metastasectomy was 41 months, and the 5-year survival rate was 51.3%. The risk factor distribution among the 3 metastatic pattern groups was insignificant. On univariate analysis, survival was significantly associated with premetastasectomy elevated levels of both carcinoembryonic antigen (CEA) and CA 19-9 and with the mediastinal or celiac lymph node status. However, the number of metastasectomies, the disease-free interval, and simultaneous versus sequential diagnosis were not significantly associated with survival (Fig 2. The multivariate analysis showed that only elevated CEA plus CA 19-9 levels were significantly associated with survival.

Conclusions.—Either simultaneous or sequential lung and liver metastases can be successfully treated with surgery. The presence of high levels of CEA plus CA 19-9 was associated with poor results of surgery.

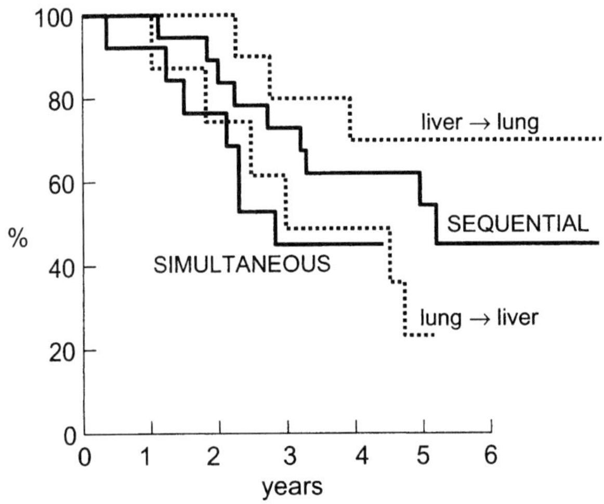

Pts at risk

simult	12	11	9	6			
seq	17		15	14	12	7	5
liver→lung	10		9		8		
lung→liver	7		6	5	4	3	2

FIGURE 2.—Kaplan-Meier survival curves. Pairwise differences between postmetastasectomy survival curves were not significant for patients who had simultaneous lung-liver vs sequential (P = .1), vs liver (P = .1), or vs lung (P = .4) as first metastatic site. *Abbreviations: Pts*, Patients; *seq*, sequential; *simult*, simultaneous. (Reprinted from Mineo TC, Ambrogi V, Tonini G, et al: Longterm results after resection of simultaneous and sequential lung and liver metastases from colorectal carcinoma. *J Am Coll Surg* 197:386-391, 2003. Copyright 2003 with permission from American College of Surgeons.)

▶ It is well recognized that surgical resection of isolated metastases in colorectal cancer can be associated with long-term survival. Data regarding resection in 2 organ sites (liver and lung) are sparse. This is a large series of patients who underwent simultaneous or metachronous resection of liver and lung metastases. These authors support that selective use of surgery for stage IV disease can be beneficial. Surgical treatment of metastatic disease need to be part of the decision-making process of patients with metastatic colorectal cancer.

P. J. Loehrer, Sr, MD

The Price Tag on Progress—Chemotherapy for Colorectal Cancer
Schrag D (Mem Sloan-Kettering Cancer Ctr, New York)
N Engl J Med 351:317-319, 2004 12–31

Background.—In the past decade, the Food and Drug Administration (FDA) has approved 5 new drugs for the treatment of metastatic colorectal cancer. The optimism encouraged by recent trial results of these newly developed therapies is tempered by the "sticker shock" that patients experience when they encounter the prices of these chemotherapy drugs. Explored were issues surrounding whether the potential clinical benefits of these new drugs are worth the financial strain they impose on patients, even when copayments are possible.

Overview.—The tremendous financial challenges facing patients beginning chemotherapy for colorectal cancer are illustrated by the example of a patient who is 170 cm tall, weighs 70 kg, and receives chemotherapy for 8 weeks. The standard regimen of fluorouracil and leucovorin (the Mayo Clinic regimen) would cost $63. In comparison, the FOLFOX regimen (fluorouracil, leucovorin, and oxaliplatin) would cost $11,889. The combination of FOLFOX and bevacizumab would cost $21,033. The near doubling of the median survival in the past decade has been accompanied by a 340-fold increase in the costs of drugs just for the first 8 weeks of treatment. In 2004, 32,000 persons in the United States will receive a diagnosis of stage IV colorectal cancer, and an additional 24,000 persons will have recurrent metastatic disease. The drug costs for an 8-week course of initial treatment for these patients will be $666 million, or they will be $1.2 billion with the addition of monoclonal-antibody therapy (Table). These costs do not include the costs of preparation, administration, and supervision or supportive medications. In the end these treatments can extend the median survival to 21 months, but they will not provide a cure.

Conclusions.—Discussions about financing cancer treatment will become more common in physicians' examination rooms in the near future, and modest gains in survival will be offset by anxiety about the financing of treatment, even for privileged, middle-class patients who have insurance coverage and copayments. It is important that as a society we explore the ethical

TABLE.—Estimated Drug Costs for Eight Weeks of Treatment for Metastatic Colorectal Cancer

Regimen	Drugs and Schedule of Administration	Drug Costs* $
Regimens containing fluorouracil		
Mayo Clinic	Monthly bolus of fluorouracil plus leucovorin	63
Roswell Park	Weekly bolus of fluorouracil plus leucovorin	304
LV5FU2	Biweekly fluorouracil plus leucovorin in a 48-hr infusion	263
Regimens containing irinotecan or oxaliplatin		
Irinotecan alone	Weekly bolus	9,497
IFL	Weekly bolus of fluorouracil plus irinotecan	9,539
FOLFIRI	LV5FU2 with biweekly irinotecan	9,381
FOLFOX	LV5FU2 with biweekly oxaliplatin	11,889
Regimens containing bevacizumab or cetuximab		
FOLFIRI with bevacizumab	FOLFIRI with fortnightly bevacizumab	21,399
FOLFOX with bevacizumab	FOLFOX with biweekly bevacizumab	21,033
Irinotecan with cetuximab	Weekly irinotecan plus cetuximab	30,790
FOLFIRI with cetuximab	FOLFIRI and weekly cetuximab	30,675

*Costs represent 95% of the average wholesale price in May 2004.

(Reprinted by permission of *The New England Journal of Medicine* from Schrag D: The price tag on progress—chemotherapy for colorectal cancer. *N Engl J Med* 351:317-319, 2004.)

questions involved in controlling access to expensive treatments that extend life by only a few weeks as well as the morality of refusing to make deliberated choices in this regard.

▶ Sometimes it is worth including papers in the YEAR BOOK that may not quite fit the typical genre. This article is one such piece of literature that I feel is a must read. The impact of our drugs on the cost of health care is clearly a pressing issue. Dr Schrag does point out the potential societal impact of high-cost therapy in an incurable setting. The benefit of therapy can be based on financial cost, which can be estimated on cost per added life-years, cost per response, or total cost of treatment for society. This article makes no decision about the proper treatments for metastatic or recurrent colon cancer—that is the physician's job. Helping define the schedule and duration of treatments as well as clarifying the population who will not benefit from treatment is also our job.

P. J. Loehrer, Sr, MD

Randomized Trial of Cytoreduction and Hyperthermic Intraperitoneal Chemotherapy Versus Systemic Chemotherapy and Palliative Surgery in Patients With Peritoneal Carcinomatosis of Colorectal Cancer

Verwaal VJ, van Ruth S, de Bree E, et al (Netherlands Cancer Inst, Amsterdam)

J Clin Oncol 21:3737-3743, 2003 12–32

Background.—Peritoneal carcinomatosis (PC) of colorectal origin is the second most frequent cause of death in patients with colorectal cancer after metastatic disease to the liver. In about 25% of patients, no other tumor locations can be found, even after a detailed diagnostic work up. It has been

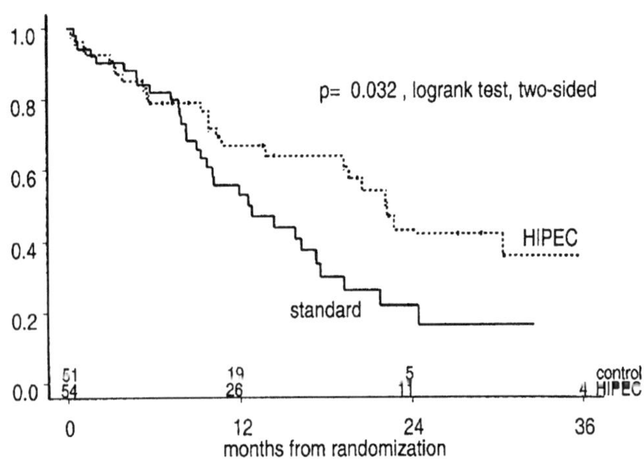

FIGURE 2.—Kaplan-Meier survival curve, comparing standard treatment to hyperthermic intraperitoneal chemotherapy (*HIPEC*). (Courtesy of Verwaal VJ, van Ruth S, de Bree E, et al: Randomized trial of cytoreduction and hyperthermic intraperitoneal chemotherapy versus systemic chemotherapy and palliative surgery in patients with peritoneal carcinomatosis of colorectal cancer. *J Clin Oncol* 21[20]:3737-3743, 2003. Reprinted with permission from the American Society for Clinical Oncology.)

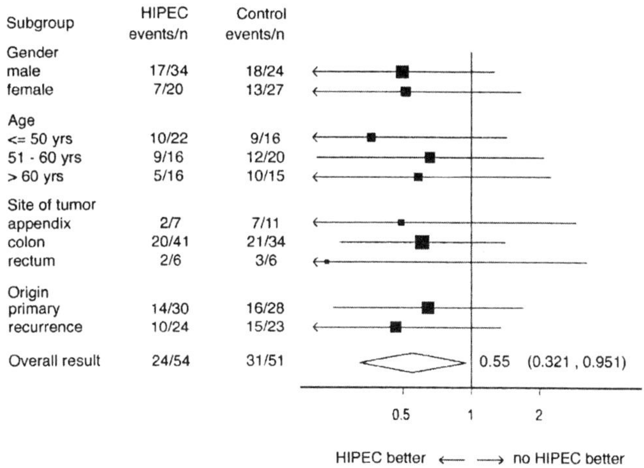

FIGURE 3.—Explorative subgroup analysis on survival of all 105 patients randomized. This Forest plot shows the hazard ratio (odds of death) for various subgroups of patients. The *size of the squares* represents the number of patients, the *horizontal lines through the squares* indicate the 99% confidence intervals (CIs). The *diamond* indicating the overall result corresponds with the 95% CI. *Abbreviation: HIPEC,* Hyperthermic intraperitoneal chemotherapy. (Courtesy of Verwaal VJ, van Ruth S, de Bree E, et al: Randomized trial of cytoreduction and hyperthermic intraperitoneal chemotherapy versus systemic chemotherapy and palliative surgery in patients with peritoneal carcinomatosis of colorectal cancer. *J Clin Oncol* 21[20]:3737-3743, 2003. Reprinted with permission from the American Society for Clinical Oncology.)

suggested that PC of colorectal origin should probably not be equated with generalized disease, but it can be a first step in dissemination, much like the situation with liver metastases of colorectal origin. This concept has been the basis of attempts to achieve long-term survival in patients with PC by combining surgery and intraperitoneal chemotherapy to eradicate microscopic residual disease. Previous uncontrolled trials have shown that aggressive cytoreduction in combination with hyperthermic intraperitoneal chemotherapy (HIPEC) is superior to standard treatment in patients with PC of colorectal cancer origin.

Methods.—One hundred five patients were randomly assigned to receive either standard treatment consisting of systemic chemotherapy with or without palliative surgery, or experimental therapy consisting of aggressive cytoreduction with HIPEC, followed by the same systemic chemotherapy regimen. Survival was the primary end point.

Results.—At a median follow-up of 21.6 months, the median survival was 12.6 months in the patients treated with standard therapy and 22.3 months in the patients treated with the experimental therapy (Fig 2). Exploratory subgroup analysis did not show any particular subgroup in which the effect of cytoreduction followed by HIPEC was better or worse compared with standard therapy (Fig 3). The treatment-related mortality in the aggressive therapy group was 8%. Most of the complications from HIPEC were related to bowel leakage (Table 2). A subgroup analysis of the HIPEC group demonstrated that patients with 0 to 5 of the 7 regions of the abdominal cavity involved by tumor at the time of the cytoreduction had a significantly better survival than patients with 6 or 7 affected regions (Fig 5). If the cytoreduc-

TABLE 2.—Major Toxicity and Complications of 48 Patients With Peritoneal Carcinomatosis Treated by Cytoreduction Followed by HIPEC

	Grade 3		Grade 4	
	No. of Patients	%	No. of Patients	%
Fever	3	6	—	—
Leukopenia	7	15	1	2
Thrombocytopenia	2	4	—	—
Neuropathy (paresis)	2	4	—	—
Pleural effusion	1	2	—	—
Pulmonary embolus (within 3 months after surgery)	—	—	2	4
Pneumonia	1	2	—	—
Renal obstruction	2	4	—	—
Anuria (acute tubular necrosis)	—	—	3	6
Cardiac arrhythmia	—	—	1	2
Heart failure	4	8	2	4
GI fistula	—	—	7	15
Pancreatitis	1	2	—	—
Catheter infections	3	6	—	—
Haemorrhage	3	6	4	8
Psychological disorders	3	6	2	4

Abbreviations: HIPEC, Hyperthermic intraperitoneal chemotherapy; *GI*, gastrointestinal.

(Courtesy of Verwaal VJ, van Ruth S, de Bree E, et al: Randomized trial of cytoreduction and hyperthermic intraperitoneal chemotherapy versus systemic chemotherapy and palliative surgery in patients with peritoneal carcinomatosis of colorectal cancer. *J Clin Oncol* 21[20]:3737-3743, 2003. Reprinted with permission from the American Society for Clinical Oncology.)

tion was macroscopically complete (R-1), the median survival was also significantly better than in patients with limited (R-2a) or extensive residual disease (R-2b).

Conclusions.—In patients with PC of colorectal origin, cytoreduction followed by HIPEC improves survival. However, the prognosis remains grave for patients with involvement of 6 or more regions of the abdominal cavity, or grossly incomplete cytoreduction.

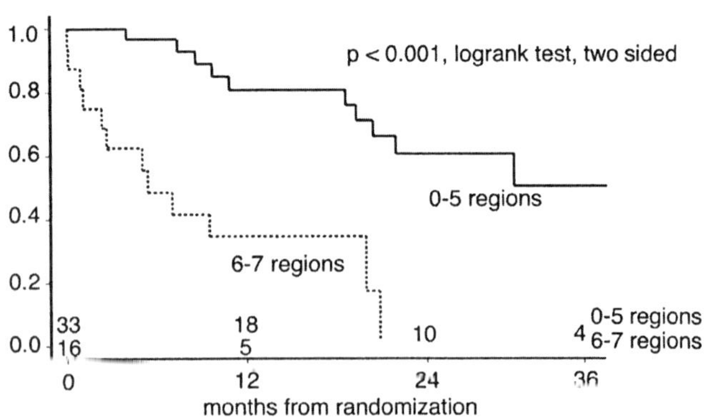

FIGURE 5.—Kaplan-Meier survival curve of 49 patients with peritoneal carcinomatosis treated by cytoreduction followed by HIPEC, comparing the number of regions with residual tumor. (Courtesy of Verwaal VJ, van Ruth S, de Bree E, et al: Randomized trial of cytoreduction and hyperthermic intraperitoneal chemotherapy versus systemic chemotherapy and palliative surgery in patients with peritoneal carcinomatosis of colorectal cancer. *J Clin Oncol* 21[20]:3737-3743, 2003. Reprinted with permission from the American Society for Clinical Oncology.)

▶ This is an interesting article from The Netherlands, which looks at carcinomatosis of the peritoneum secondary to colorectal cancer. One hundred five patients were randomly assigned to receive either standard treatment consisting of systemic chemotherapy with 5-fluorouracil and leucovorin, with or without additional palliative surgery, versus experimental therapy consisting of aggressive cytoreductive surgery followed by hyperthermia and intraperitoneal chemotherapy with mitomycin C. The hyperthermia was said to consist of an influx into the peritoneal cavity at 41°C to 42°C. Once the temperature achieved 40°C, the mitomycin C was added. The experimental treatment appeared to have some advantage, although the key thing in a study like this is to see which patients do not relapse. Unfortunately, the only data given are for survival, which is obviously important, but which can be affected by a host of different issues, including subsequent treatments. It would have been very helpful had the authors given a time to progression curve, but unfortunately that is absent. It is not a surprise that the more sites of involvement of the peritoneum, the worse the prognosis, although the definition of a "region" is unclear. In any event, it is food for thought.

The toxicity of this experimental approach is not trivial, and it is worthwhile pointing out that not only did patients develop fevers, leukopenia, and thrombocytopenia, but also a significant number developed renal obstruction, heart failure, fistulas, hemorrhage, and infection. It really does not appear to be something for the faint of heart.

E. Glatstein, MD

Phase II Trial of Cetuximab in Patients With Refractory Colorectal Cancer That Expresses the Epidermal Growth Factor Receptor

Saltz LB, Meropol NJ, Loehrer PJ Sr, et al (Mem Sloan-Kettering Cancer Ctr, New York; Fox Chase Cancer Ctr, Philadelphia; Indiana Univ, Indianapolis; et al)

J Clin Oncol 22:1201-1208, 2004 12–33

Background.—Early stage colorectal cancer is often curable with surgery, but unresectable metastatic disease is uniformly fatal. Palliative treatment is centered on the use of chemotherapy with various antineoplastic agents, but there are no established treatment options with demonstrated efficacy once a patient's cancer becomes refractory to these agents. The antitumor activity and toxicity of single-agent cetuximab were evaluated in patients with chemotherapy-refractory colorectal cancer whose tumors express the epidermal growth factor receptor (EGFr).

Methods.—This phase II, nonrandomized, open-label, multicenter trial enrolled 57 patients with EGFr expression demonstrated on formalin-fixed paraffin embedded tumor tissue by immunohistochemical staining. The patients were required to have received irinotecan, either alone or in a combination regimen, and to have demonstrated clinical failure on this regimen. Cetuximab was administered weekly by IV infusion. The first dose of 400 mg/m^2 was administered over a 2-hour period. Weekly doses were then given at a dose of 250 mg/m^2 over a 1-hour period.

Results.—The most commonly encountered grade 3 to 4 adverse events were an acnelike skin rash, predominantly of the face and upper torso (86% with any grade, 9% with grade 3), and a composite of asthenia, fatigue, malaise, or lethargy (56% with any grade, 9% with grade 3). Grade 3 allergic reactions developed in 2 patients (3.5%), who had to leave the study. A third patient had a grade 3 allergic reaction that resolved, and the patient continued in the study. Diarrhea and neutropenia were not dose limiting in any patient. A partial response was obtained in 5 patients, and 21 patients had stable disease or minor responses. The median survival in the previously treated patients with chemotherapy-refractory colorectal cancer was 6.4 months.

Conclusions.—Once-weekly use of cetuximab showed modest activity and was well tolerated as a single agent in patients with chemotherapy-refractory colorectal cancer whose tumors express the EGFr. The use of cetuximab in conjunction with first-line and adjuvant treatments in persons with refractory colorectal cancer will be evaluated in future studies.

▶ This is a simple, straightforward phase II trial that demonstrates that cetuximab does indeed have single-agent activity in recurrent colorectal cancer. This, together with the European trial (see Abstract 12–18), was the basis for approval of this drug in this country. It is unclear whether patients who are EGFr negative will respond to this drug, as they were not included in this trial. An ongoing study is currently evaluating this population, but it would appear that response did not correlate with intensity of staining.

Ultimately, the role of cetuximab as part of *first-line* therapy needs to be discerned.

P. J. Loehrer, Sr, MD

Cetuximab Monotherapy and Cetuximab Plus Irinotecan in Irinotecan-Refractory Metastatic Colorectal Cancer

Cunningham D, Humblet Y, Siena S, et al (Royal Marsden Hosp, London; Université Catholique de Louvain, Brussels; Ospedale Niguarda Ca' Granda, Milan, Italy; et al)

N Engl J Med 351:337-345, 2004 12–34

Introduction.—The epidermal growth factor receptor (EGFR), which participates in signaling pathways that are deregulated in cancer cells, is relevant in colorectal cancer (CRC) because expression or upregulation of the EGFR gene occurs in 60% to 80% of cases. Cetuximab is a chimeric immunoglobulin G1 monoclonal antibody that specifically blocks EGFR. The efficacy of cetuximab in combination with irinotecan was compared with cetuximab alone in patients with metastatic CRC refractory to treatment with irinotecan.

Methods.—A total of 329 patients whose disease had progressed during or within 3 months after treatment with an irinotecan-based regimen were randomly assigned to treatment with either cetuximab and irinotecan (at the same dose and schedule as in a prestudy regimen; 218 patients) or cetuximab monotherapy (111 patients). In the presence of disease progression, the addition of irinotecan to cetuximab was allowed. Tumor response was assessed radiologically. Patients were evaluated for time to tumor progression, survival, and treatment side effects.

Results.—The response rate was significantly higher in the combination therapy versus the monotherapy group (22.9% [95% confidence interval {CI}, 17.5-29.1%] vs 10.8% [95% CI, 5.7-18.1%]; $P = .007$). The median time to disease progression was significantly greater in the combination therapy versus control groups (4.1 vs 1.5 months; $P < .001$). The median survival was 8.6 versus 6.9 months, respectively, in the combination therapy and controls groups ($P = .48$). Toxic effects were more common in the combination therapy group; severity and incidence were similar to those expected for irinotecan alone.

Conclusion.—Cetuximab has clinically significant activity administered along or in combination with irinotecan in patients with irinotecan-refractory CRC.

▶ This study gives credence to the similarly designed trials by Saltz and his colleagues (Abstract 12–33).[1,2] These trials together demonstrate single-agent activity for cetuximab that ultimately led to the approval in this country by the Federal Drug Administration. The data also suggest an additive effect of cetuximab plus irinotecan in patients previously treated with irinotecan. Unlike HER2 blockade with trastuzumab in metastatic breast cancer, there is no apparent relation with EGFR staining in tissue and response to cetuximab. Patients who were EGFR negative on staining (representing approximately 30% of all patients) were not treated in this trial and are currently being studied as part of another ongoing trial. The proper integration of cetuximab as part of primary therapy remains to be discerned.

P. J. Loehrer, Sr, MD

References

1. Saltz L, Rubin MS, Hochster HS, et al: Cetuximab (IMC-C225) plus irinotecan (CPT-11) is active in CPT-11 refractory colorectal cancer that expresses epidermal growth factor receptor [abstract]. *Prog Proc Am Soc Clin Oncol* 20:3a, 2001.
2. Saltz LB, Meropol NJ, Loehrer PJ Sr, et al: Phase II trial of cetuximab in patients with refractory colorectal cancer that expresses the epidermal growth factor receptor. *J Clin Oncol* 22:1201-1208, 2004.

13 Endocrine Cancer

Early Malignant Progression of Hereditary Medullary Thyroid Cancer

Machens A, for the European Multiple Endocrine Neoplasia (EUROMEN) Study Group (Martin-Luther-Universität Halle-Wittenberg, Halle, Germany; et al)

N Engl J Med 349:1517-1525, 2003 13–1

Introduction.—An age-related progression from C-cell hyperplasia to medullary thyroid cancer is linked with assorted germ-line mutations in the rearranged during transfection (RET) proto-oncogene that could be used to identify the optimal time for prophylactic surgery. The pace of early malignant progression to hereditary thyroid carcinoma was examined among asymptomatic carriers of RET gene mutations in the multicenter European Multiple Endocrine Neoplasia investigation.

Methods.—A standardized questionnaire was completed by eligible patients who had evidence of an RET point mutation in the germ line, were 20 years of age or younger, were clinically asymptomatic, and had undergone total thyroidectomy after genetic verification of the RET point mutation. Patients with medullary thyroid carcinomas of over 10 mm in the greatest diameter and distant metastasis were excluded.

Results.—A total of 207 patients from 145 families were identified. A significant age-associated progression was noted from C-cell hyperplasia to medullary thyroid carcinoma and, ultimately, nodal metastasis in patients whose RET mutations were grouped according to the extracellular- and intracellular-domain codons affected and in those with the codon 634 genotype (Table 2). No lymph node metastases were observed in patients younger than 14 years of age. The age-associated penetrance was not affected by the type of amino acid substitution encoded by the various codon 634 mutations. The codon-specific differences in the age at diagnosis of cancer and the familial incidence of concomitant adrenal and parathyroid involvement indicate that the risk of progression was based on the transforming potential of the individual RET mutation.

Conclusion.—These data contribute initial guidelines for the timing of prophylactic thyroidectomy in asymptomatic carriers of RET gene mutations.

TABLE 2.—Progression to Medullary Thyroid Carcinoma in the First 2 Decades of Life, According to the Position of the Rearranged During Transfection Codon Domain

Thyroid Pathological Findings	No. of Patients*	Mean Age (95% CI)	Sequence of Progression	Mean Change in Age (95% CI)	P Value	
					Pairwise†	Overall‡
		yr		yr		
Extracellular-domain condons§	172					<0.001
Normal	7	10.0 (6.7 to 13.3)	Progression to C-cell hyperplasia	−1.7 (−5.2 to 1.8)	0.77	
C-cell hyperplasia	47	8.3 (7.0 to 9.6)	Progression to medullary thyroid carcinoma N0	1.9 (0.4 to 3.4)	0.07	
Medullary thyroid carcinoma						
N0	111	10.2 (9.3 to 11.0)	Progression to N1	6.9 (3.6 to 10.3)	<0.001	
N1	7	17.1 (13.9 to 20.4)	—			
Intracellular-domain condons‖	31					0.005
Normal	4	9.0 (4.8 to 13.2)	Progression to C-cell hyperplasia	2.2 (−2.4 to 6.8)	0.59	
C-cell hyperplasia	19	11.2 (9.3 to 13.1)	Progression to medullary thyroid carcinoma N0	5.4 (1.9 to 8.9)	0.01	
Medullary thyroid carcinoma						
N0	8	16.6 (13.7 to 19.6)	Progression to N1	—	—	
N1	0	—	—			

*Four carriers of the M918T genotype who had node-negative medullary thyroid carcinoma were excluded.

†Values were adjusted for all pairwise comparisons within 1 factor according to the Tukey-Kramer test (Kramer CY: Extension of multiple range tests to group means with unequal numbers of replications. *Biometrics* 12:307-310, 1956) (adjacent pathologic groups).

‡Overall the *P* values were calculated with the use of 1-way analysis of variance.

§Extracellular-domain codons are 609, 611, 620, 630, and 634.

‖Intracellular-domain codons are 768, 790, 791, 804, and 891.

Abbreviations: CI, Confidence interval; *NO*, no nodal involvement; *NI*, nodal involvement.

(Reprinted by permission of *The New England Journal of Medicine* from Machens A, for the European Multiple Endocrine Neoplasia (EUROMEN) Study Group: Early malignant progression to hereditary medullary thyroid cancer. *N Engl J Med* 349:1517-1525, 2003.)

▶ The multiple endocrine neoplasia syndrome and medullary carcinoma of the thyroid are rare entities cared for in specialty centers. However, this article provides an interesting example of the power of molecular genetics to allow preventive therapies to be tailored to an individual's level of risk. The development of predictive testing for RET germ-line mutations to allow precise identification of individuals at risk for medullary carcinoma and multiple endocrine neoplasia–2 syndrome was a major clinical advance.

This study provides evidence that the specific RET mutation that is present is associated with the speed of progression to carcinoma. Clinically, this translates into a recommendation for prophylactic thyroidectomy before age 5 for children with mutations in high-risk codons. For those with other mutations, current consensus guidelines recommend prophylactic surgery between the ages of 5 and 10 years.[1] Information such as this would be extremely valuable in planning the timing of preventive interventions for a wide range of genetically mediated malignancies.

M. Morrow, MD

Reference

1. Brandi ML, Gagel RF, Angeli A, et al: Guidelines for diagnosis and therapy of MEN type 1 and type 2. *J Clin Endocrinol Metab* 86:5658-5671, 2001.

14 Pediatric Cancer

Leukemia

Genotoxicity of Therapeutic Intervention in Children With Acute Lymphocytic Leukemia

Rice SC, Vacek P, Homans AH, et al (Univ of Vermont, Burlington)

Cancer Res 64:4464-4471, 2004 14–1

Background.—The number of childhood cancer survivors is growing. The genotoxic effects of chemotherapy in this population are unclear. The genotoxic effects of antineoplastic therapy in children were investigated.

Methods.—One hundred thirty peripheral blood samples were obtained from 45 children with acute lymphocytic leukemia at diagnosis and during and after treatment. The changes in the frequency of somatic mutations at the *HPRT*-reporter gene were analyzed.

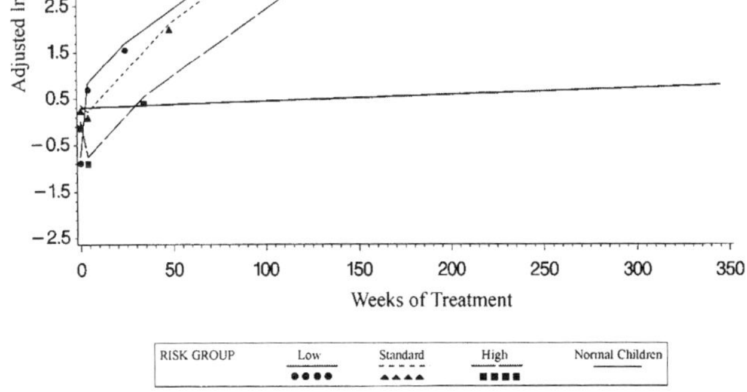

FIGURE 3.—Estimated longitudinal effects of antineoplastic therapy on somatic mutant frequency (*Mf*) in children treated for acute lymphocytic leukemia. (Courtesy of Rice SC, Vacek P, Homans AH, et al: Genotoxicity of therapeutic intervention in children with acute lymphocytic leukemia. *Cancer Res* 64:4464-4471, 2004.)

Findings.—A significant increase in mean *HPRT* somatic mutations occurred in each phase of treatment, independent of the risk group treatment protocol used. The 200-fold increase in mean somatic mutations was still increased years after treatment completion (Fig 3). No significant difference was observed in the genotoxicity of each risk group treatment modality, despite differences in the compositional and clinical toxicity related to the protocols.

Conclusions.—Combination chemotherapy used in the treatment of acute lymphocytic leukemia in children is quite genotoxic. Such therapy may result in an increased somatic mutational load that may increase the risk for the development of multifactorial diseases, especially second malignancies.

▶ The mutagenic effects of radiation therapy and exposure to chemotherapy have been well documented for many years. There is considerably less information, however, on the cumulative frequencies of mutations during the course of therapy, particularly therapies considered to be relatively safe and well tolerated. This is certainly the case for the treatment of children with acute lymphocytic leukemia (ALL). The study by Rice et al generates some question as to the ultimate safety of such treatment approaches. Their study measured the frequency of somatic mutations of *HPRT* reporter gene in the T lymphocytes of children with low-, standard-, and high-risk ALL on Pediatric Oncology Group protocols. Surprisingly, the observations show an approximately 200-fold increase in the mean mutation frequency compared with control subjects over the course of therapy. Further, the increase in mutation frequency continued to occur during all phases of therapy and did not decrease to control group baseline levels after cessation of treatment. The results also show no significant difference in mutational frequency among the different risk groups, although the numbers within each group were probably not large enough to detect small differences. These results demonstrate the genotoxic consequences of ALL therapy, at least for this genetic locus, and raise significant questions in terms of whether children with ALL have predisposition for increased genotoxic affects of even low-dose chemotherapy and how subgroups with specific genotypes with known increased drug sensitivity are affected. Finally, although the functional consequences of these results are unclear, we should take to heart that even these seemingly well-tolerated and safe therapies may have significant long-term genotoxic sequelae. This should continue to motivate us to develop less genotoxic, curative therapies, even in a disease where victory has mostly been already declared.

R. J. Arceci, MD, PhD

Establishment of a Pediatric Oncology Program and Outcomes of Childhood Acute Lymphoblastic Leukemia in a Resource-Poor Area

Howard SC, Pedrosa M, Lins M, et al (St Jude Children's Research Hosp, Memphis, Tenn; Instituto Materno Infantil de Pernambuco, Recife, Brazil; Univ of Tennessee, Memphis)

JAMA 291:2471-2475, 2004 14–2

Introduction.—The cure rate for childhood acute lymphoblastic leukemia (ALL) varies substantially between developed and developing countries. The effect of a multidisciplinary team approach and protocol-based therapy on the event-free survival (EFS) of children with ALL in an area with limited resources was evaluated in a retrospective cohort investigation.

Methods.—The medical records were reviewed for outcomes in 375 children with ALL diagnosed between 1980 and 2002 in a pediatric hospital in the resource-poor city of Recife, Brazil. Eighty-three patients had ALL diagnosed in the early period between 1980 and 1989 in the absence of a dedicated pediatric unit, protocol-based therapy, specially educated nurses, 24-hour on-site physician coverage, and ready access to an ICU. Seventy-eight patients were treated (all according to protocol) during the middle period of July 1994 to March 1997. During the recent period between April 1997 to December 2002, 214 children were treated according to protocol in a dedicated pediatric oncology unit staffed 24 hours by both pediatric oncology nurses and oncologists. Improvements were achieved gradually during the middle period and were completed during the recent period.

Results.—The 5-year EFS improved steadily over time: 32% (95% CI, 21%-43%) in the early period, 47% (95% CI, 36%-58%) in the middle period, and 63% (95% CI, 55%-71%) in the recent period. The probability of cause-specific treatment failure in the early, middle, and late periods, respectively, within 1 year of diagnosis was 14%, 3.8%, and 3.3%, respectively, for relapse; 6.0%, 12%, and 9.8%, respectively, for death from infection; 2.4%, 13%, and 4.2%, respectively, for death from noninfectious toxicity; and 16%, 1.3%. 0.5%, respectively, for abandonment of therapy.

Conclusion.—The treatment of children with ALL in a dedicated pediatric oncology unity that used a comprehensive multidisciplinary team approach, protocol-based therapy, and local support and funding is linked with improved outcome in a resource-poor area.

▶ More than 80% of children in the world with cancer live in developing countries and have an overall cure rate for ALL of less than 40%. This is in comparison with the approximately 20% of children with ALL in developed countries who have an 80% cure rate. Several important questions arise out of these disparate numbers, including the precise causes for the differences as well as how the gaps in cure rates might be closed. This article describes a systematic analysis of some of the reasons for the poor cure rates in developing countries but also maps out the results of several, sequential interventional strategies. Nearly 400 children with ALL were tracked from 1980 to 2002. Survival was determined during periods of early intervention (1980-1989), middle period

(1994-1997), and a more recent period (1997-2002). During each period, significant interventions were made, with particular emphasis on early and correct diagnosis, early initiation of therapy, improved supportive care measures particularly with improved transfusion delivery, maintenance treatment drug compliance, a standardized protocol, improved nutrition, lodging, and transportation. These interventions resulted in an improvement from 325 EFS of 32% in the early period to 63% in the most recent period. Although one can question the need of some of the interventions, such as a dedicated pharmacy for pediatric oncology—something some centers in countries like the United States do not have—most of the changes were both practical and achievable. These types of model interventions should provide hope that more children with cancer throughout the world can benefit from improved care with the use of a standard armamentarium of drugs. A more difficult challenge will be how to achieve similar improvements in more difficult cancers that require integration of multidisciplinary medical specialties such as surgery, radiation therapy, and oncology.

R. J. Arceci, MD, PhD

Reassessment of the Prognostic Significance of Hypodiploidy in Pediatric Patients With Acute Lymphoblastic Leukemia

Raimondi SC, Zhou Y, Mathew S, et al (St Jude Children's Research Hosp, Memphis, Tenn; Univ of Tennessee, Memphis)

Cancer 98:2715-2722, 2003 14–3

Background.—Hypodiploidy, occurring in 6% to 7% of children with acute lymphoblastic leukemia (ALL), is defined as the presence of 45 chromosomes or less in leukemic cells. The cytogenetic characteristics of hypodiploid leukemic cells in children with this rare form of ALL were investigated. Whether subdividing the hypodiploid category serves a prognostic purpose was also explored.

Methods and Findings.—The cytogenetic records of 979 children with ALL treated at 1 center between 1984 and 1999 were reviewed. The leukemic cells of 67 patients (6.8%) contained a modal number (MN) of 45 chromosomes or less. The MN was 45 in 57 children and less than 45 in 10 children. Cells with an MN of 45 had a whole chromosome missing in 19 children, which was a sex chromosome in 12. In 33 patients, leukemic cells with an MN of 45 contained dicentric chromosomes formed from chromosome 9p in 55%, 12p in 18%, and both in 21%. Thirty-nine percent of 28 evaluable B-lineage cases with an MN of 45 had the *ETV6-CBFA2* fusion. The event-free survival rate at 5 years was 20% in patients with hypodiploid leukemic cells with an MN of less than 45 compared with 74.9% in those with an MN of 45 or greater (Fig 2). This difference was significant.

Conclusions.—Low hypodiploidy, defined as leukemic cells with an MN of less than 45, should be considered a high-risk feature in children with ALL. Subdividing hypodiploid groups into those with an MN of less than 45 and those with an MN of 45 may be sufficient for prognostic evaluation.

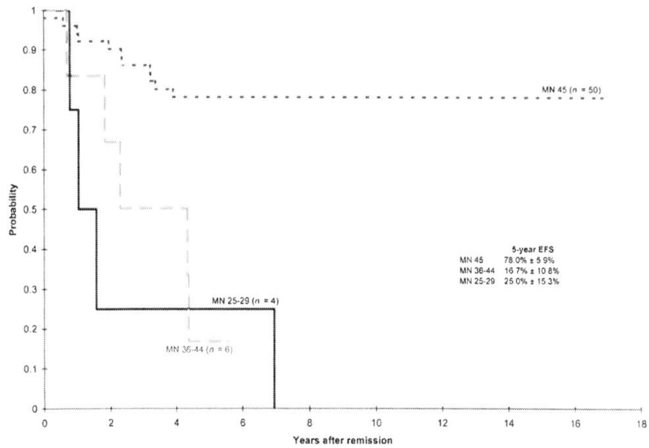

FIGURE 2.—Event-free survival (*EFS*) and 5-year EFS estimates for patients in hypodiploid ALL subgroups. (Courtesy of Raimondi SC, Zhou Y, Mathew S, et al: Reassessment of the prognostic significance of hypodiploidy in pediatric patients with acute lymphoblastic leukemia. *Cancer* 98:2715-2722, 2003. Copyright 2003 American Cancer Society. Reprinted by permission of Wiley-Liss, Inc, a subsidiary of John Wiley & Sons, Inc.)

▶ Cytogenetic changes, particularly chromosomal translocations, play a critical prognostic role in ALL. In ALL, karyotypic ploidy abnormalities are also strongly prognostic. For example, hyperdiploid leukemic blasts confer the best prognosis, and patients with near haploid karyotypes have a dismal prognosis. However, there is clearly heterogeneity in the degree of ploidy changes. In the case of hyperdiploid blasts, trisomies of subsets of chromosomes take on the greatest impact on prognosis. Hypodiploid blasts, that is, with fewer than 45 chromosomes, often display additional chromosomal changes. In 63% of the patients with hypodiploid blasts, a sex chromosome was missing, and in 55% of cases a dicentric chromosome derived from chromosome 9p was observed. These data suggest that specific chromosomes are more likely to be lost or be involved in chromosomal changes. The event-free survival rate for the hypodiploid cases was less than 45% compared with just under 75% for other patients. These results help to confirm the poor prognosis for hypodiploid ALL, which should not be treated on conventional ALL protocols; they may best be treated with allogeneic bone marrow transplantation. In addition, the molecular basis of why these hypodiploid leukemias have such a poor prognosis remains a mystery.

R. J. Arceci, MD, PhD

Survival Variability by Race and Ethnicity in Childhood Acute Lymphoblastic Leukemia

Kadan-Lottick NS, Ness KK, Bhatia S, et al (Yale Univ, New Haven, Conn; Univ of Minnesota, Minneapolis; City of Hope Natl Med Ctr, Duarte, Calif)
JAMA 290:2008-2014, 2003 14–4

Background.—The most common childhood cancer in the United States is acute lymphoblastic lymphoma (ALL), which accounts for 25% of all cancers in patients under 20 years of age. At 1 time ALL was a uniformly fatal disease, but treatment advances in recent decades have yielded a 5-year survival probability of greater than 80%. However, variability in survival outcome across racial and ethnic groups has been identified in most, but not all, clinical research studies. Some studies have reported poorer survival among minority children, whereas others have reported equivalent survival across race and ethnicity in the modern, risk-stratified treatment era. The relationship between race/ethnicity and survival in a large, population-based analysis of incident ALL cases in the United States was investigated.

Methods.—The study group was composed of 4952 patients in whom ALL was diagnosed from 1973 to 1999 at the age of 19 years or younger. Cases of ALL were identified from 9 population-based registries of the National Cancer Institute's Surveillance, Epidemiology, and End Results Program. Survival probabilities were compared among several racial and ethnic cohorts, including white, black, Hispanic, Asian/Pacific Islander, and American Indian/Alaskan Native children. Kaplan-Meier curves and proportional hazard ratios from Cox regression analysis were calculated to account for treatment era (1973 to 1982, 1983 to 1989, and 1990 to 1999), age at diagnosis (<1 year, 1 to 9, and 10 to 19 years), and sex.

Results.—There was improvement in overall 5-year survival probabilities with each successive treatment era, but differences in race/ethnicity persisted. For the most recent treatment period (1990 to 1999), 5-year survival was 84% for white children, 81% for Asian/Pacific Islander children, 75% for black children, and 72% for both American Indian/Alaskan Native children and Hispanic children. The largest difference by race/ethnicity was found in children in whom the disease was diagnosed between ages 1 and 9 years. After adjustment for treatment era, sex, and age at diagnosis, children of black, Hispanic, and American Indian/Alaskan Native descent had hazard ratios of 1.50, 1.83, and 1.90 compared with white children.

Conclusions.—The indication from these findings is that black, Hispanic, and American Indian/Alaskan Native children with ALL continue to have poorer survival than white and Asian/Pacific Islander children. There is a need for additional studies to clearly elucidate the social and biological factors involved in these differences in outcome, including any differences in pharmacokinetics associated with chemotherapeutic agents.

► The results of this study stand in contrast to those from Pui et al,[1] which concluded that there was no difference in outcome for black versus white children with ALL. The study by Kadan-Lottick et al comes to quite different conclusions. Their study represents a larger number of patients from multiple centers belonging to the national pediatric cooperative clinical trials. The time span was from 1973 to 1999 compared with the 1991 to 1998 time frame of the Pui et al study. The Kadan-Lottick results show improved survival over time. In the more modern era (1990 to 1999), 5-year survival for black children was 75%, for American Indian/Alaskan Native children 72%, for Asian/Pacific Islander children 81%, and for white children 84%. The differences, albeit relatively small, were significant in that poorer survival was observed for black, Hispanic, and Native American children compared with white and Asian patients. The greatest significant difference was observed in the group of patients aged 1 to 9 years. The authors of both articles raise important differences in the 2 studies to account for the different conclusions such as sample size, biased population from a single institution versus a national assessment, improved compliance with therapy from a single institution, and differences in therapeutic approach. These issues are not merely academic, as they have an impact on the potential for future risk stratification or alternative therapeutic approaches. A reasonable request would be for both groups to get together and analyze their data together to try to get to the truth of the matter.

R. J. Arceci, MD, PhD

Reference

1. Pui CH, Sandlund JT, Pei D, et al: Results of therapy for acute lymphoblastic leukemia in black and white children. *JAMA* 290:2001-2007, 2003.

Results of Therapy for Acute Lymphoblastic Leukemia in Black and White Children

Pui C, Sandlund JT, Pei D, et al (St Jude Children's Research Hosp, Memphis, Tenn; Univ of Tennessee, Memphis)
JAMA 290:2001-2007, 2003 14–5

Background.—Several studies have reported racial and ethnic differences in survival of adult cancer patients, with minority or underprivileged groups demonstrating poorer long-term results. These findings have been attributed to various causes, including the presence of more advanced disease at diagnosis, comorbid conditions, cancer types with unfavorable biological features, and lower socioeconomic status, which results in decreased access to effective therapies or poor compliance with treatment. In the most common childhood cancer, acute lymphoblastic lymphoma (ALL), black children treated from 1960 to 1990 consistently had worse outcomes than did white children treated during the same period. However, an exception to these outcomes was found among a cohort of ALL patients treated from 1984 to 1992 at St Jude's Children's Research Hospital in Memphis, Tennessee. At this institution, black children with ALL had a 5-year survival rate of 77% compared with 80% for white children. The clinical outcomes of therapy for black and white children with ALL treated at this institution were compared.

Methods.—A retrospective analysis was conducted of 412 children and adolescents (68 black, 338 white, and 6 of other races) with newly diagnosed ALL who were treated consecutively at a pediatric cancer center. The patients were enrolled from December 1991 to July 1998 in successive Total Therapy studies, regardless of race, ethnicity, or ability to pay, and they received risk-directed therapy according to stringent criteria. The remission-induction therapy was followed by 120 weeks of risk-assigned postremission therapy, including reinduction treatment, pulses of high-dose methotrexate, and early intrathecal chemotherapy.

Results.—The black children were significantly more likely than the white children to have higher-risk prognostic features and less likely to have hyperdiploid blast cells, which is a favorable prognostic factor in childhood ALL. However, there was no significant difference in clinical outcome between the 2 groups. The 5-year event-free and overall survival rates were 80.7% and 86.2% for black children versus 79.4% and 85% for white children. The lack of a racial effect on long-term outcome of therapy persisted after adjustment on multivariate Cox regression analysis for sex, age, presenting leukocyte count, leukemic cell DNA index, immunophenotype, and CNS status.

Conclusions.—Access to effective therapy is the most significant factor accounting for differences in outcome for black versus white children with acute lymphoblastic leukemia. With equal access to effective antileukemic therapy, the same high rate of cure can be expected among both black and white children with ALL.

▶ Poorer outcome has been documented in several studies for minority and/or underprivileged groups of adult and pediatric patients with cancer compared with white and not underprivileged patients. While some of the these discrepancies have been attributed to differences in the care received, other studies have suggested that even with the same care, minority group patients, particularly black children, have a worse outcome than white patients. To this end, the results reported by Pui et al are of considerable importance. They retrospectively examined a cohort of patients with ALL treated from 1991 to 1998. They identified 68 black children, representing about 16% of their total patient population with ALL during that same time period. All patients received the same treatment. Black children were found to more commonly present with higher risk features such as higher initial white blood cell counts, T lymphocyte immunophenotype and the t(1;19) translocation. The black children also had fewer good prognostic features such as hyperdiploid leukemic blasts. Nevertheless, there were no significant outcome differences in the black versus white children, with both groups achieving an approximately 85% 5-year overall survival rate. Although this report is retrospective in nature and, therefore, potentially flawed by bias, the results are encouraging and strongly suggest that black children, even though many were from lower socioeconomic groups than white children, can share the same good outcome as other children. Of note, however, these results stand in contrast to reports from the Pediatric Oncology Group and the Children's Cancer Group, which have shown decreased event-free and overall survival for black children with ALL compared to white children. The reason for this discrepancy is not known, but clearly an important area for further investigation and comparative analysis.

R. J. Arceci, MD, PhD

Outcome of Childhood Acute Promyelocytic Leukemia With All-*Trans*-Retinoic Acid and Chemotherapy

de Botton S, Coiteux V, Chevret S, et al (Hôpital Avicenne, Bobigny, France, et al)

J Clin Oncol 22:1404-1412, 2004 14–6

Background.—Acute promyelocytic leukemia (APL) is characterized by blast cells; t(15;17) translocation leading to a fusion between the *PML gene*, situated in 15q, and the *RARα* gene, situated in 17q; and specific coagulopathy. The efficacy of a treatment combining all-*trans*-retinoic acid (ATRA) and chemotherapy in childhood APL was investigated.

Methods.—Thirty-one children with newly diagnosed APL enrolled in the APL93 trial were treated with ATRA combined with or followed by daunorubicin–cytarabine. The children were then assigned randomly to no maintenance, intermittent ATRA, continuous chemotherapy, and intermittent ATRA plus continuous chemotherapy.

Findings.—All but 1 child (97%) achieved complete remission (CR). Four children (13%), all of whom obtained CR, had ATRA syndrome. Headaches occurred in 39% of the children, and signs of pseudotumor cerebri occurred in 16%. Twenty-three percent of the patients had a relapse. None of the 8 patients receiving ATRA plus chemotherapy during maintenance had a relapse. All children with a relapse were able to obtain a second CR. At 43 to more than 96 months, 22 children remained in first CR. After 17 to 66 months, 6 were in second CR. Three children died. The 5-year event-free survival rate was 71%; the relapse rate was 27%; and the overall survival rate was 90%.

Conclusions.—The combination of ATRA and chemotherapy for induction and probably also for maintenance therapy yields as good outcomes in children with APL as in adults with this disease. This treatment strategy is the reference first-line therapy for both children and adults with APL.

▶ The similarities and differences between different types of leukemia in children compared with adults have profound implications for testing new antileukemic therapies targeted to shared molecular pathways. This study on APL, in which the same treatment protocol was used in children and adults, nicely demonstrates that, while differences certainly exist in the presentation and toxicity profiles, the use of therapy directed to the t(15;17) fusion product that characterizes this leukemia and that is shared by children and adults results in very similar outcomes. This type of result lends considerable support to the concept that the target, not the age of the patient, is the issue. Of course, age-specific aspects of pharmacologic metabolism, treatment-related toxicity, and the differences in the care of children and adults remain the work of age-specific specialists. Nevertheless, it is important to use such examples of target equivalency to increase the testing of new and potentially improved agents earlier in children, on the basis of biology, not just age.

R. J. Arceci, MD, PhD

Thioguanine Offers No Advantage Over Mercaptopurine in Maintenance Treatment of Childhood ALL: Results of the Randomized Trial COALL-92

Harms DO, for the COALL Study Group (Children's Univ Hosp, Hamburg, Germany; Children's Univ Hosp, Düsseldorf, Germany; Children's Univ Hosp, Munich, Germany; et al)

Blood 102:2736-2740, 2003 14–7

Background.—Mercaptopurine (MP) has become the standard agent for maintenance treatment in patients with acute lymphoblastic leukemia (ALL). To date, thioguanine (TG) has been used only to treat acute myeloid leukemia and relapsed ALL. Both agents are prodrugs that have to be converted intracellularly to 6-thioguanine nucleotides (TGNs) for cytostatic activity. Compared with 6-MP, TG is converted to TGN in fewer steps. It has also been shown to be more cytotoxic in equimolar doses in vitro. In the German cooperative study group for childhood acute lymphoblastic leukemia (COALL), the clinical efficacy of TG was compared with that of MP in the maintenance treatment of childhood ALL.

Methods.—Five hundred twenty-one patients were enrolled in the randomized multicenter trial. By random assignment, 474 received a daily oral dose of MP or TG during maintenance treatment. The median observation time was 6.6 years.

Findings.—The probability of event-free survival was 79% among MP recipients and 78% among the TG recipients. The TGN levels of TG recipients were 7 times greater than those of the MP recipients, but TG treatment did not improve outcomes. Furthermore, TG had a toxicity profile of prolonged myelosuppression with marked thrombocytopenia, which made this agent more difficult to use.

Conclusions.—TG did not seem to be more effective than MP in maintenance treatment in children with ALL. In addition, the toxicity of TG was troublesome. Thus, MP should remain the maintenance treatment of choice in this patient population.

▶ TG and 6-MP are 2 drugs that date back to the beginning of attempts to treat childhood leukemia. Among the potential advantages to using TG are data showing a more direct conversion to TGNs compared with conversion of 6-MP to active metabolites within the leukemic blasts and a correlation of blast TGN concentrations with relapses, as well as an increased in vitro cytotoxicity at lower concentrations of TG compared with 6-MP against leukemic blasts. Based on such information, the COALL-92 study postulated that TG would improve outcomes for children with ALL. To answer the question, they randomly assigned patients to receive either TG or 6-MP orally and daily during maintenance therapy. A 91% compliance with randomization was achieved. The results demonstrated that TG did not improve outcomes but, interestingly, produced more prolonged myelosuppression and thrombocytopenia. The study was not designed to detect less than a 10% difference in the 2 arms, but these results are important and will likely lead to 6-MP remaining as the drug of choice for maintenance in the near future.

R. J. Arceci, MD, PhD

Increasing Mixed Chimerism Is an Important Prognostic Factor for Unfavorable Outcome in Children With Acute Lymphoblastic Leukemia After Allogeneic Stem-Cell Transplantation: Possible Role for Pre-emptive Immunotherapy?

Bader P, Kreyenberg H, Hoelle W, et al (Univ of Tübingen, Germany; Univ Children's Hosp, Essen, Germany; Univ Children's Hosp, Duesseldorf, Germany; et al)

J Clin Oncol 22:1696-1706, 2004 14–8

Background.—Children with acute forms of leukemia showing increasing mixed chimerism (MC) after allogeneic stem-cell transplantation have been shown to have a significantly elevated risk of a relapse. A prospective multicenter study was done to determine whether a relapse of acute lymphoblastic leukemia (ALL) could be determined in advance by chimerism analysis and whether withdrawing immunosuppression and/or infusing low-dose donor lymphocytes in patients with increasing MC can improve outcomes.

Methods and Findings.—One hundred sixty-three children with ALL underwent serial and quantitative analysis of chimerism. A fluorescent-based short-tandem-repeat-polymerase chain reaction was used. Complete chimerism (CC) or low-level MC was found in 101 patients. Forty-six patients

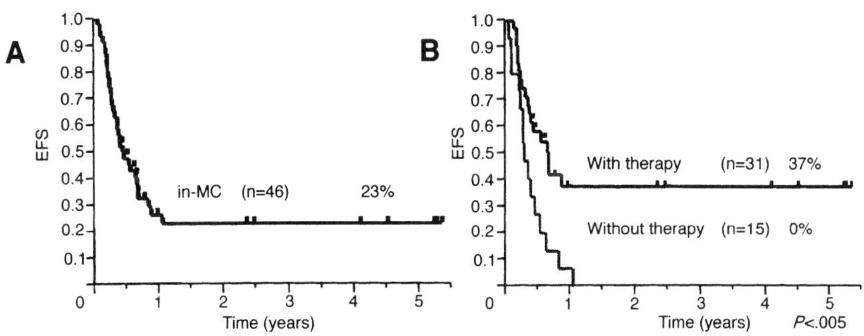

FIGURE 3.—Kaplan-Meier analysis of event-free survival (EFS) in patients with increasing mixed chimerism (MC). Patients with increasing MC (*in-MC*) who received additional therapy (**A**, n = 31) and patients with increasing MC who did not receive additional treatment (**B**, n = 15). (Courtesy of Bader P, Kreyenberg H, Hoelle W, et al: Increasing mixed chimerism is an important prognostic factor for unfavorable outcome in children with acute lymphoblastic leukemia after allogeneic stem-cell transplantation: Possible role for pre emptive immunotherapy? *J Clin Oncol* 22:1696-1706, 2004. Reprinted with permission from the American Society of Clinical Oncology.)

had increasing MC, and 16 patients had declining MC. A relapse was significantly more common in patients with increasing MC than in those with CC or low-level MC or in those with declining MC. Overall, the probability of 3-year event-free survival (EFS) was 54%. For patients with CC or low-level MC, the EFS was 66%; for those with declining MC, 66%; and for those with increasing MC, 23%. Thirty-one of 46 patients with increasing MC received immunotherapy. The EFS estimated in this group was 37%, which was significantly greater than the EFS in patients who did not receive immunotherapy (0%; $P < .001$; Fig 3).

Conclusions.—Children with ALL at the highest risk of a relapse can be identified by serial analysis of chimerism. In the absence of immunotherapy, the 3-year EFS was 0% in children with increasing MC. With identification by serial chimerism analysis, an overt relapse may be prevented in a substantial number of these patients.

▶ The outcomes of children with ALL who relapse after allogeneic bone marrow transplantation has been particularly poor. Options have included withdrawal of immunosuppression, giving donor lymphocyte infusions, and reinduction therapy followed by a second transplant if the relapse occurs 6 to 12 months after the first transplant. By closely monitoring the emergence of MC as detected molecularly by polymerase chain reaction amplification of allelic differences and early removal of graft versus host disease prophylaxis (ie, cyclosporine) and/or donor lymphocyte infusions, Bader et al report that 37% of their patients are alive and without evidence of leukemia compared with 0% of those not so treated (see Fig 3 in text). In addition, among patients who have decreasing MC, CC, or low-level MC, the survival rate is 66% compared with 23% for those with increasing MC overall. This is an important article, although it is not without some significant problems. First of all, this is not a prospective randomized trial; therefore, there may be inherent bias, although the differences in the groups are quite large. It would have been more useful to have more information on the patients and their type of ALL, as well as to have some more detailed data and recommendations on the frequency of monitoring for molecular minimal residual disease. The minimal residual disease test was also relatively insensitive—only 1 recipient cell in 100 donor cells—and is an area worth improving. Controlling for the number of donor lymphocytes among the centers would have strengthened the study. Last, relapse was uniform for patients who received transplants in CR3, with 1 exception—a patient who experienced graft rejection. These caveats do not, however, completely take away from the importance of this article, which should provide other investigators with the foundation on which to do early monitoring of chimerism followed by immunologic intervention.

R. J. Arceci, MD, PhD

Pilot Study of Idarubicin-Based Intensive-Timing Induction Therapy for Children With Previously Untreated Acute Myeloid Leukemia: Children's Cancer Group Study 2941

Lange BJ, Dinndorf P, Smith FO, et al (Children's Hosp of Philadelphia; Food and Drug Administration, Rockville, Md; Cincinnati Children's Hosp, Ohio; et al)

J Clin Oncol 22:150-156, 2004 14–9

Background.—Randomized studies of adults with acute myeloid leukemia have shown that idarubicin (IDA) produces a higher remission rate and longer remission duration than does daunorubicin (DNR). The Children's Cancer Group Pilot Study CCG-2941 investigated the feasibility of substituting 4 mg of DNR with 1 mg of IDA in intensive-timing DNR-based induction therapy (DNR/DNR).

Methods.—Sixty-five patients were initially enrolled in the study. Two courses of dexamethasone, cytarabine, 6-thioguanine, etoposide, and IDA (IDA/IDA) were administered on days 1 through 3 and 10 through 14. Toxicity prompted substitution of IDA with DNR (IDA/DNR) on days 10 through 14 in an additional 28 patients enrolled in the study. Outcomes were compared with the outcomes of patients treated with intensive timing in CCG-2891.

Findings.—After 2 courses of induction, treatment-related mortality rate did not differ significantly among the 3 regimens: 14% in the IDA/IDA group, 7% in the IDA/DNR group, and 9% in the DNR/DNR group. In the first course of CCG-2941 IDA/IDA therapy, 11% of patients were withdrawn compared with 5% in the IDA/DNR group and 1.5% in CCG-2891. Compared with the CCG-2891 protocol, the DNR/DNR and IDA/IDA protocols increased mean length of stay in the hospital by 7 days and mean duration of course 1 by 1 week. In addition, the risk of grade 3 or 4 hyperbilirubinemia was 18% and 5%, respectively. Toxicity of IDA/DNR did not differ from that of DNR/DNR in CCG-2891. The mean day 7 marrow blast percentages in CCG-2941 and CCG-2891 were 11.4% and 21.1%, respectively. The CCG-2941 and CCG-2891 protocols were similar in remission induction, survival, and event-free survival rates.

Conclusions.—These data indicate that the excessive toxicity and withdrawals associated with the CCG-2941 protocol outweigh the potential benefits of early response with IDA. However, when DNR replaced IDA in the second cycle of each induction course, toxicity approximated that of DNR/DNR in CCG-2891. Thus, IDA/DNR merits further study.

▶ Intensification of treatment, either by dose or timing, has proven to be an important advance in the treatment of children with acute myeloid leukemia. The CCG-2941 study thus aimed at replacing presumed equitoxic doses of DNR with IDA to determine the feasibility of such a change but also with the hope that the longer metabolite half-life of IDA, its better CNS penetration, and the manner in which it is handled by drug resistance mechanisms would translate into improved outcomes. Thus, CCG-2941 built on the intensively timed

CCG-2891 study in which the 2 courses were both with DNR (DNR/DNR) to 2 courses with IDA (IDA/IDA). Unfortunately, the intensively timed IDA/IDA regimen was stopped after only 65 patients were enrolled because of toxicity, including prolonged periods of neutropenia, increased days in the hospital, hyperbilirubinemia, and patient withdrawals. However, the day 7 bone marrow leukemic blast percentage was significantly lower in the CCG-2941 study than in the CCG-2891 study when compared retrospectively. This result is consistent with other reports showing increased antileukemic activity of IDA compared with DNR. To decrease early toxicity of the IDA/IDA regimen, the CCG-2941 was modified to include IDA only on the first of the 2 courses (IDA/DNR). This regimen was better tolerated and showed no increased toxicity compared with the DNR/DNR regimen of CCG-2891. Although a pilot study, this article raises some important aspects about clinical trials and leukemia therapy. Certainly, the most effective antileukemic agent available is not particularly useful if toxicity is too great. In addition, early withdrawals from a trial can have a major impact on the overall outcome analyses. Last, it is unclear what role IDA will play in the future of COG. The current COG pilot for acute myeloid leukemia is based primarily on the Medical Research Council developed in Great Britain and does not use IDA. However, subsequent Medical Research Council trials, as well as those from the Berlin-Frankfurt-Munster cooperative group, include IDA. It is unclear when the next opportunity to test IDA in COG will be.

R. J. Arceci, MD, PhD

Outcome in Children With Relapsed Acute Myeloid Leukemia After Initial Treatment With French Leucémie Aiquë Myéloïde Enfant (LAME) 89/91 Protocol of the French Society of Pediatric Hematology and Immunology

Aladjidi N, Auvrignon A, Leblanc T, et al (Univ Hosp Ctrs of Bordeaux, France)

J Clin Oncol 21:4377-4385, 2003 14–10

Background.—Among children with acute myeloid leukemia (AML), complete remission (CR) rates are between 75% and 90% and long-term event-free survival rates have increased to between 40% and 51%. The main cause of treatment failure is relapse, which develops in 40% of patients who had a CR. Among these children, the 2-year overall survival (OS) is usually less than 20%. A retrospective study was undertaken to determine whether a second CR (CR2) is attainable for these children and which postremission consolidation therapy is best suited to these cases.

Methods.—Relapse developed in 106 of 308 children enrolled in a multicenter prospective protocol. Twenty-one received allogenic HLA-identical bone marrow transplantation (BMT) and 85 underwent chemotherapy after the first CR (CR1). The various protocols chosen by the treating institutions were followed in seeking CR2. A curative strategy was offered to most patients, with a 9% rate of purely palliative treatments.

Results.—Seventy-one percent of the patients had a CR2 after reinduction therapy. BMT was performed in 78% of the patients in CR2. A 33% 5-year OS rate was achieved in all 106 patients, with a disease-free survival (DFS) rate of 45% for children in CR2. Nine percent of the children had lethal toxicity after the first reinduction course and 15% after BMT. Transplantation patients had the highest rate of toxic mortality for retreatment of relapsing AML, toward the high end of a range from 7% to 50%. Half of the patients alive after BMT had moderate-to-severe long-term toxicity develop. When CR1 lasted over 12 months, the 5-year OS rate was 54%, but when CR1 was less than 12 months, it was only 24%. If maintenance therapy was given after CR1, the 5-year OS rate was lower (12%) than when chemotherapy without maintenance therapy (40%) or HLA-identical BMT was given (52%). The best results were obtained when high or intermediate doses of cytarabine plus anthracycline or the fludarabine, cytarabine, and granulocyte colony–stimulating factor regimen was used for therapy. No significant difference in 5-year DFS rate was linked to the source of the BMT. For matched sibling-donor BMT, the rate was 60%, for autograft 47%, and for alternative-donor BMT 44%. Age 1 year or younger was a strong predictor of poor outcome after relapse. Differences in outcome related to karyotype that were present with the initial diagnosis carried through for the relapsing cases.

Conclusions.—The results achieved (33% 5-year OS rate and 45% DFS rate) were comparable with those obtained in German and British research groups. Cure was accomplished in a third of the children who had relapsing AML when aggressive first-line therapy was used. Children with relapse require the same intensive strategy of CR2 reinduction and marrow transplantation regardless of whether the relapse is extramedullary or medullary. Therapeutic options include further intensified schedules with alterations considered to handle multidrug resistance, immunomodulatory approaches, or the use of anti-CD33 monoclonal antibodies. Optimal reinduction regimen and megadose chemotherapy require further study, as do the late effects of these treatment strategies.

▶ The cure rate for children with newly diagnosed AML has continued to improve such that approximately 50% are currently able to be cured. Unfortunately, the overall outcome for patients with relapsed AML remains poor, although there are subgroups of patients who indeed can be cured following relapse. Keys to being able to cure such patients include the ability to achieve a CR2 by using intensive reinduction therapy usually followed by some type of allogeneic, and less commonly autologous, transplant. Such approaches have achieved an overall cure rate of less than 40% with the lowest survival in patients relapsing on or relatively close to finishing their up-front treatment. The study by Aladjidi et al reports similar results in a group of 106 patients who relapsed after intensive up-front therapy. The overall survival is 33% but considerably better for patients with a CR1 of more than 12 months (54%); patients with a CR1 duration of less than 12 months was only 24%. An unexpected result from this study was that an allogeneic transplant in CR1 did not adversely affect the outcome of patients compared with patients who only received chemotherapy. There is no obvious explanation for this observation, as most evaluations have shown that survival after a posttransplant relapse is usually significantly worse. Further, they showed that survival was worse for patients who relapsed after receiving low-dose maintenance chemotherapy, which included 18 months of low-dose 6-mercaptopurine and cytarabine. This is presumably because of the development of increased resistance after chronic, long-term exposure to chemotherapy in AML. There was no difference in 5-year DFS for patients receiving a matched sibling-donor BMT (60%), autologous BMT (47%), or alternative-donor BMT (44%), although the reasons for failure differed with increased treatment-related deaths being found in the allogeneic BMT groups. This study demonstrates at the very least that in a group of patients uniformly treated with modern intensive chemotherapy for AML, a significant percentage can be cured. Nevertheless, that cure rate is not sufficiently good to conclude that we do not have a major challenge still in front of us.

R. J. Arceci, MD, PhD

Solid Tumors

Profiling and Functional Annotation of mRNA Gene Expression in Pediatric Rhabdomyosarcoma and Ewing's Sarcoma

Baer C, Nees M, Breit S, et al (Univ Children's Hosp, Heidelberg, Germany; Heinrich-Heine-Univ, Düsseldorf, Germany; Children's Hosp of Los Angeles)
Int J Cancer 110:687-694, 2004 14–11

Introduction.—The specific relationship of fusion genes with alveolar rhabdomyosarcoma (aRMS) and Ewing's sarcoma (EWS) indicates that chimeric oncoproteins have a causative role in the development of these pediatric sarcomas. Both of these tumors share an unfavorable prognosis and the presence of characteristic oncogenic fusion transcripts, which distinguishes these tumors from other, more common small round blue cell tumors. The diagnostic classification of these tumors is often complicated by the highly similar appearance in routine histology. Additional molecular markers could substantially enhance tumor classification. Affymetrix oligonucleotide microarrays (Affymetrix Inc, Santa Clara, Calif) were used to analyze messenger RNA (mRNA) gene expression patterns of 12 primary pediatric RMS and 11 EWS, which belong to the small round blue cell tumors.

Methods.—Tumor samples were analyzed for tumor-specific fusion transcripts. Statistical microarray data analysis was conducted. Quantitative real-time polymerase chain reaction (PCR) was performed with the use of the LightCycler system (Roche Diagnostics, Penzberg, Germany) as an independent approach to evaluating relative gene expression and validating the microarray expression data.

Results.—A combination of 3 independent statistical approaches (*t* test, SAM, K-nearest neighborhood analysis) provided 101 highly significant probe sets that clearly discriminate between EWS and RMS. Novel marker transcripts were identified that have not previously been linked with either RMS or EWS; they included CITED2, glypican 3, and cyclin DI. Expression levels for selected candidate genes were confirmed via real-time, reverse-transcription PCR. To distinguish biologically meaningful trends, functional annotations were assigned to 946 genes differentially expressed between EWS and RMS (*t* test). Twenty-eight, 9, 23, 22, and 11 genes, respectively, involved in protein biosynthesis and complex assembly, lipid metabolism, energy generation, and mRNA processing showed significantly higher expression in EWS.

Conclusion.—Functional annotation of tumor-specific genes demonstrates detailed insights into tumor biology and differentiation-specific expression patterns and provides important clues associated with the possible cellular origin of these pediatric tumors.

▶ Although several studies have examined mRNA expression patterns in sarcomas by microarray analysis, this study provides several new and important additions to the field of expression profiling of sarcomas. The results certainly define subsets of genes characteristic of RMS compared with EWS, but, importantly, additional functional pathway-oriented subsets were also defined. These subsets include such areas as cell cycle control and proliferation, DNA repair, complex assembly, lipid metabolism, and others. This type of approach allows smaller differences to carry more significance than just quantitative differences in expression in that if smaller expression increases occur in several members of a pathway, then one can conclude that entire pathway is unregulated. This type of analysis thus can lead to a deeper understanding of not only the physiology of a cancer, but also the cellular origins. Thus, microarray analysis can be taken from an assessment of marker gene differences to true physiologic pathway interrogation.

R. J. Arceci, MD, PhD

Failure Pattern and Factors Predictive of Local Failure in Rhabdomyosarcoma: A Report of Group III Patients on the Third Intergroup Rhabdomyosarcoma Study

Wharam MD, Meza J, Anderson J, et al (Children's Oncology Group, Arcadia, Calif; Stanford Univ, Calif; Johns Hopkins Univ, Baltimore, Md; et al)

J Clin Oncol 22:1902-1908, 2004 14–12

Background.—More than half of children with rhabdomyosarcoma (RMS) undergo subtotal resection or biopsy only of the primary tumor; thus, radiotherapy is the definitive method for local control. The success of radiotherapy in such patients is essential for reducing local failures and improved survival rates. The patterns of treatment failure and patient, tumor, and radiation factors predicting local failure were investigated in children receiving radiotherapy for RMS in the third Intergroup Rhabdomyosarcoma Study.

Methods.—Of the 1062 children enrolled in the study, 472 had group III disease and were eligible for the current study. Group III disease was defined as gross residual disease after biopsy or initial surgery and no distant metastases. Of this group, 405 underwent radiotherapy and were included in the analysis.

Findings.—The estimated cumulative incidence rates at 5 years were 19% for total local failure, 2% for total regional nodal failure, and 11% for total distant failure. The probability of death from toxic effects or an unknown recurrence type at 5 years was estimated to be 4%. The best predictor of an increased risk of total local failure was lymph node involvement. A total radiotherapy dose over the prescribed range of 41.4 to 50.4 Gy had no significant effect on the risk of local failure. Overall, the estimated 5-year failure-free survival rate was 70%, and the overall survival rate was 78%.

Conclusions.—The main type of relapse in children undergoing radiotherapy for group III RMS is a local failure. Lymph node involvement at diagnosis predicts a greater risk of local and distant treatment failure in this patient population.

► Whereas metastatic disease was the primary type of treatment failure in patients with RMS in the initial Intergroup Rhabdomyosarcoma Study (IRS) trials, subsequent trials have seen local failure rates take on an increasingly important outcome. This study helps to define some of the risk factors associated with local failure. Although no association with the dose of radiation was identified when radiotherapy was delivered as prescribed in the protocol, the presence of tumor-positive lymph nodes was predictive of a significantly increased risk of local failure.

The estimated 5-year survival rate for group III patients was 70%, which yields an approximately 30% relapse rate. The estimated 5-year cumulative incidence of total local failure was 19%, which was similar to the results of IRS-II (22%) but possibly higher than the 13% observed in IRS-IV. The IRS-V study is attempting to test the hypothesis that incorporating surgery after induction chemotherapy and followed by local radiotherapy will reduce the local recurrence rate. Another lesson reestablished from this study is that the initial response to chemotherapy positively affects survival. The IRS-III study ran from 1984 to 1991; these results were just published in 2004, when nearly all events had occurred by year 5. For progress to be made in childhood cancer in as rapid a manner as possible, it should be mandatory that the results be reported in a timely fashion.

R. J. Arceci, MD, PhD

Histone Deacetylase Inhibitors Induce Growth Suppression and Cell Death in Human Rhabdomyosarcoma In Vitro

Kutko MC, Glick RD, Butler LM, et al (Sloan Kettering Inst, New York; Cornell Univ, New York)

Clin Cancer Res 9:5749-5755, 2003 14–13

Background.—Research has demonstrated the efficacy of a group of histone deacetylase inhibitors (HDACIs) in suppressing the growth of a variety of transformed cell lines in vivo and in vitro. The effects of 2 of these agents, suberoylanilide hydroxamic acid (SAHA) and suberoyl-3-

aminopyridineamide hydroxamic acid (pyroxamide), on growth suppression in rhabdomyosarcoma (RMS) cells were investigated.

Methods.—Dose–response experiments with SAHA and pyroxamide were performed on 2 RMS cell lines, the embryonal RD and alveolar RH30B. Doses of SAHA and pyroxamide ranged from 0.25 to 3 μM and from 1.25 to 20 μM, respectively.

Findings.—Both agents produced a dose-dependent decline in the viable cell number as well as an increase in the percentage of dead cells over time. Western blot analysis showed that RMS cells exposed to SAHA and pyroxamide had an accumulation of acetylated histones with increasing doses. When cells were cultured with concentrations of SAHA and pyroxamide that successfully inhibited cell growth and initiated cell death in the 2 RMS cell lines, an induction of p21/WAF1 occurred at 15 and 24 hours. Flow cytometry showed an increase in nuclei with a hypodiploid or sub-G_1 fraction with increasing doses of SAHA and pyroxamide over time, which is a finding consistent with DNA fragmentation and cell death by apoptosis.

Conclusions.—In these in vitro experiments, pyroxamide and SAHA induced growth suppression and cell death in human RMS. Cells exposed to either agent showed accumulation of acetylated histones and induction of p21/WAF1 expression.

► The development of more effective and less toxic anticancer drugs remains a major challenge in oncology, particularly in pediatric oncology, in which few agents have been approved for children with cancer. This article represents a very nice extension of basic laboratory work focused on transcriptional therapy using HDACIs. The primary function of HDACIs is to deacetylate nucleosomal core histones, which results in decreased histone acetylation, which, in turn, is associated with compaction and decreased transcription of chromatin. This article shows that exposure to either of the 2 HDACIS, SAHA or pyroxamide, results in increased acetylation of the histone H3, induction of the cell cycle arrest protein, p21/WAF21, decreased growth, and increased levels of apoptosis. These agents, particularly SAHA, are being actively studied in early phase clinical trials in patients, which makes the identification of tumor targets particularly important. The presented data would be stronger with additional cell lines and xenograft data, but this article may provide a hint that RMS would be a potentially good tumor type to therapeutically target.

R. J. Arceci, MD, PhD

Efficacy of Topotecan and Cyclophosphamide Given in a Phase II Window Trial in Children With Newly Diagnosed Metastatic Rhabdomyosarcoma: A Children's Oncology Group Study

Walterhouse DO, Lyden ER, Breitfeld PP, et al (Children's Mem Med Ctr, Chicago; Nebraska Med Ctr, Omaha; Duke Univ, Durham, NC; et al)

J Clin Oncol 22:1398-1403, 2004 14–14

Background.—The outcomes of childhood metastatic rhabdomyosarcoma (RMS) are poor, and little improvement has been seen in the past 3 decades. Strategies investigated to improve outcomes have included dose intensification of cyclophosphamide and the addition of agents known to be active—doxorubicin, cisplatin, dacarbazine, and etoposide—to conventional vincristine, dactinomycin, and cyclophosphamide (VAC). The current study determined the antitumor activity and toxicity of topotecan administered immediately after cyclophosphamide as window therapy, then combined with conventional agents, in children with newly diagnosed RMS.

Methods.—Sixty-one patients younger than 21 years with a recent diagnosis of metastatic RMS or undifferentiated sarcoma were enrolled in the study. Patients received window therapy at weeks 0 to 6 with topotecan, 0.75 mg/m^2 daily for 5 days every 21 days, immediately after cyclophosphamide, 250 mg/m^2 daily for 5 days every 21 days (TC). Patients showing objective improvement, a partial response, or a complete response to TC continued to be treated with these agents combined with vincristine (VTC), alternating courses of VTC with VAC between weeks 6 and 41. Patients with no response to TC or with progressive disease after TC were given VAC only. In all patients, radiotherapy was administered to sites of unresected disease between weeks 15 and 21.

Findings.—The overall response rate to TC, including partial responses and complete responses, was 47%. An early response correlated with a tumor size of 5 cm or smaller. The main toxic effect associated with TC was myelosuppression. Overall, the 3-year disease-free survival rate was 10%, and the survival rate was 20%. Patients receiving VTC–VAC and those receiving VAC only had similar toxicity profiles.

Conclusions.—The administration of topotecan after cyclophosphamide is active against newly diagnosed RMS. The toxicity profile is acceptable. However, overall and disease-free survival rates continue to be disappointing in children with metastatic disease at RMS diagnosis.

▶ This study presents important and instructive lessons. The first is the continued use of upfront windows in high-risk patients with newly diagnosed disease. The ethics of using upfront drug testing windows has been debated over the years, but a consensus was developed that provided for their use in particularly high-risk patients with very poor outcomes. Certainly, patients with metastatic RMS and undifferentiated sarcomas qualify, with survival rates in the range of 20% or less. The window therapy tested in this trial included topotecan and cyclophosphamide, based on empirical preclinical data showing enhanced activity of the combination, presumably because of the increased DNA damage associated with the combination of a topoisomerase I inhibitor and an alkylating agent.

A phase 2 trial showed reasonable activity, which, in turn, led to window therapy for patients with newly diagnosed disease. The results showed a 47% overall response rate, which was essentially the same as a previous window treatment that used topotecan alone. This was clearly a disappointing result. Those patients that responded to the upfront window therapy had an improved but still extremely poor survival rate compared with those who did not show a response. For patients who did not respond to window therapy, standard VAC-based therapy was given. Thus, half the patients received what would be considered to be standard therapy, which has a known survival outcome of 20% or less.

One must ask whether alternative experimental approaches could not be used in this group. This would potentially affect a comparative study arm, but standard therapy associated with such a poor survival rate must be carefully considered. No biological correlative studies were presented in this article to attempt to confirm at least the proposed mechanism of action of combining the 2 drugs. This would have been particularly useful.

Last, it is of interest that the initiation of the study in April of 1996 and the publication of the manuscript in April 2004 represent nearly a decade. In this light, one must ask what therapeutic advances were achieved. A final twist in this study was that responders to upfront therapy had a better outcome than did nonresponders, which is in contrast to the results of the previous topotecan upfront window trial, which showed no difference in outcomes between responders and nonresponders to window therapy.

There is no obvious explanation for this result. Upfront window treatments in patients with sarcomas have been part of the cooperative group trials since the late 1980s. All the window trials have involved relatively conventional agents, and little to no biological mechanisms have been reported as a result of these window trials. As the authors point out, the overall outcome in this group of patients remains extremely poor, and improvements will "likely depend on a better understanding of tumor biology and the development of therapies based specifically on molecular genetic defects in the tumors." Although this is true and such agents are available, investigators will need to quickly move forward not just with the clinical testing of the efficacy of these agents but also with the actual determination of whether they are working as predicted by their biological mechanisms.

R. J. Arceci, MD, PhD

Association Between Telomerase Activity and Outcome in Patients With Nonmetastatic Ewing Family of Tumors

Ohali A, Avigad S, Cohen IJ, et al (Schneider Children's Med Ctr of Israel, Petah Tikva; Tel Aviv Univ, Israel)

J Clin Oncol 21:3836-3843, 2003 14–15

Introduction.—At the time of diagnosis of Ewing's sarcoma (ES), about 25% of patients have detectable metastatic disease; most may have micrometastases undetectable by conventional methods. Telomeres are specialized structures at the end of eukaryotic chromosomes that protect chromosomes from DNA degradation, end-to-end fusions, rearrangements, and chromosome loss. A decrease in telomere length has been reported in a wide range of human cancers. Progressive telomere shortening contributes to genomic instability. Telomerase is regarded as a molecular marker for malignancy. Telomere activity (TA) as a prognostic factor at diagnosis and as a marker for minimal residual disease during therapy and follow-up in nonmetastatic Ewing family of tumors (EFT) were examined.

Methods.—Primary tumor specimens and 97 peripheral blood (PBL) samples from 31 patients with EFT were evaluated for TA via the Telomeric Repeat Amplification Protocol (TRAP assay). The telomerase catalytic subunit (human telomerase reverse transcriptase gene expression) was assessed via quantitative reverse transcriptase polymerase chain reaction (RT-PCR). Telomerase length was ascertained by Southern blotting. The presence of the EFT chimeric transcripts was examined via RT-PCR. Correlations with progression-free survival (PFS) were assessed.

Results.—At diagnosis, TA in primary tumors were not associated with outcome. During therapy and follow-up, highly significant correlations were seen between high TA in PBL samples and adverse prognosis ($P <$ .0001). No patients with low TA progressed at long-term follow-up (median, 60 months) and a PFS of 100%. In 9 patients, high TA actually predicted relapse long before overt clinical relapse. Patients with high TA and positive RT-PCR experienced the most adverse outcome; PFS of 20% ($P =$ .0025). Telomerase activity was a better prognostic factor than RT-PCR and histopathologic response at surgery.

Conclusion.—It appears that TA is a significant prognostic variable. It is superior to the established clinical prognostic parameters during therapy and tumor surveillance. It may be that TA used in combination with RT-PCR could represent a new risk classification.

▶ The identification of new and more accurate prognostic factors is an important area of investigation in oncology. Such work is fueled by the belief that early detection of relapse with minimal residual disease or the prediction at diagnosis of high- and low-risk groups will allow for alternative therapeutic interventions. The EFT is characterized by the presence of unique translocations involving chromosome 22 and resulting in fusion messenger RNA transcripts that can be used to detect minimal residual disease (MRD) by RT-PCR. Another approach to the detection of MRD is to measure gene products that are particularly elevated in tumor cells but not in normal hematopoietic cells. TA has been shown to be essential for maintenance of telomere length which, in turn, has a significant impact on tumorigenesis. This study by Ohali et al measures TA in primary tumor specimens and in PBL mononuclear cell samples from patients with nonmetastatic ES during therapy and follow-up. They find no significant correlation of outcome with TA in the primary tumor specimens, but a strong correlation of detectable TA with poor outcome. The TA appeared a stronger predictor of poor outcome than even the detection of fusion transcripts, which are known to be specific for the tumor cells. There are several caveats for such a study. First, the numbers of patients examined was quite small and the issues of potential bias are not possible to rule out. The detection of the TA was not actually shown to arise from circulating tumor cells, as this would take isolation of such tumor cells and direct in situ measurements. Thus, it is unclear from which cells the TA being measured actually derives. Thus, we are left with a potentially very interesting observation and correlation, but one that also begs for more specific documentation of cell type TA expression as well as increased numbers of patients being analyzed.

R. J. Arceci, MD, PhD

Coamplification of *DDX1* Correlates With an Improved Survival Probability in Children With *MYCN*-Amplified Human Neuroblastoma

Weber A, Imisch P, Bergmann E, et al (Univ of Marburg, Germany)

J Clin Oncol 22:2681-2690, 2004 14–16

Background.—An aggressive subtype of human neuroblastoma with a poor clinical outcome can be identified by amplifying the *MYCN* oncogene at chromosome 2p24-25. Previous studies have reported differences in amplicon structure and coamplification of genes telomeric and centromeric to the *MYCN* oncogene. However, a relevant role for gene coamplification in the pathogenesis of neuroblastoma has not been determined.

Methods.—Ninety-eight primary neuroblastoma tumors with *MYCN* amplification for coamplification of 7 additional genes at chromosome 2p24-25 were analyzed. These were *DDX1, NAG, NSE1, LPIN1*, EST-*AA581763*, *SMC6*, and *SDC1*. The amplification status of the target genes in relation to a reference gene on chromosome 2q was determined with the use of 2 semiquantitative multiplex polymerase chain reactions. In addition, the messenger RNA (mRNA) expression pattern of coamplified genes was analyzed in a subgroup of tumors.

Findings.—The frequency of gene coamplification on 2p24-25 in neuroblastomas directly correlated with the physical distance to *MYCN*. Coamplification was associated with an upregulated *DDX1* and NAG gene expression. By coamplifying the *DDX1* gene within 400 kilobases telomeric to *MYCN*, a subset of advanced neuroblastomas with a more favorable outcome could be identified. A high level of *DDX1* expression correlated with a trend toward better survival probability.

Conclusions.—*DDX1* coamplification appears to be associated with a better prognosis and improved survival probability in patients with *MYCN*-amplified neuroblastomas. Further information is needed to help develop possible treatment approaches influencing *DDX1*.

► The amplification of the N-*myc* or *MYCN* proto-oncogene has long been associated with a poor prognosis in children with neuroblastomas. However, *MYCN*-amplified tumors are not always fatal and present a variable clinical response to therapy. The article by Weber et al attempts to provide a molecular explanation for this phenomenon by further defining the genes and their level of coamplification within the same amplicon as *MYCN*. Their results show increased frequency of coamplification of genes closest to *MYCN*. They further show that *DDX1* coamplification and increased mRNA expression are associated with a subgroup of *MYCN*-amplified tumors that have an improved prognosis (see Fig 3 in original article). By further defining the amplicon associated with *MYCN* gene amplification as well as differences in clinical outcomes, this article helps to possibly explain the heterogeneity of neuroblastomas. Now it will be particularly important to further define how or why increased *DDX1* gene copy numbers and expression lead to a better prognostic group. Confirmation in larger studies will also be important.

R. J. Arceci, MD, PhD

Early Molecular Response of Marrow Disease to Biologic Therapy Is Highly Prognostic in Neuroblastoma

Cheung IY, Lo Piccolo MS, Kushner BH, et al (Mem Sloan-Kettering Cancer Ctr, New York)

J Clin Oncol 21:3853-3858, 2003 14–17

Background.—The repeated application of anti-GD2 immunotherapy after myeloid effector activation with granulocyte-macrophage colony-stimulating factor (GM-CSF) is a promising treatment strategy for stage 4 neuroblastoma. The use of early marrow response as a prognostic indicator is especially relevant for patients unlikely to benefit from this treatment. The transcript levels of patients with GD2-positive neuroblastoma undergoing 3F8/GM-CSF therapy were measured.

Methods.—Eighty-six patients with stage 4 neuroblastoma older than 1 year at diagnosis were included. Thirty-three were classified as in complete remission or very good partial remission, 33 as primary refractory, 10 as secondary refractory, and 10 as having progressive disease. Bone marrow samples were collected before and after therapy for GD2 synthase mRNA analysis by real-time reverse transcriptase polymerase chain reaction. Response and survival analyses were performed on posttreatment samples before the third cycle 1.8 months after study entry.

Findings.—The pretreatment marrow samples demonstrated GD2 synthase mRNA in 42%, 52%, 60%, and 80% of the 4 clinical groups, respectively. Corresponding median transcript levels were 10, 16.6, 26.5, and

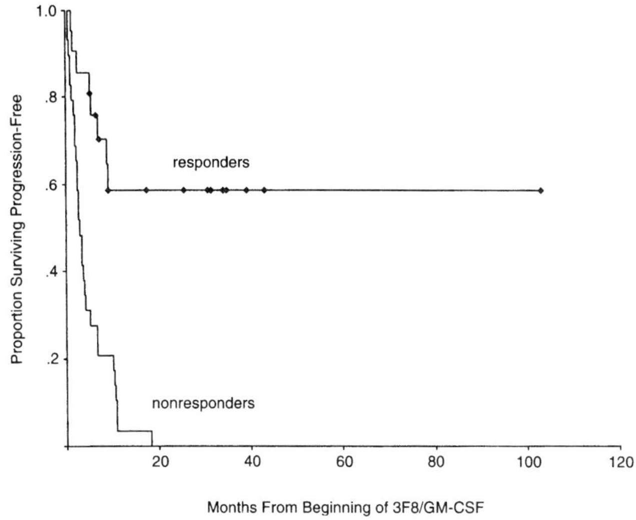

FIGURE 2.—Relation between progression-free survival and early molecular response in 74 patients treated with 3F8/GM-SCF and assessed before cycle 3 ($P < .0001$). (Courtesy of Cheung IY, Lo Piccolo MS, Kushner BH, et al: Early molecular response of marrow disease to biologic therapy is highly prognostic in neuroblastoma. *J Clin Oncol* 21:3853-3858, 2003. Reprinted with permission from the American Society of Clinical Oncology.)

87.2. After antibody plus GM-CSF, this marker became negative in 77% of those in complete or very good partial remission, 45% of those with primary refractory disease, 25% with secondary refractory disease, and in none with progressive disease. Responders and nonresponders differed significantly in progression-free survival rate. Molecular responders in the group with minimal residual disease had a significantly lower risk of progression at a median 29.8-month follow-up (Fig 2).

Conclusions.—These data show that GD2 synthase mRNA is a sensitive indicator of neuroblastoma response in the bone marrow. This marker is particularly useful in patients with minimal residual disease. It may also be useful as an early predictor of resistance to antibody plus GM-CSF immunotherapy.

▶ Advanced stage neuroblastoma continues to have an overall poor outcome, although some advances have been made, such as the introduction of autologous bone marrow transplantation and the use of cis-retinoic acid. Nevertheless, treatment-refractory metastatic disease remains a significant obstacle to cure in many children. The introduction of anti-GD2 antibody therapy, augmented with GM-CSF, represents a potential new approach to treatment. In the study by Cheung et al, it is shown that the clearance of bone marrow of neuroblastoma cells, as assayed by a sensitive reverse-transcription polymerase chain reaction technique, detected GD2 synthase mRNA in children treated with anti-GD2 antibody, and GM-CSF is strongly predictive of progression-free survival. These data, although not randomized for treatment with or without anti-GD2 antibody and GM-CSF, provide evidence that such treatment may provide a surrogate marker for patients with an improved outcome compared with those who do not clear their minimal residual disease.

R. J. Arceci, MD, PhD

Localised and Unresectable Neuroblastoma in Infants: Excellent Outcome With Low-Dose Primary Chemotherapy

Rubie H, for the Neuroblastoma Study Group of the Société Française d'Oncologie Pédiatrique (SFOP) (Hôpital des Enfants, Toulouse, France; et al)

Br J Cancer 89:1605-1609, 2003 14–18

Background.—Almost one third of the cases of neuroblastoma are diagnosed in children younger than 1 year of age. Half of the patients have localized disease at presentation, which requires gross surgical excision for cure. The outcomes of unresectable disease are not as good as for resectable disease unless secondary radical excision can be performed. The efficacy of low-dose chemotherapy in infants with localized and unresectable neuroblastoma was reported.

Methods.—One hundred thirty-four infants with localized neuroblastoma were enrolled in the study between 1995 and 1999. Thirty-nine had unresectable neuroblastoma without N-*myc* amplification. Twenty-eight had no threatening symptoms and were eligible to receive chemotherapy per protocol, consisting of low-dose cyclophosphamide, 5 $mg^{-1}kg\ day^{-1}$ for 5 days, and vincristine, 0.05 $mg\ kg^{-1}$ at day 1, repeated 1 to 3 times every 2 weeks until surgical excision could be safely performed. No therapy was provided postoperatively.

Findings.—Fifty percent of the 28 patients undergoing chemotherapy for unresectable neuroblastoma had an objective response. The remainder had no response and were given second-line chemotherapy. In 38 patients undergoing surgery, including 14 after chemotherapy alone, resection was complete in 23. Four patients had local relapses. At a median follow-up of 55 months, survival and event-free survival were 100% and 90%, respectively.

Conclusions.—Primary low-dose chemotherapy without anthracyclines is effective in approximately half of infants with unresectable NB and no N-*myc* amplification. Excellent survival rates can be achieved without jeopardizing long-term outcomes, even in nonresponding patients receiving the standard regimen.

▶ The treatment of localized and unresectable neuroblastoma in infants remains a controversial area. Because spontaneous regression of the neuroblastoma has been observed in infants, some investigators have proposed a watch-and-see approach. Such studies have usually involved relatively few patients. Other series have used multiagent chemotherapy with excellent results in terms of response and respectability as well as overall outcome. Nevertheless, there was significant short-term morbidity associated with the regimens and concern over the possibility of long-term adverse sequelae. In the present study patients with localized, unresectable neuroblastoma who were stable and not having neurologic deterioration were treated with low-dose cyclophosphamide (5 mg/kg/d for 5 days) and vincristine (0.05 mg/kg on day 1). This low-dose combination was repeated 2 to 3 more times every 2 weeks until surgical resection was performed. Approximately half of the patients showed significant enough response to allow complete resection and the overall and event-free survival for the entire group of 100% and 90%, respectively. At the very least, this study demonstrates that relatively low-dose chemotherapy can convert half of infants with localized, unresectable neuroblastoma without N-*myc* amplification to a respectable status, a critical outcome for disease control in most of these patients.

R. J. Arceci, MD, PhD

Localized Pelvic Neuroblastoma: Excellent Survival and Low Morbidity With Tailored Therapy—The 10-Year Experience of the French Society of Pediatric Oncology

Leclair M-D, Hartmann O, Heloury Y, et al (Hôpital Mère-Enfant, Nantes, France; Institut Gustave Roussy, Villejuif, France; CHRU Dupuytren, Limoges, France; et al)

J Clin Oncol 22:1689-1695, 2004 14–19

Background.—Only 5% of all neuroblastomas (NBs) occur in the pelvis. The prognosis of pelvic NBs is considered good, but it is not known whether an extra-abdominal location influences the outcome. The outcomes and morbidity in children treated for localized pelvic NBs were reported.

Methods.—All 47 consecutive cases of localized pelvic NBs in children included in 2 French multicenter, prospective studies conducted between 1990 and 1999 were reviewed. Clinical and radiologic evidence was analyzed to determine whether the tumors could be resected. In cases considered unresectable, preoperative primary chemotherapy was administered, consisting of combinations of carboplatin plus etoposide or vincristine plus cyclophosphamide and doxorubicin.

Findings.—At the completion of therapy, 66% of the children were in complete remission. Seven children (15%) had long-term neurologic sequelae, and, in 3, the sequelae were directly attributed to surgery. Forty-four patients were still alive after a median 48 months. A local relapse occurred in 6 children, of whom 4 had subsequent remission. Projected 5-year overall and event-free survival rates were 93% and 84%, respectively. The survival rates of children treated with preoperative chemotherapy were comparable to those undergoing primary surgery, at 80% and 88%, respectively. The extent of surgical resection did not appear to affect outcomes.

Conclusions.—Children with localized pelvic NBs have an excellent survival rate. The efficacy of preoperative chemotherapy suggests that patients should be screened carefully for primary surgery. The risk of neurologic impairment during radical excision needs to be balanced against the good outcomes for children with minimal residual cancer.

▶ A pelvic presentation is infrequent in NBs but has been reported to have a relatively good prognosis. One of the major issues involved in the treatment of such patients is the high incidence of significant adverse sequelae resulting from surgical attempts at complete resection of minimal residual disease. The importance of this careful retrospective review of patients with pelvic NBs is that it shows an excellent outcome for patients with complete resection or with minimal residual disease after surgery. Furthermore, patients who received preoperative chemotherapy had outcomes similar to those treated with primary surgery (80% and 88%, respectively). These results suggest that primary surgery should be the approach for such patients whenever possible, and, although complete resection should be the goal, leaving minimal residual disease is preferable to producing adverse postoperative functional complications with the aim of completely removing these tumors.

R. J. Arceci, MD, PhD

Loss of Caspase-8 Protein Expression Correlates With Unfavorable Survival Outcome in Childhood Medulloblastoma

Pingoud-Meier C, Lang D, Janss AJ, et al (Univ Children's Hosp of Zurich, Switzerland; Children's Hosp of Philadelphia)

Clin Cancer Res 9:6401-6409, 2003 14–20

Background.—A recent study of medulloblastoma cell lines demonstrated that resistance to tumor necrosis factor (TNF)-related apoptosis-inducing ligand-induced apoptosis correlated with loss of caspase-8 mRNA expression because of aberrant gene methylation. In addition, loss of caspase-8 mRNA expression has been reported in a subset of primary medulloblastoma. Primary medulloblastoma samples were investigated to determine whether loss of caspases is associated with survival outcome.

Methods.—Tumor samples were obtained from 77 children with well-characterized medulloblastoma and paraffin embedded for analysis. Immunohistochemistry was used to assess protein expression of the key initiator caspase-8 and caspase-9. Expression levels of caspase-8 and caspase-9 were compared with apoptosis indexes, clinical variables, and survival outcomes.

Findings.—Weak caspase-8 expression was detected in 16% of the medulloblastoma samples and weak caspase-9 expression in 24%. Weak caspase-8 expression significantly and independently predicted unfavorable progression-free survival outcomes (Fig 1). This variable was more predictive than standard clinical factors. However, expression of caspase-9 was not a prognostic indicator. When caspase-8-deficient medulloblastoma cells were treated with interferon-γ, there was a dose-dependent restoration of caspase-8 mRNA and protein expression and restoration of TNF-related apoptosis-inducing ligand sensitivity.

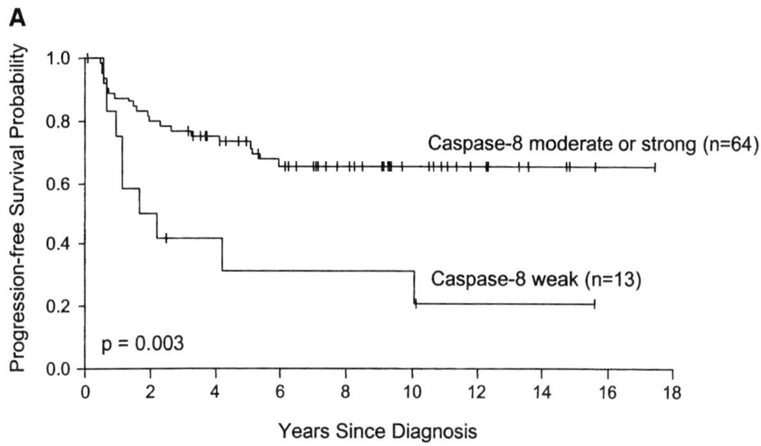

FIGURE 1.—Caspase-8 protein expression and survival. Kaplan-Meier curves show probability of progression-free survival in terms of levels of expression of caspase-8 protein determined by immunohistochemistry. Survival curves were analyzed by log-rank test. (Courtesy of Pingoud-Meier C, Lang D, Janss AJ, et al: Loss of caspase-8 protein expression correlates with unfavorable survival outcome in childhood medulloblastoma. *Clin Cancer Res* 9:6401-6409, 2003.)

Conclusions.—Loss of initiator caspase-8 appears to correlate with unfavorable survival outcomes in children with medulloblastoma. Restoring caspase-8 with interferon-γ therapy may be a novel experimental treatment for such patients.

► The regulation of cell death pathways in cancer is an important component of therapeutic success or failure. In particular, regulators of apoptosis, such as the caspase family of effector proteins, are fundamental to tumor cell killing. Previous reports have shown that that there is downregulation of the critically important caspase-8 in a variety of solid tumors. This decreased expression is sometimes due to epigenetic silencing of the caspase-8 promoter, thus leading to decreased ability of a cell to undergo apoptotic death. The study by Pingoud-Meier et al shows that decreased caspase-8 expression, as detected semiquantitatively by immunohistochemical methods, is strongly correlated with a worse outcome in patients with medulloblastoma. While the numbers of patients are relatively small and this is a retrospective study, the results are particularly interesting in light of the ability of interferon-γ to upregulate caspase-8 in medulloblastoma cell lines. If confirmed on more cell lines or xenograft models, these observations would certainly be a reasonable foundation on which to build future clinical testing.

R. J. Arceci, MD, PhD

Progression-Free Survival in Children With Optic Pathway Tumors: Dependence on Age and the Quality of the Response to Chemotherapy—Results of the First French Prospective Study for the French Society of Pediatric Oncology

Laithier V, Grill J, Le Deley M-C, et al (Institut Gustave Rousy, Villejuif, France; Univ Hosp, Besançon, France; Roger Salengro Hosp, France; et al)
J Clin Oncol 21:4572-4578, 2003 14–21

Introduction.—Optic pathway tumors (OPTs) account for 5% of childhood brain tumors, with about 65% arising in children younger than 5 years of age. OPTs are typically low-grade astrocytomas, yet their behavior is highly unpredictable. It can range between spontaneous regression to progressive visual and neurologic impairment culminating in death. Because of long-term radiation-induced side effects, chemotherapy has been proposed to postpone or avoid radiotherapy (RT), particularly in young children. A strategy focused on avoiding RT during first-line treatment in children with progressive OPT by exclusively administering multiagent chemotherapy during 16 months was evaluated in 85 children in a multicenter nationwide trial.

Methods.—Between 1990 and 1998, 85 children with progressive OPT underwent chemotherapy every 3 weeks alternating procarbazine plus carboplatin, etaposide plus cisplatin, and vincristine plus cyclophosphamide. On relapse or progression, second-line chemotherapy was authorized before recourse to RT.

Results.—The objective response rate (partial response [PR] + complete response [CR]), 5-year progression-free survival (PFS), overall survival, and 5-year RT-free survival rates were 42%, 34%, 89%, and 61%, respectively. Multivariate analysis of the 85 patients who entered the trial showed that factors linked with the risk of disease progression were age younger than 1 year at diagnosis ($P = .47$) and absence of neurofibromatosis type 1 (NF1) ($P = .035$). Multivariate analysis of the 74 patients who remained in the trial after the first cycle of chemotherapy showed that factors linked with the risk of disease progression were age younger than 1 year at diagnosis ($P = .0053$) and no objective response to chemotherapy ($P = .0029$). Three-year PFS was 44% in infants 1 year or younger and 55% in children over age 1 year. The 3-year PFS was 53% in the absence of an objective response to chemotherapy, compared with 68% after a PR or CR.

Conclusion.—A significant percentage of children with OPT can avoid RT after prolonged chemotherapy. Overall survival and visual function were not compromised because of deferring irradiation with chemotherapy protocols.

► The clinical behavior of OPTs represents an often difficult clinical situation in terms of how best to treat patients at diagnosis and progression. These tumors, while usually low-grade gliomas, can regress or progress, the latter situation leading to visual impairment and loss as well as death. Because OPTs often affect young children as well as patients with NF1, avoidance of radiotherapy whenever possible is desirable. In this prospective study by Laithier et al, 85 children with OPTs were monitored for outcome, risk factors, and response to chemotherapy. Patients were observed until progression at which time they were treated with 3 rounds of chemotherapy, including procarbazine and carboplatin (course A), etoposide and cisplatin (course B), and vincristine and cyclophosphamide (course C). A 42% objective response rate was observed to chemotherapy resulting in an overall survival rate of 89% at 5 years. Importantly, the 5-year RT-free survival rate was 61%, indicating that there are indeed subgroups of patients who may avoid RT. The greatest risk factors for progression included age less than 1 year and NF1. Of note is that even though patients responded to chemotherapy, all patients eventually progressed, usually within 3 years after starting treatment. Thus, chemotherapy may be looked upon as a method to delay radiation, but not curative. Improving chemotherapeutic approaches or novel alternatives remains an important future challenge for these patients.

R. J. Arceci, MD, PhD

Outcome of Children With Centrally Reviewed Low-Grade Gliomas Treated With Chemotherapy With or Without Radiotherapy on Children's Cancer Group High-Grade Glioma Study CCG-945

Fouladi M, Hunt DL, Pollack IF, et al (St Jude Children's Research Hosp, Memphis, Tenn; Univ of Pittsburgh, Pa; Children's Hosp of Pittsburgh, Pa; et al)

Cancer 98:1243-1252, 2003 14–22

Background.—Approximately one third of all childhood CNS tumors are low-grade gliomas. The outcomes of children undergoing chemotherapy and radiotherapy on the Children's Cancer Group high-grade gliomas protocol diagnosed with low-grade gliomas on post hoc pathologic review were reported. Clinical and biologic features associated with prognosis were identified.

Methods.—Two hundred fifty children with high-grade gliomas were enrolled in the study between 1995 and 1991. Children older than 24 months with intracranial lesions were randomly assigned to the control regimen, consisting of lomustine, vincristine, and prednisone, or to the experimental regimen, the "8 drugs in 1 day" regimen. Children younger than 24 months and those with primary spinal cord tumors were nonrandomly placed in the experimental regimen group. Seventy patients reclassified as having low-grade gliomas were the focus of the analysis. The 42 boys and 28 girls had a median age of 7.7 years. The median follow-up was 10.4 years.

Findings.—The progression-free survival (PFS) rate at 5 years was 63%, and overall survival was 79%. In the rest of the cohort, PFS and overall survival rates were 19% and 22%, respectively. Children younger than 24 months, those with fibrillary astrocytoma, and those with posterior fossa tumors had a significantly lower 5-year PFS. Compared with children with low-grade gliomas treated with contemporary chemotherapy-alone approaches, the remainder had a modest improvement in PFS with no improvement in overall survival rates.

Conclusions.—Aggressive front-line combined chemotherapy does not appear to produce a survival advantage in children with centrally reviewed low-grade gliomas. The current study underscores the importance of central pathologic review in large multicenter studies of children with gliomas.

▶ The management of children with primary CNS malignancies remains an immense challenge both in terms of delivering effective treatment as well as reducing adverse late sequelae. The study by Fouladi et al is interesting in this regard because it raises important issues of accurate pathologic review. Their analysis focuses on patients treated on the high-grade gliomas protocol CCG 945 who actually were diagnosed with low-grade gliomas on post hoc central pathologic review. Patients greater than 24 months of age were randomized to receive lomustine, vincristine, and prednisone (the standard regimen) or a more intensive "8 drugs in 1 day" regimen (the experimental regimen). Patients younger than 24 months of age received the experimental regimen. The results show that the outcome was not different between the standard and more intensive experimental regimen, strongly suggesting that this type of strategy is not the proper direction to follow in future trials. As expected, young age (younger patients did worse than older patients), histology (high-grade gliomas did worse than low-grade gliomas), and location (hemispheric tumors had better prognosis than posterior fossa tumors) were all important prognostic factors. In contrast to previous reports, p53 expression level or mutations were not correlated with outcome. MIG-1 labeling index also was not associated with a particular outcome. This report is important for several reasons, including the demonstration that intensification did not alter outcome and the importance of several prognostic factors. One of the most interesting aspects of the findings is the reclassification of 28% of patients who were initially diagnosed and treated as if they had high-grade gliomas but were subsequently believed to have low-grade gliomas. This raises important ethical and legal issues, but also the importance of correct pathologic diagnosis in the conduct of clinical trials. Unfortunately, it is not clear what the answers are to these questions.

R. J. Arceci, MD, PhD

Patterns of Failure Using a Conformal Radiation Therapy Tumor Bed Boost for Medulloblastoma

Wolden SL, Dunkel IJ, Souweidane MM, et al (Mem Sloan-Kettering Cancer Ctr, New York)

J Clin Oncol 21:3079-3083, 2003 14–23

Background.—The most common malignant brain tumor in children is medulloblastoma. Traditionally, treatment for medulloblastoma has included surgery followed by craniospinal radiation therapy with a high-dose boost to the entire posterior fossa (PF). In recent years, the practice of delivering high-dose radiation therapy to the entire PF in this patient population has been challenged. The patterns of failure for patients with medulloblastoma receiving a conformal tumor bed boost rather than a boost to the entire PF were determined.

Methods.—Thirty-two consecutive patients with newly diagnosed medulloblastoma at 1 center were enrolled in the study between 1994 and 2002. Median age was 9 years, with a range of 3 to 34 years. Twenty-seven patients were judged to have standard-risk disease and 5 to have high-risk disease. All received a conformal boost to the tumor bed along with craniospinal radiation therapy. Craniospinal doses ranged from 23.4 to 39.6 Gy. Total tumor bed doses ranged from 54 to 59.4 Gy. In addition, 28 patients underwent chemotherapy. Median follow-up was 56 months.

Findings.—Relapses occurred in 6 patients during follow-up, 5 outside the PF and 1 within the PF outside the high-dose boost volume. At 5 years, the actuarial disease-free survival rate was 84% and the overall survival rate was 85%. Freedom from PF failure was 100% at 5 years and 86% at 10 years. Freedom from distant failure at 5 years was 84%. There was a trend toward improvement when full-dose craniospinal radiation, 36 to 39.6 Gy, was applied compared with a reduced dose of 23.4 Gy.

Conclusions.—Critical structures are significantly spared through the use of conformal treatment to the tumor bed in patients with medulloblastoma. The PF failure rate in the current study is comparable to failure rates associated with treatment of the entire PF. A phase III trial is now needed to further investigate this approach.

▶ The development of conformal radiation approaches for CNS tumors has been viewed as a major hope for reducing PF radiation exposure in children with medulloblastoma, thus potentially resulting in reduced adverse short- and long-term adverse toxicities. The report by Wolden et al provides encouraging data from a pilot study in which 32 patients with newly diagnosed medulloblastoma received a conformal boost of radiation to the tumor bed in conjunction with craniospinal radiation. Although not a randomized comparison with patients who received radiation to the entire PF, the results are promising. They show a 5-year disease-free survival rate of 84% and a 100% freedom from PF failure at 5 years and 86% at 10 years. There was a suggestion that patients who received full-dose craniospinal radiation had an improved survival than patients receiving a reduced dose of craniospinal radiation. While such data appear to be encouraging, this study was not designed to directly and prospectively compare conformal dosing to entire PF treatment, thus compromising any definitive conclusions. One might therefore ask whether an alternative strategy would be to perform the randomized trial with strict stopping rules for evidence of increased local or distant relapse rates. This study is now being performed in the Children's Oncology Group, unfortunately years after conformal approaches have been readily available.

R. J. Arceci, MD, PhD

Intravenous RNA Interference Gene Therapy Targeting the Human Epidermal Growth Factors Receptor Prolongs Survival in Intracranial Brain Cancer

Zhang Y, Zhang Y, Bryant J, et al (Univ of California, Los Angeles; California and Armagen Technologies, Inc, Santa Monica)

Clin Cancer Res 10:3667-3677, 2004 14–24

Introduction.—The human epidermal growth factor (EGFR) has an oncogenic role in solid cancer, including brain cancer. The ability of a weekly IV injection of nonviral gene therapy that causes RNA interference (RNAi) of EGFR gene expression to prolong survival in mice with intracranial human brain cancer was examined.

Methods.—Human U87 gliomas were implanted in the brain of adult scid mice. Weekly IV gene therapy was initiated on day 5 after implantation of 500,000 cells. An expression plasmid encoding a short hairpin RNA (shRNA) directed at nucleotides 2529-2557 within the human EGFR messenger RNA was encapsulated in pegylated immunoliposomes, which were targeted to brain cancer with 2 receptor-specific monoclonal antibodies (MAbs): the murine 83-14 MAb to the human insulin receptor and the rat 8D3 to the mouse transferrin receptor.

Results.—In cultured glioma cells, the delivery of the RNAi expression plasmid resulted in a 95% suppression of EGFR function, as determined by measurement of thymidine incorporation or intracellular calcium signaling. Weekly IV RNAi gene therapy caused decreased tumor expression of immunoreactive EGFR and an 88% increase in survival time of mice with advanced intracranial brain cancer.

Conclusion.—Weekly IV nonviral RNAi gene therapy directed against the human EGFR is a new therapeutic approach to silencing oncogenic genes in solid cancers. This is possible using a nonviral gene transfer technology that delivers liposome-encapsulated plasmid DNA across cellular barriers with receptor-specific targeting ligands.

► We are always proposing the need for novel, targeted, less toxic, and more effective therapies. The report by Zhang et al presents an intriguing approach to cancer treatment by combining several different strategies rather than just one. Their interest is in high-grade brain cancers, but their approach may be applicable in a variety of other settings. The first take advantage of inhibitory shRNAs designed to downregulate EGFR expression. They clone this shRNA into an expression vector for transduction into tumor cells. The expression could have a tumor-specific promoter if desired. Their delivery system is a pegylated immunoliposome that has monoclonal antibodies against the human insulin receptor and the murine transferring receptor. Thus, this "smart bomb" has targeting selectivity at several levels providing a potentially useful approach to cancer treatment, especially for tumors restricted in particular anatomic compartments such as brain tumors. Although this technology may be in its early phases, there should be considerable excitement about such clever, truly novel therapeutic approaches.

R. J. Arceci, MD, PhD

Microarray-Based Screening for Molecular Markers in Medulloblastoma Revealed *STK15* as Independent Predictor for Survival

Neben K, Korshunov A, Benner A, et al (Deutsches Krebsforschungszentrum, Heidelberg, Germany; NN Burdenko Neurosurgical Inst, Moscow)
Cancer Res 64:3103-3111, 2004 14–25

Background.—Medulloblastoma is one of the most common CNS malignancies in children. Despite aggressive multimodal treatment, 5-year survival rates associated with this primitive neuroectodermal tumor of the cerebellum approach only 50% to 60%. Candidate genes predicting overall survival were sought in children with medulloblastomas.

Methods.—Gene expression profiling analysis was conducted in 35 newly diagnosed medulloblastomas. The 9 most promising candidate genes were then evaluated with the use of immunohistochemical analysis and fluorescence in situ hybridization on tumor tissue microarrays representing 180 tumors.

Findings.—Fifty-four genes with expression levels predictive of unfavorable survival rates were identified. Positive staining for STK15, stathmin 1, and cyclin D1 correlated with an unfavorable overall survival rate. By contrast, cyclin B1, DAXX, Ki-67, MYC, NRAS, and p53 did not have a significant effect. Compared with clinical variables such as sex, age, metastatic stage, the extent of tumor resection, the use of chemotherapy, and the tumor grade, positive STK15 staining was an independent prognostic indicator for overall survival. Additional gene copy numbers of *MYC* and *STK15* predicted poor survival rates.

Conclusions.—In this study, the combination of gene expression profiling with tissue microarray experiments enabled identification of a series of candidate genes predicting survival in cases of medulloblastoma. Genes associated with cell proliferation, transcription, and, especially, mitosis as pathomechanisms of medulloblastoma warrant further investigation.

► Medulloblastomas remain a significant problem for children, both in terms of survival as well as adverse late sequelae. In addition to identifying very high-risk patients for whom alternative therapeutic approaches could be used, defining prognostic indicators might also allow reduced therapy in some children, thus potentially avoiding treatment-related toxic effects. Neben et al performed an extensive analysis of RNA expression patterns using microarray analysis on 35 newly diagnosed medulloblastoma specimens. Importantly, they confirmed differences in RNA expression using tissue microarray immunohistochemical analysis on 185 additional specimens. Positively detected by immunohistochemical analysis, cyclin D1, STK15 and stathmin all correlated with a poor prognosis. Interestingly, although MYC expression was not associated with a poor outcome, additional gene copy numbers of *MYC* did show such an association, which suggests that other genes amplified with *MYC* might be responsible for the association with poor survival. These data need to be confirmed, particularly on an independent data set, but this study provides an excellent starting point for a better definition of risk grouping in patients with medulloblastomas in addition to or in replacement of conventional staging procedures.

R. J. Arceci, MD, PhD

Late Effects

Risk of Secondary Leukemia After a Solid Tumor in Childhood According to the Dose of Epipodophyllotoxins and Anthracyclines: A Case-Control Study by the Société Française d'Oncologie Pédiatrique

Le Deley M-C, Leblanc T, Shamsaldin A, et al (Institut Gustave-Roussy, Villejuif, France; Hôpital Saint-Louis, Paris; INSERM Unit 521, Villejuif, France; et al)

J Clin Oncol 21:1074-1081, 2003 14–26

Background.—An increased risk of leukemia has been reported in patients treated with high cumulative doses of epipodophyllotoxins weekly or twice weekly in childhood. Secondary leukemias have also been reported after anthracycline treatment. The risk of secondary leukemia as a function of the dose of epipodophyllotoxins and anthracyclines was estimated.

Methods.—The risk of secondary leukemia or myelodysplasia after a solid tumor in childhood was investigated by survey sent to all French regional cancer registries and all investigators in a pediatric oncology professional society in France. The case-control study included 61 patients with leukemia and 196 matched control subjects. The 2 groups were compared for characteristics of the first cancer, the patient's family history of cancer, and treatment.

Findings.—In a multivariate analysis, only 2 factors were found to increase the risk of leukemia: the type of the first tumor and exposure to epipodophyllotoxins and anthracyclines. Risk was increased in patients who had had Hodgkin's disease (relative risk, 6.4) and in those with osteosarcoma (relative risk, 5.0). Patients receiving 1.2 to 6 g/m^2 of epipodophyllotoxins or greater than 170 mg/m^2 anthracyclines had a leukemia risk 7-fold higher than those receiving lower doses or none of these drugs. In patients receiving more than 6 g/m^2 of epipodophyllotoxins, the risk of leukemia was multiplied by 197. Exposure to alkylating agents or radiotherapy did not appear to increase leukemia risk.

Conclusions.—These data provide further evidence that epipodophyllotoxins and anthracyclines increase the risk of secondary leukemia in patients surviving a solid tumor in childhood. The mutagenic effects of these drugs must be minimized by decreasing cumulative doses without compromising therapeutic benefits.

► The development of secondary leukemias due to exposure to treatment in patients with solid tumors is a tragic outcome. Thus, a better understanding of the risks for developing these secondary leukemias is extremely important. The study by Le Deley et al presents some relevant data on this issue. They conducted a case-control study on children who developed leukemia after being treated for a variety of solid tumors. In a multivariate analysis, they found that the type of initial malignancy (ie, Hodgkin's disease and osteosarcoma) and the exposure to epipodophyllotoxins and anthracyclines were the 2 strongest risk factors. Doses of anthracyclines of more than 170 mg/m^2 of doxorubicin or equivalent resulted in a 7-fold relative risk. The relative risk associated with greater than 6 g/m^2 of epipodophyllotoxins was 197. Unfortunately, this study was not able to distinguish the consequences of cumulative dose versus schedule for epipodophyllotoxin use and risk. Of interest, no association was observed for exposure to alkylating agents or radiation exposure. Clearly, the results indicating increased risk for patients with Hodgkin's disease and osteosarcoma strongly suggest a predisposition, which should be an area of important future investigations. Further, the cumulative doses generating increased risk of secondary leukemia of epipodophyllotoxins and, particularly, anthracyclines are often reached during treatment regimens. These results should stimulate investigators to continue to search for ways to reduce or eliminate the need for such exposures through the identification of efficacious, nongenotoxic agents.

R. J. Arceci, MD, PhD

High Risk of Subsequent Neoplasms Continues With Extended Follow-up of Childhood Hodgkin's Disease: Report From the Late Effects Study Group

Bhatia S, Yasui Y, Robison LL, et al (City of Hope Natl Med Ctr, Duarte, Calif; Univ of Minnesota, Minneapolis; Royal Manchester Children's Hosp, England; et al)

J Clin Oncol 21:4386 4394, 2003 14–27

Background.—The Late Effects Study Group investigation of a cohort of 1380 children with Hodgkin's disease (HD) diagnosed between 1955 and 1986 has been previously reported. The current update of that study focused on the pattern and incidence of subsequent neoplasms (SNs) during extended follow-up.

Methods.—The patients were diagnosed between 0.3 and 16.9 years of age, with a median of 11.7 years. The median age at latest follow-up was 27.8 years. Patients were followed up for a median of 17 years.

Findings.—By the latest follow-up, 103 additional SNs had been diagnosed, for a total of 212 SNs since the initial diagnosis. The risk of developing SNs in the cohort, compared with the general population, was increased 18.5 fold. The cumulative incidence of any second malignancy occurring at 20 years was 10.6%, increasing to 26.3% by 30 years. The cumulative incidence of solid malignancies at 20 years was 7.3%, rising to 23.5% at 30

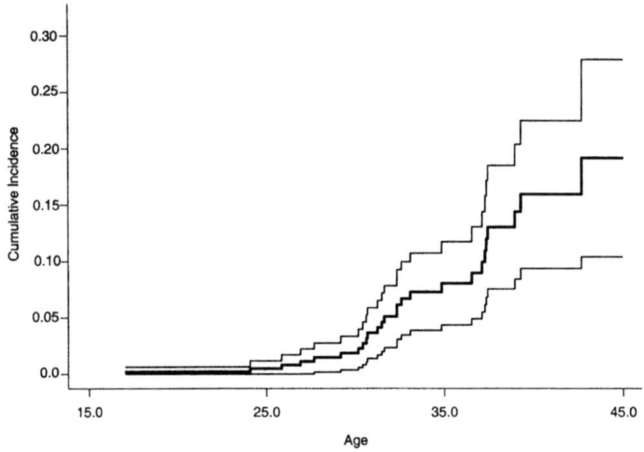

FIGURE 2.—Cumulative incidence (*middle line*) of breast cancer as a function of age of cohort of female survivors of Hodgkin's disease, with 95% confidence intervals (*upper and lower curves*). (Courtesy of Bhatia S, Yasui Y, Robison LL, et al: High risk of subsequent neoplasms continues with extended follow-up of childhood Hodgkin's disease: Report from the Late Effects Study Group. *J Clin Oncol* 21:4386-4394, 2003. Reprinted with permission from the American Society of Clinical Oncology.)

years. The most common solid malignancy was breast cancer, with a standardized incidence ratio (SIR) of 56.7 (Fig 2). Bone tumors had an SIR of 37.1; thyroid cancer, 36.4; colorectal cancer, 36.4; and lung cancer, 27.3. Gastric cancers had an SIR of 63.9. Young age at HD diagnosis and receipt of radiation-based therapy were risk factors for solid tumors. A third neoplasm developed in 32 patients, the cumulative incidence approaching 21% 10 years from the diagnosis of second malignancy.

Conclusions.—Further follow-up of this large cohort of HD survivors has revealed an increasing occurrence of known radiation-associated solid tumors, such as breast and thyroid cancers. In addition, epithelial neoplasms common in adults emerged at a younger age in the cohort than in the general population. Thus, ongoing surveillance of this high-risk population is necessary.

► While updates of previous study results are usually not worth taking much notice of, the report by Bhatia et al presents some important results in terms of secondary malignancies in patients treated for HD. This update at 30 years of 1380 children treated for HD diagnosed between 1955 and 1986 shows the continued increased in the frequency of radiation-related solid tumors, particularly breast cancer. At 30 years, the cumulative incidence of developing a second cancer is 26.3%, increased from 10.6% observed at 20 years' follow-up. The same previous risk factors were again identified as young age at the time of diagnosis and the use of a radiation-based treatment. Of further interest, the risk of leukemia reached a plateau at 14 years and showed an approximately 2% 30-year cumulative incidence compared with solid tumors, which continue to show an increased cumulative incidence now reaching 23.5% at 30 years. A great deal has changed in the treatment of patients with HD over the last 50 years. It will therefore be critically important to evaluate patients treated with more modern approaches to determine whether we are in fact improving the overall outcome of patients with this usually very curable cancer.

R. J. Arceci, MD, PhD

Cancerous Stem Cells Can Arise From Pediatric Brain Tumors

Hemmati HD, Nakano I, Lazareff JA, et al (California Inst of Technology, Pasadena; Univ of California, Los Angeles)

Proc Natl Acad Sci U S A 100:15178-15183, 2003 14–28

Introduction.—The cellular origin of pediatric brain tumors (PBTs) is not known. It is possible that they derive from self-renewing multipotent neural stem cells. Pediatric brain tumor and nontumor human brain specimens from patients undergoing neocortical resections for intractable epilepsy were evaluated to determine whether different PBTs, including medulloblastomas and gliomas, contain cells with properties similar to neural stem cells.

Findings.—Tumor-derived progenitors form neurospheres that can be passaged at clonal density; they have the ability to self-renew. Under conditions promoting differentiation, individual cells are multipotent, giving rise to both neurons and glia, in proportions that demonstrate the tumor of origin. Unlike normal neural stem cells, tumor-derived progenitors have an unusual ability to proliferate; these sometimes differentiate into abnormal cells with multiple differentiation markers. Gene expression analysis showed that both whole tumors and tumor-derived neurospheres express several gene characteristics of neural and other stem cells, including CD133, *Sox2*, musashi-1, *bmi-1*, maternal embryonic leucine zipper kinase, and phosphoserine phosphatase, with variation from tumor to tumor. After grafting to neonatal rat brains, tumor-derived neurosphere cells migrate, generate neurons and glia, and continue to proliferate for more than 4 weeks.

Conclusion.—PBTs contain neural stem-like cells with altered characteristics that may augment tumorigenesis. This may have important implications for treatment concerning specific targeting of stem-like cells within brain tumors.

► The identification of self-renewing cancer stem cells was initially described in the hematopoietic malignancies, particularly in chronic myelogenous and acute myelogenous leukemia. This type of work arose as part of the basic laboratory investigations leading to the identification of normal hematopoietic stem cells. Although the existence of self-renewing stem cells for solid tumors was first proposed in the 1970s, only recently has definitive data on their identification in a variety of solid tumors been characterized. The report from Hemmati et al now describes multipotential and replicative precursor cells for medulloblastoma and gliomas. These studies also demonstrate that these cells have characteristic RNA and protein expression patterns supporting their early lineage status and relation, but not identity, to normal neural stem-like cells. These results are not just important in terms of deepening our understanding of the development of brain tumors, but should also help focus therapeutic approaches on the proper cellular targets.

R. J. Arceci, MD, PhD

Prognosis of Child Recipients of Hematopoietic Stem Cell Transplantation Requiring Intensive Care

Lamas A, Otheo E, Ros P, et al (Hosp Ramón y Cajal, Madrid)

Intensive Care Med 29:91-96, 2003 14–29

Background.—Eleven percent to 40% of bone marrow transplant (BMT) recipients have been reported to need critical care because of the severity of complications after transplantation. Prognostic factors in children requiring critical care after receiving hematopoietic stem cell transplantation from blood or bone marrow were determined.

Methods.—Of 151 children undergoing BMT at 1 center between 1991 and 2000, 44 (29.1%) were admitted to the pediatric ICU a total of 49 times. This cohort was retrospectively analyzed.

Findings.—Thirty-four children, representing 69.4% of all pediatric ICU admissions, required mechanical ventilation (MV). Thirty-one children died, for an overall mortality rate of 70.4%. The death rate was 76.5% in children requiring MV and 50% in those not requiring MV. In a univariate analysis, factors correlating significantly with death were male sex, older age, acute graft versus host disease grades III or IV, severe hemorrhagic cystitis, a diagnosis of lung injury, the need for MV or renal replacement therapy, respiratory failure, cardiovascular failure, gastrointestinal failure, and the failure of 3 or more organs. In a multivariate analysis, independent predictors of death were the presence of acute graft versus host disease grades III or IV, male sex, severe hemorrhagic cystitis, and the failure of 3 or more organs.

Conclusions.—In this series, nearly one third of children undergoing BMT required pediatric ICU admission. The mortality rate among these patients is high. However, some complications are reversible with critical care support. Certain clinical parameters are useful for establishing prognosis and optimizing resource use.

► The prognosis of children undergoing BMT who go to the ICU is usually believed to be grave. However, the factors contributing to that poor outcome are not always clear. Lamas et al examined a cohort of 44 children undergoing BMT who required care in the ICU. The overall mortality rate was high at 70% and most significantly correlated with multiorgan failure, grades III or IV graft versus host disease, and hemorrhagic cystitis. Such information raises several important issues. First, this type of information may be quite helpful in decision making for such patients, their families, and their caretakers when it comes to decisions regarding escalation of care. Second, these data point out that 30% of patients have a much better chance of survival. Third, advances in the prevention of transplant-related complications are likely to be the key to survival, unless new approaches of caring for these severely ill children are developed after the complications have already established themselves.

R. J. Arceci, MD, PhD

The Effect of Dexrazoxane on Myocardial Injury in Doxorubicin-Treated Children With Acute Lymphoblastic Leukemia

Lipshultz SE, Rifai N, Dalton VM, et al (Univ of Miami, Fla; Univ of Rochester, New York; Children's Hosp Boston; et al)

N Engl J Med 351:145-153, 2004 14–30

Background.—Doxorubicin chemotherapy is effective against acute lymphoblastic leukemia (ALL) in children, but it also injures myocardial cells. Dexrazoxane is a free-radical scavenger that may protect the heart from doxorubicin-related damage. Whether dexrazoxane reduced such injury was investigated.

Methods.—A total of 101 children with ALL were assigned to doxorubicin only, 30 mg/m^2 body surface area every 3 weeks for 10 doses; 105 children were assigned to dexrazoxane, 300 mg/M^2, followed immediately by doxorubicin. Serum cardiac troponin T were measured serially in 76 and 82 patients in the dexrazoxane and doxorubicin groups, respectively. A total of 2377 serum samples (mean per patient, 15.1) were acquired before, during, and after doxorubicin treatment.

Findings.—Overall, 35% of patients had increases in troponin T. Children receiving doxorubicin only were more likely to have elevated troponin T concentrations than children receiving dexrazoxane and doxorubicin (50% and 21%, respectively). Thirty-two percent of doxorubicin recipients had extremely elevated troponin T levels compared with 10% of children in

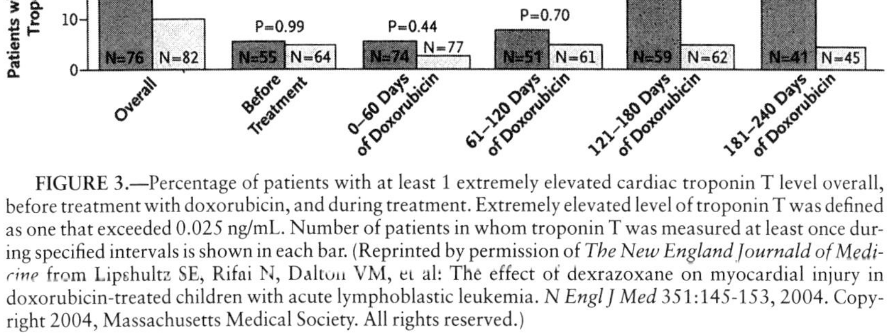

FIGURE 3.—Percentage of patients with at least 1 extremely elevated cardiac troponin T level overall, before treatment with doxorubicin, and during treatment. Extremely elevated level of troponin T was defined as one that exceeded 0.025 ng/mL. Number of patients in whom troponin T was measured at least once during specified intervals is shown in each bar. (Reprinted by permission of *The New England Journald of Medicine* from Lipshultz SE, Rifai N, Dalton VM, et al: The effect of dexrazoxane on myocardial injury in doxorubicin-treated children with acute lymphoblastic leukemia. *N Engl J Med* 351:145-153, 2004. Copyright 2004, Massachusetts Medical Society. All rights reserved.)

the dexrazoxane and doxorubicin group (Fig 3). In both treatment groups, the event-free survival rate at 2.5 years was 83%.

Conclusions.—Dexrazoxane appears to prevent or decrease cardiac injury associated with doxorubicin therapy in children with ALL. A smaller proportion of children receiving dexrazoxane and doxorubicin had increased troponin T than children receiving doxorubicin alone. The addition of dexrazoxane does not appear to compromise the antileukemic efficacy of doxorubicin. A longer follow-up is needed to establish the effects of dexrazoxane on echocardiographic results at 4 years and on event-free survival.

► The prevention of both short- and long-term treatment-related toxicities continues to be a major goal of improving the treatment of patients with cancer. This report is a randomized study testing the ability of the antioxidant agent dexrazoxane to serve as a cardioprotectant in children with high-risk ALL exposed to anthracyclines. Cardiac damage was measured by using the surrogate marker troponin T. Thirty-five percent (55 of the 158 patients) had elevated troponin T levels. The results show that patients who received dexrazoxane were less likely (21%) to have elevated troponin T levels than those who did not receive dexrazoxane (50%). The study also shows no difference in event-free survival between the 2 groups, although the follow-up is still relatively short and it is unclear that the curves have reached plateau. In addition, approximately 20% of patients were eliminated from the analysis because samples for troponin T levels were not available. It is also of some interest why the elevations in troponin T levels were significant in comparing groups only after 60 days of treatment and not earlier. While troponin T levels are commonly used to measure cardiac damage, it is unclear if the differences in levels measured in this trial will be clinically relevant. Thus, critical issues will be whether in this study future clinical outcomes in terms of cardiac function and leukemia cure rates are different between the 2 groups. This will clearly be an important study group of patients to follow and hear about for a long time.

R. J. Arceci, MD, PhD

Long-term Event-Free Survival After Intense Chemotherapy for Ewing's Family of Tumors in Children and Young Adults

Kolb EA, Kushner BH, Gorlick R, et al (Mem Sloan-Kettering Cancer Ctr, New York)

J Clin Oncol 21:3423-3430, 2003 14–31

Background.—Ewing's family of tumors (EFTs) include bone and soft tissue sarcomas mostly affecting children and young adults. The potential of high-dose, short-term chemotherapy to improve long-term event-free survival in patients with EFTs was investigated.

Methods.—Between 1991 and 2001, 68 previously untreated patients were enrolled in the prospective trial. All patients were newly diagnosed as having EFTs. Disease was local-regional in 44 patients at diagnosis. The remaining 24 had distant metastases at presentation. Treatment consisted of 7 cycles of chemotherapy. In cycles 1, 2, 3, and 6, cyclophosphamide 2100 mg/m^2 per day was given on days 1 and 2, with a 72-hour continuous infusion of doxorubicin, 75 mg/m^2, and vincristine, 2 mg/m^2, beginning on day 1. In cycles 4, 5, and 7, ifosfamide, 1800 mg/m^2 per day, and etoposide, 100 mg/m^2 per day, were given on 5 consecutive days.

Findings.—Patients with local-regional disease at diagnosis had an 82% event-free survival (EFS) at 4 years. Overall survival was 89%. For patients with distant metastases, the 4-year EFS rate was 12%, with an overall survival of 17.8%. Disease progressed during treatment in 4 patients with distant metastases and in none of those with local-regional disease.

Conclusions.—Intensive chemotherapy for local-regional EFTs in children and young adults can produce sustained EFS and overall survival rates. Unfortunately, this approach is not very effective in patients with metastatic disease.

▶ The use of adjuvant chemotherapy in patients with localized sarcomas has been an important key to the eradication of micrometastatic disease and the overall success of treatment. However, patients with more advanced disease have not benefited nearly as much, and their outcome remains grim. Alternative approaches to therapy, particularly using intensification of chemotherapy timing and dosing, have therefore been tried. The study by Kolb et al attempts to use high-dose, short-term intensified chemotherapy for patients with EFT that was locoregional or metastatic. As with other such studies, the outcome for patients with locoregional disease had a very good outcome overall with 89% survival at 4 years. However, patients with overt metastatic disease had a 17.8% 4-year survival. These results, along with those of other reports, strongly argue for a significant paradigm shift in the approach to therapy for patients with metastatic EFT. Such strategies could certainly utilize a conventional chemotherapy backbone but should begin to include novel biologic agents and immunotherapeutic approaches. Too many years have gone by testing different approaches with conventional therapy, resulting in the same poor outcomes to justify further studies of this type in this very high-risk group of patients.

R. J. Arceci, MD, PhD

Enalapril to Prevent Cardiac Function Decline in Long-term Survivors of Pediatric Cancer Exposed to Anthracyclines

Silber JH, Cnaan A, Clark BJ, et al (Children's Hosp of Philadelphia; Univ of Pennsylvania, Philadelphia; Children's Hosp Cincinnati, Ohio; et al)

J Clin Oncol 22:820-828, 2004 14–32

Background.—Almost 70% of all children with a malignancy survive in the long term. However, this impressive cure rate relies on intensive treatments associated with significant side effects. An estimated half of all patients exposed to anthracyclines subsequently have cardiac abnormalities.

Whether enalapril, an angiotensin-converting enzyme, can prevent deterioration in cardiac function in long-term survivors of childhood cancer was investigated.

Methods.—One hundred thirty-five long-term survivors of pediatric malignancies were enrolled in the randomized, double-blind, controlled clinical trial. All participants had at least 1 cardiac abnormality identified after their exposure to anthracycline. Sixty-nine participants were assigned to enalapril and 66 to placebo. The mean ages in these 2 groups were 17.8 and 18.9 years, respectively. The median follow-up was 2.8 years, ranging from 2 weeks to 6.1 years.

Findings.—The 2 treatment groups did not differ in rate of change in maximal cardiac index per year. In the first treatment year, however, the rate of change in left ventricular end-systolic wall stress (LVESWS) was higher in the enalapril recipients than in the placebo recipients. This difference persisted over the course of the study, leading to a 9% decrease in estimated LVESWS by year 5 in patients taking enalapril. Six of the 7 patients who had to leave the study because of cardiac deterioration were initially in the placebo group. One of these patients subsequently died of heart failure. Adverse effects associated with enalapril were dizziness or hypotension in 22% and fatigue in 10%.

Conclusions.—Enalapril in these long-term childhood cancer survivors exposed to anthracycline reduced LVESWS in the first year of treatment. This decrease was maintained over the study period. Enalapril therapy did not affect exercise performance. Clinicians must weigh the theoretical benefits of LVESWS reduction against the potential adverse effects associated with angiotensin-converting enzyme inhibitors.

► The risk of cardiac damage and clinical heart failure after exposure of patients, particularly children, with anthracyclines for the treatment of cancer remains a major concern. Because of the significant concerns over heart failure in patients receiving anthracyclines, strategies to reduce the dose or the use of cardioprotectants during anthracycline exposure have been tested. However, despite the exploration of such strategies, significant numbers of patients continue to require anthracyclines as a component of curative treatment. The study by Silber et al attempts to reduce the long-term adverse affects of anthracycline exposure with the use of the angiotensin-converting enzyme inhibitor enalapril. They performed a randomized, double-blind, controlled trial comparing enalapril to placebo in 135 long-term survivors of pediatric cancer who had had at least 1 cardiac problem after anthracycline exposure. While they documented an early and sustained decrease in LVESWS in the enalapril-treated group, this finding did not translate into a significant reduction in clinical heart failure. And although more patients were observed in the placebo group who experienced 2 consecutive declines in cardiac performance, requiring intervention by their cardiologists, this did not reach statistical significance. Thus, even though this trial should have been designed and carried out with the ability to provide a definitive answer as to whether enalapril did or did not improve clinical cardiac outcome in this group of patients, it instead concluded that LVESWS varied, but that there was insufficient statistical power and long-term follow-up to determine answers to the more important clinical outcome questions. This is not a trial or academic criticism, in that enalapril has significant side-effects that could adversely influence the quality of life of these patients. This study also demonstrates that surrogate markers may provide nice outcome data for publication, but they may not be the definitive answers predicting clinical outcome, the only important outcome for patients.

R. J. Arceci, MD, PhD

Change in Neurocognitive Functioning After Treatment With Cranial Radiation in Childhood

Spiegler BJ, Bouffet E, Greenberg ML, et al (Hosp for Sick Children, Toronto)
J Clin Oncol 22:706-713, 2004 14–33

Background.—CNS tumors, the most common solid tumors in childhood, account for 20% of all malignancies in children. Most of these tumors need radiation therapy for effective control. The pattern of stability and change of neurocognitive functioning over time in irradiated survivors of posterior fossa (PF) tumors was investigated.

Methods.—Thirty-four children treated for malignant PF tumors were followed up with serial clinical neuropsychologic examinations. Thirty patients had medulloblastoma and 21 had ependymoma. Treatment consisted of reduced doses of cranial radiation in 12 patients and standard doses of cranial radiation in 21, all with additional boosts to the PF. One child received PF radiation only.

Findings.—The patients demonstrated a 2- to 4-point decline annually in intelligence scores. Intellectual function dropped quickly in the first few years after therapy and more gradually thereafter. The children were also found to have significant decreases in visual-motor integration, visual memory, verbal fluency, and executive functioning. Verbal memory and receptor vocabulary did not appear to decline.

Conclusions.—Multiple neurocognitive domains appear to decline in children undergoing radiation therapy for PF tumors. The mechanism by which cranial radiation causes such impairment may by understood by examining factors that contribute to the general decrease in functioning but relative stability in specific domains.

► The adverse effects of radiation therapy on the developing CNS have been documented for many years. Unfortunately, in many instances radiation therapy is the only means to a cure, particularly for young patients with high-grade brain tumors. However, detailed and comprehensive studies of neurocognitive functioning over time have been rare. This is why the report by Spiegler et al is of considerable importance. In a group of 34 children with malignant PF tumors, they chronologically studied a variety of functional outcomes, including intelligence quotient. They observed an initial rapid early decrease in intellectual function within the first several years after radiation therapy followed by a more gradual yearly decline over subsequent years. The greatest effect was on intelligence quotient, but other variables such as executive functioning were also affected. No significant changes were observed in visual memory or receptive vocabulary. Although a larger sample size would have significantly added to the study, the results are important in that they demonstrate the pace or rate of decline after radiation therapy over a long period. These data also serve as an important lesson to treating physicians that frequent and long-term follow-up of detailed neurocognitive functioning in children receiving cranial radiation is critical. Last, these data underscore the immense need of finding effective alternatives to radiation therapy.

R. J. Arceci, MD, PhD

Miscellaneous

In Children and Adolescents, the Pharmacodynamics of High-Dose Busulfan Is Dependent on the Second Alkylating Agent Used in the Combined Regimen (Melphalan or Thiotepa)

Bouligand J, Boland I, Valteau-Couanet D, et al (Institut Gustave Roussy, Villejuif, France)

Bone Marrow Transplant 32:979-986, 2003 14–34

Background.—High systemic exposure to busulfan is strongly related to the occurrence of hepatic veno-occlusive disease (HVOD) after a busulfan-cyclophosphamide regimen (BU+CY). The pharmacodynamics of high-dose busulfan combined with either melphalan (BU+MEL) or thiotepa (BU+TTP) followed by autologous stem cell transplantation were determined in children and adolescents with a malignant solid tumor.

Methods.—Forty-five patients, aged a median 6.3 years, were included. Oral busulfan was administered at a total dose of 600 mg/m^2. Twenty-five received BU+MEL and 20 received BU+TTP.

Findings.—The incidence of HVOD in the BU+MEL group and the BU+TTP group was 44% and 25%, respectively. Patients in the BU+TTP group in whom HVOD developed had a significantly greatly area under the curve at 0 to 6 hours after dose 13 compared with patients who did not. In the BU+MEL group, patients with and without HVOD did not differ in their systemic exposure to busulfan.

Conclusions.—No correlation is shown between busulfan exposure and liver toxicity with BU+MEL. This may be caused by a drug interaction between busulfan and melphalan through a glutathione-*S*-transferase/glutathione pathway. Further research is needed.

▶ Some aspects of medicine we take for granted until experimental evidence leads us to a different conclusion. Busulfan is most commonly used as a part of the standard preparative regimen for bone marrow transplantation in combination with cyclophosphamide. Over the past several years, the determination of individualized pharmacokinetic data for busulfan has proven to be both safer and more efficacious in terms of antileukemic activity. By modifying the dosing of busulfan depending on a patient's metabolism of the drug, one can reduce the risk of severe HVOD. Little information has been provided, however, when busulfan is combined with other agents such as melphalan or thiotepa, also commonly used in the transplant setting. In the study by Bouligand et al, pharmacokinetic and toxicity data were determined for both melphalan and thiotepa when used in combination with busulfan. The results showed that important differences exist. For example, the incidence of HVOD was 44% with BU+MEL and 25% with BU+TTP. Although the expected correlation of greater busulfan area under the curve with HVOD was observed with thiotepa, no difference was observed in busulfan area under the curve with those patients who developed HVOD when melphalan was used, suggesting a distinct interaction. The importance of these results is that one cannot assume that combining busulfan with other alkylating agents will necessarily translate into the same toxicity outcome or efficacy profile. It is always worth testing such new combinations from a pharmacokinetic and clinical perspective.

R. J. Arceci, MD, PhD

Randomized Controlled Trial of Once- Versus Thrice-Daily Tobramycin in Febrile Neutropenic Children Undergoing Stem Cell Transplantation

Sung L, Dupuis LL, Bliss B, et al (Univ of Toronto; Hosp for Sick Children, Toronto)

J Natl Cancer Inst 95:1869-1877, 2003 14–35

Background.—The benefits of aminoglycoside antibiotics in the treatment of febrile neutropenia have been reported in many patient populations. However, data on its safety and toxicity for children undergoing stem cell transplantation are lacking. This patient group is at especially high risk of aminoglycoside-related toxicity and infectious morbidity. The relative nephrotoxicity and efficacy of a single daily dose or 3 daily doses of tobramycin were investigated in pediatric recipients of stem cell transplants.

Methods.—Sixty children were enrolled in the double-blind, randomized controlled study between October 2000 and November 2002. All study subjects were 18 years of age or younger and had fevers and neutropenia during stem cell transplantation. Twenty-nine children received IV tobramycin daily, and 31 received IV tobramycin every 8 hours. Tobramycin was combined with piperacillin or ceftazidime in all patients. Doses of tobramycin were adjusted to obtain pharmacokinetic targets.

Findings.—A modified intent-to-treat analysis demonstrated that the mean maximal percent increase in the serum creatinine level was 32% in children receiving the once daily dose and 51% in those receiving 3 doses daily. Among patients assessable for efficacy, 46% in the once-daily dose group and 19% in the thrice-daily dose group survived febrile neutropenia without modifications in antibacterial treatment. One child in each group died.

Conclusions.—A single daily dose of tobramycin appears to be safer than tobramycin delivered every 8 hours in children with febrile neutropenia during stem cell transplantation. The once-daily dose also appears to be more effective. Thus, 1 dose of tobramycin per day should be prescribed for children with febrile neutropenia, including those undergoing stem cell transplantation.

▶ Finding ways to reduce the toxic effects of supportive care, particularly antimicrobial treatments, in severely immunocompromised patients, remains an important challenge. One approach to reducing the nephrotoxic effects of aminoglycoside antibiotics is to deliver them once a day rather than 2 or 3 times a day. The once-daily dosing has been shown to be less toxic, involve less nursing time and resources, and be as efficacious as thrice-daily dosing in patients with cancer.

The study by Sung et al examines this question in a particularly high-risk population of patients who underwent bone marrow transplantation. They performed a "mostly" blind, randomized controlled trial of once- versus thrice-daily tobramycin administration in febrile children with neutropenia undergoing bone marrow transplantation. Two investigators not involved in direct patient care were aware of the dosing regimens for each group so that adjustments could be made in the tobramycin dosing to achieve similar levels in both groups of patients. The analysis showed that the once-daily dosing was less nephrotoxic and equally efficacious in terms of infectious outcomes than the thrice-daily dosing. This study, therefore, provides justification for once-daily dosing of tobramycin in oncology patients as well as in those undergoing bone marrow transplantation.

R. J. Arceci, MD, PhD

Cognitive Outcome of Long-term Survivors of Multisystem Langerhans Cell Histiocytosis: A Single-Institution, Cross-Sectional Study

Nanduri VR, Lillywhite L, Chapman C, et al (Inst of Child Health and Great Ormond Street Hosp, London; Royal Hosp for Sick Children, Edinburgh, Scotland, United Kingdom)

J Clin Oncol 21:2961-2967, 2003 14–36

Background.—Langerhans cell histiocytosis (LCH) has been associated with damage to the CNS, including the cerebellum, as well as to the hypothalamopituitary axis. Neuropsychologic deficits have been reported. Cognitive function in 1 cohort of LCH survivors was systematically assessed.

Methods.—Twenty-eight long-term survivors of multisystem LCH were included in the study. Mean age was 15.1 years. Intelligence, memory and learning, language, and academic level were assessed.

Findings.—The patients' mean intelligence quotient (IQ) did not differ significantly from that of the general population. However, the ranges were wide. CNS involvement was a significant risk factor for lower scores. Patients with CNS involvement had lower verbal, performance, and full-scale IQs than patients with no CNS involvement. Even after adjustment for the effects of reduced full-scale IQ, specific deficits were noted in patients with CNS involvement.

Conclusions.—Significant cognitive deficits may develop in long-term survivors of multisystem LCH, especially those with CNS involvement. Formal, repeated neuropsychologic evaluation should be a part of the long-term follow-up of LCH survivors. Such an approach will allow deficits to be detected early and appropriate supportive measures explored.

▶ Although the etiology of LCH remains unclear, an increasing appreciation for the variability of the short- and long-term clinical manifestations is becoming evident. In particular, the development of CNS disease leading to cerebellar ataxia and neurocognitive deficits is now recognized as a serious and often progressive consequence of having LCH and not related to treatment. The report by Nanduri et al documents detailed observations on a variety of neurocognitive outcomes in patients with CNS involvement. They show that these patients have significantly lower verbal IQ, performance IQ, and full-scale IQ scores than patients without CNS involvement or those who only have diabetes insipidus. Of note is that 28% of the 28 long-term survivors of LCH had some evidence of clinical or radiographic CNS involvement. These results strongly suggest that patients with CNS involvement have a significant adverse neurocognitive outcome. Because no effective therapy has been developed for the treatment of this type of involvement, the best approach may ultimately be in the up-front treatment of newly diagnosed patients that will prevent adverse CNS sequelae.

R. J. Arceci, MD, PhD

Association Between Surgical Margins and Long-term Outcome in Advanced Hepatoblastoma

Dicken BJ, Bigam DL, Lees GM (Univ of Alberta, Edmonton, Canada)

J Pediatr Surg 39:721-725, 2004 14–37

Background.—In many patients with newly diagnosed hepatoblastomas, the disease at presentation is unresectable. Neoadjuvant treatment has increased resectability rates, but many patients are left with tumors of borderline resectability. Whether favorable outcomes can be obtained, even when resection margins are less than 1 cm, thus avoiding the need for liver transplantation, was investigated.

Methods and Findings.—Twenty-three children undergoing surgical resection for hepatoblastomas between 1981 and 2003 were included in the study. At the latest follow-up, 78% were alive with no evidence of a recurrence. Resection margins were 1 cm or greater in 56.5% and less than 1 cm in 43.5%. These 2 groups did not differ significantly in survival rates. The survival rate was significantly worse among the 13 patients seen with synchronous pulmonary metastatic disease. Subgroup analysis with adjustment for pulmonary metastatic disease verified that margins of less than 1 cm did not significantly alter the survival rate.

Conclusions.—Survival rates are equivalent for children with surgical resection margins of less than 1 cm and surgical resection margins of 1 cm or greater after treatment for advanced hepatoblastomas. Small resection margins allow preservation of key structures, obviating the need for liver transplantation in this patient population.

▶ Complete surgical resection has been one of the keys to curing hepatoblastomas. This approach has sometimes resulted in the need to perform a liver transplantation if greater than 1-cm surgical margins could not be achieved. Determining whether greater than 1-cm margins were, in fact, necessary for a cure was the goal of this retrospective analysis of surgical margins and outcomes in patients with hepatoblastomas. Although the numbers are relatively small, the data show no significant difference between margins of less than 1 cm and margins of greater than 1 cm, when adjustment was made for the presence of pulmonary metastases. These data may help to guide the aggressiveness of surgery in cases in which complete but less than 1-cm margins are achieved and liver transplantation is considered.

R. J. Arceci, MD, PhD

Regulatory Approvals of Pediatric Oncology Drugs: Previous Experience and New Initiatives

Hirschfeld S, Ho PTC, Smith M, et al (Food and Drug Administration, Rockville, Md; NIH, Bethesda, Md; GlaxoSmithKline, Philadelphia)
J Clin Oncol 21:1066-1073, 2003 14–38

Background.—The Food and Drug Administration (FDA) has approved more than 100 drugs to treat malignancies, including approximately 30 that are currently used in children. Fifteen of these agents have been labeled for pediatric use. The FDA experience with approvals of new drugs for childhood cancers was reviewed. New regulatory initiatives directed at pediatric oncology were also discussed.

Methods and Findings.—Archival FDA documents and the published literature were retrospectively analyzed. The 15 agents approved by the FDA for pediatric oncology indications are L-asparaginase, approved for the treatment of leukemias; cyclophosphamide for leukemias, lymphomas, neuroblastomas, and retinoblastoma; cytarabine for acute nonlymphocytic leukemia; dactinomycin for Wilms' tumor, rhabdomyosarcoma, choriocarcinoma, testicular carcinoma, Ewing's sarcoma, and sarcoma botryoides; daunorubicin and mercaptopurine for acute lymphocytic leukemia (ALL); doxorubicin for Wilms' tumor, neuroblastoma, soft tissue sarcomas, Hodgkin's disease, other malignant lymphomas, and leukemias; lomustine for brain tumors and Hodgkin's lymphoma; methotrexate for ALL, meningeal leukemia, osteosarcoma, and non Hodgkin's lymphomas; procarbazine for Hodgkin's lymphoma; thioguanine for acute nonlymphocytic leukemia; teniposide for refractory childhood ALL; tretinoin for acute promyelocytic leukemia; vinblastine for histiocytosis, testicular germ cell carcinomas, and Hodgkin's lymphoma; and vincristine for acute leukemias, lymphomas, Wilms' tumor, rhabdomyosarcoma, and neuroblastoma. Between 1980 and

2001, 6 agents have been submitted to the FDA for cancer treatment in children. In 1990, teniposide was approved for the treatment of ALL in children. In the mid 1980s, daunorubicin and methotrexate were approved as supplements in the treatment of ALL and osteosarcoma, respectively. The remaining 3 applications were not approved, including vindesine for ALL in 1980, teniposide for neuroblastoma in 1981, and 5-azacytidine for AML in 1983. Reasons for failure to approve agents for pediatric indications include the small numbers of patients in studies, lack of appropriate controls, and failure to demonstrate benefits to the patients. Regulations to address the general lack of adequate labeling of drugs for children have been issued since 1979, a reflection of the FDA's concern about the paucity of submissions for pediatric oncology indications. Potential reasons for the lack of new submissions for pediatric oncology drug treatments include the small size of the market for such drugs compared with the market for adults with cancer and perceived barriers to performing research in children. Approval criteria are performance of controlled trials, prospective data collection, and inclusion of disease-appropriate end points.

Conclusions.—More than 100 drugs have received FDA approval for the treatment of malignancies, but only 15 have pediatric use information in their labeling. Regulatory initiatives are in place in an attempt to promote the development of cancer drugs for children.

▶ The development, testing, and approval for anti-cancer drugs in children have been major challenges for pediatric oncology. The report by Hirschfeld et al delineates the problems and some of the potential solutions. Certainly, history has much to teach us in this regard. While more than 100 anti-cancer drugs have been approved by the FDA, only 15 have pediatric use information in their labeling, and these 15 are, except for tretinoin for acute promyelocytic leukemia, relatively old and currently conventional therapy. In addition to the expected problems of small market and ethical issues of doing early phase clinical trials in children, several other important problems with approval of pediatric indications are enumerated. In particular, some of the most important reasons for failure to receive approvals for pediatric indications included too few patients treated to ensure statistical significance, lack of appropriate controls, and failure to demonstrate benefit, possibly related to the numbers of patients or study design. Although those of us involved in testing new agents in pediatric patients with cancer have a difficult job, we have no one but ourselves to scold when new agents are not properly tested such that approval is granted based on the appropriate weight of the scientific evidence. This report is an excellent learning tool and reminder of what is needed and how best to proceed with federal regulatory agencies involved in patient protection and new drug approvals.

R. J. Arceci, MD, PhD

Comparison of the Informed Consent Process for Randomized Clinical Trials in Pediatric and Adult Oncology

Simon CM, Siminoff LA, Kodish ED, et al (Case Western Reserve Univ, Cleveland, Ohio)

J Clin Oncol 22:2708-2717, 2004 14–39

Introduction.—Properly informing and gaining consent of potential research subjects is an important ethical safeguard in the ongoing search for new and improved cancer therapies. The goals of informed consent are similar for both pediatric and adult oncology, yet the care environments for these 2 groups are different in significant ways that may impact how treatment goals are interpreted and met in reality. The informed consent processes for phase III pediatric and adult oncology randomized clinical trials were compared to identify any significant differences between these 2 processes.

Methods.—Of 219 decision makers evaluated, 79 were from the adult trial and 140 from the pediatric trial (36.1% and 63.9%, respectively). Research subjects in both investigations were observed and audiotaped in conversation with their oncologists. Cancer patients or their surrogates were interviewed afterward to elicit data regarding: consent issues, demographic background, and other key variables.

Results.—Significant differences between the adult and pediatric informed consent processes for cancer clinical trials were seen. Adult oncology decision makers were usually more fully informed and more actively engaged by their oncologists. Pediatric decision makers were given more information concerning survival, cure, randomization, and voluntariness. The pediatric disclosure process was significantly longer in pediatric versus adult oncology patients (78.76 min vs 54.73 min; $P < .001$). Comprehension difficulties were more common among pediatric decision makers.

Conclusion.—Ongoing efforts to improve the ethical framework of clinical cancer research need to consider the key differences between pediatric and adult oncology informed consent. Future trials are needed to explore the differences between adult and pediatric informed consent processes in oncology.

► It is self-evident that children are different than adults. However, less clear is whether the adult decision makers for children are different than adults making decisions for themselves when it comes to clinical trials and informed consent for cancer treatment. Simon et al attempt to capture some of the similarities and differences in the consent process that occurs in pediatric versus medical oncology. Based primarily on an interview data collection method, several differences were observed, particularly in the level of understanding of information (better in the adult group) or more information supplied on outcomes, randomization, and voluntariness (better in pediatric group) between the 2 groups. It would have been interesting if the study had controlled more for age of the subjects as the pediatric decision makers were significantly younger than those in the adult group. More information on what the perception of the physicians actually doing the consent would also have been important to see. We are, in a sense, left with the perceptions of the individuals granting the consent, with less information of what actually happened in the interactions. Nevertheless, this type of study is important and should help us refine the consenting process without, hopefully, making it yet more complex.

R. J. Arceci, MD, PhD

15 Cancer Therapies

Phase 1 Study of TLK286 (Telcyta) Administered Weekly in Advanced Malignancies

Rosen LS, Laxa B, Boulos L, et al (Univ of California, Los Angeles; Telik, Inc, Palo Alto, Calif)

Clin Cancer Res 10:3689-3698, 2004 15–1

Introduction.—TLK286 (Telcyta) is a novel glutathione analog prodrug created to undergo activation of GST P1-1, an enzyme overexpressed in many human malignancies. Brief exposure to TLK286 induces apoptosis in cultured human cells mediated by induction of the stress-response pathway. The dose-limiting toxicities, maximum tolerated dose, and pharmacokinetics of TLK286 administered weekly were examined in a phase I investigation.

Methods.—Thirty-seven patients with a variety of advanced malignancies were treated with IV TLK286 administered weekly over a 30-minute period in escalating doses of 60 to 90 mg/m^2. A treatment cycle was 3 weekly treatments. Patients underwent tumor evaluations on day 43; those with clinical benefit continued treatment until disease progression or unacceptable toxicity. The World Health Organization criteria was used to evaluate safety.

Results.—Patients received 111 cycles of TLK286 at 8 dose levels (median, 3 cycles; range, 1-16 cycles). TLK286 administered weekly at 960 mg/m^2 was well tolerated and there were no dose-limiting toxicities. The TLK286-associated toxicities included grade 1 to 2 nausea and vomiting, fatigue, and anemia. Nine of 31 assessable patients continued therapy beyond 43 days (median, 5 cycles; range, 3-16 cycles) and had durable stable disease or minor tumor regression. An optimized 2-compartment model was used to describe pharmacokinetic characteristics of TLK286. Mild to moderate renal or hepatic organ dysfunction did not influence elimination of TLK286.

Conclusion.—TLK286 was well tolerated when administered weekly at doses up to 960 mg/m^2. The safety and antitumor activity seen in a broad range of cancer types supports phase II disease activity trials of TLK286 administered weekly at 960 mg/m^2.

► TLK286 (Telcyta) is a modified glutathione analog converted by glutathione S-transferase into 2 electrophilic molecules that activate the stress-response pathway leading to apoptosis. One of the more interesting aspects of Telcyta is its apparent ability to reverse resistance to the platinum compounds when given in combination with them. This phase I study demonstrates that the drug can be given safely and is well tolerated. Other studies have suggested activity of the agent in a variety of tumors both as a single agent and in combination with a platinum compound. In particular, if this agent can indeed reverse resistance to the platinums, it has significant potential in such tumors as ovarian carcinoma and carcinoma of the lung, among others.

J. T. Thigpen, MD

Genetic Variants in the *UDP-glucuronosyltransferase 1A1* Gene Predict the Risk of Severe Neutropenia of Irinotecan

Innocenti F, Undevia SD, Iyer L, et al (Univ of Chicago)

J Clin Oncol 22:1382-1388, 2004 15–2

Background.—Severe toxicity is commonly observed in cancer patients receiving irinotecan. The risk of severe and potentially fatal toxicity might be predicted by investigating the genetic variation of irinotecan disposition. UDP-glucuronosyltransferase 1A1 (*UGT1A1*) catalyzes the glucuronidation of the active metabolite SN-38. The association between the prevalence of severe toxicity and *UTG1A1* genetic variation was prospectively evaluated.

Methods.—The study group was composed of 66 cancer patients with advanced disease refractory to other treatments. The patients received irinote-

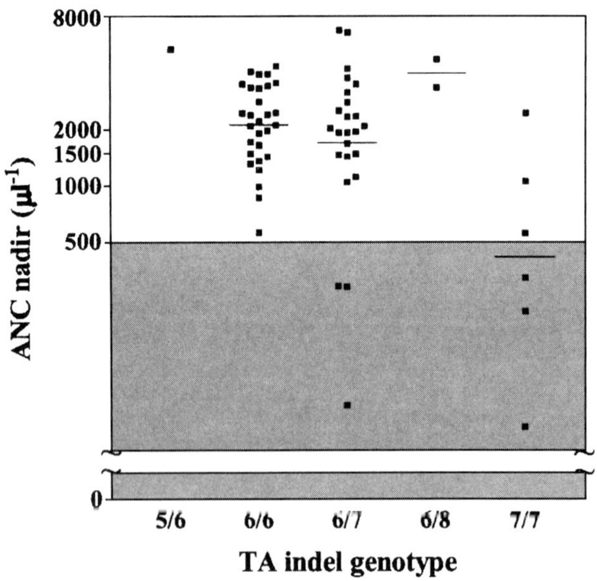

FIGURE 1.—Correlation between absolute neutrophil count (*ANC*) nadir (log scale) and TA indel genotype. *Bars* represent means. *Shaded area* represents ANC levels of grade 4 neutropenia. The 7/8 patient was not assessable for neutropenia. (Courtesy of Innocenti F, Undevia SD, Iyer L, et al: Genetic variants in the *UDP-glucuronosyltransferase 1A1* gene predict the risk of severe neutropenia of irinotecan. *J Clin Oncol* 22:1382-1388, 2004. Reprinted with permission from the American Society of Clinical Oncology.)

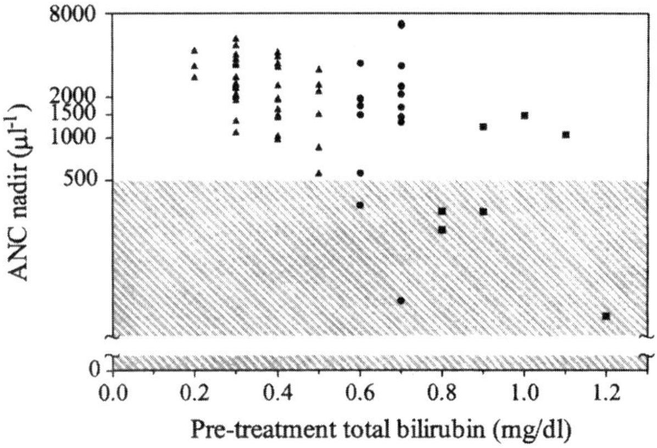

FIGURE 3.—Correlation between absolute neutrophil count (*ANC*) nadir (log scale) and pretreatment total bilirubin levels. *Shaded area* represents ANC levels of grade 4 neutropenia. *Triangles*, <0.6 mg/dL; *circles*, 0.6 to 0.7 mg/dL; *squares*, ≥0.8 mg/dL. (Courtesy of Innocenti F, Undevia SD, Iyer L, et al: Genetic variants in the *UDP-glucuronosyltransferase 1A1* gene predict the risk of severe neutropenia of irinotecan. *J Clin Oncol* 22:1382-1388, 2004. Reprinted with permission from the American Society of Clinical Oncology.)

can 350 mg/m^2 every 3 weeks. Toxicity and pharmacokinetic data were measured during cycle 1, and *UGT1A1* variants were genotyped.

Results.—The prevalence of grade 4 neutropenia was 9.5%. Grade 4 neutropenia was much more common in patients with the TA indel 7/7 genotype (3 of 6 patients; 50%) compared with 6/7 (3 of 24 patients; 12.5%) and 6/6 (0 of 29 patients; 0%) (Fig 1). There was a significant association between the TA indel genotype and the absolute neutrophil count nadir (Fig 3). The relative risk of grade 4 neutropenia was 9.3 for the 7/7 patients compared with the rest of the patients. Pretreatment total bilirubin levels were significantly higher in patients with grade 4 neutropenia compared with patients without grade 4 neutropenia. The −3156G>A variant seemed to distinguish different phenotypes of total bilirubin with the TA indel genotypes. The −3156 genotype and the SN-38 area under the concentration versus time curve were significant predictors of neutropenia (absolute neutrophil count nadir; $r^2 = 0.51$).

Conclusions.—The *UGT1A1* genotype and total bilirubin levels were found to be strongly associated with severe neutropenia and thus could be used for identification of cancer patients with a predisposition to the severe toxicity of irinotecan. Further evaluation is required of the hypothesis that the −3156G>A variant is a better predictor of *UGT1A1* status than the previously reported TA indel.

▶ Irinotecan is a key component in the treatment of colorectal cancer and other malignancies. The principal side effects, diarrhea and neutropenia, can be severe in up to one third of patients, which include fatalities in approximately 5%. SN-38 is the active metabolite of irinotecan and is primarily responsible for the therapeutic and toxic profile of the drug. SN-38 is inactivated through glucuronidation by *UGT1A1*, which is also responsible for the glucuronidation of bilirubin.

This trial sought to describe the association of toxicity with *UGT1A1* genetic variation. Indeed, this genotype and total bilirubin were strongly associated with neutropenia and may be used as a molecular marker to identify potential toxicity. Given the increasing number of drugs available for the treatment of metastatic colorectal cancer, defining the optimal drugs and schedules is clearly important. This is an emerging field that will have a definite impact.

P. J. Loehrer, Sr, MD

16 Cancer Biology

Large-Scale Meta-analysis of Cancer Microarray Data Identifies Common Transcriptional Profiles of Neoplastic Transformation and Progression

Rhodes DR, Yu J, Shanker K, et al (Univ of Michigan, Ann Arbor; Inst of Bioinformatics, Bangalore, India; Johns Hopkins Univ, Baltimore)

Proc Natl Acad Sci U S A 101:9309-9314, 2004 16–1

Introduction.—Several trials have used DNA microarrays to identify the gene expression signatures of human cancer, but the critical characteristics of these often unmanageable large signatures remain elusive. To address this, a statistical method (metaprofiling) was developed that identifies and evaluates the intersection of multiple gene expression signatures from a diverse collection of microarray datasets.

Findings.—Forty published cancer microarray datasets were obtained and analyzed that comprised 38 million gene expression measurements from more than 3700 cancer samples. From this, a common transcription profile was characterized that is universally activated in most cancer types relative to normal tissues from which they arose, likely reflecting essential transcriptional characteristics of neoplastic transformation. A transcriptional profile commonly activated in various types of undifferentiated cancer was also characterized, indicating common molecular mechanisms by which cancer cells progress and avoid differentiation. These transcription profiles were validated on independent datasets.

Conclusion.—By integrating microarray data and analysis from several cancer types, it was possible to characterize a metasignature of neoplastic transformation, thereby defining a transcriptional program that is nearly always activated in cancer, regardless of cell of origin. This universal activation indicates that these genes may be crucial to carcinogenesis and likely represent the convergence of a number of transforming mechanisms in a variety of contexts. The universal overexpression suggests that these genes may act as attractive therapeutic targets.

▶ Rhodes et al collected and analyzed 40 published cancer microarray datasets, comprising 38 million gene expression measurements from more than 3700 cancer examples. The authors were able to characterize a profile that is universally activated in most cancers, suggesting common molecular events that result in neoplastic transformation. This information will allow scientists to narrow their focus on a smaller number of genes for study and to define as therapeutic targets.

N. H. Hanna, MD

Antitumor Efficacy of Intermittent Treatment Schedules With the Rapamycin Derivative RAD001 Correlates With Prolonged Inactivation of Ribosomal Protein S6 Kinase 1 in Peripheral Blood Mononuclear Cells

Boulay A, Zumstein-Mecker S, Stephan C, et al (Novartis Pharma AG, Basel, Switzerland; Friedrich Miescher Inst for Biomedical Research, Basel, Switzerland)

Cancer Res 64:252-261, 2004 16–2

Background.—Potent antiproliferative effects have been noted with everolimus (RAD001), which is an orally bioavailable derivative of rapamycin. This antibiotic inhibits cytokine-driven lymphocyte proliferation and the proliferation of cells derived from human tumors and grown in culture or as tumors in animals. Thus, RAD001 is being developed for use in immunosuppression to prevent allograft rejection and therapeutically against human cancer. The antitumor activity of RAD001 was assessed in a pancreatic tumor model (CA20948 syngeneic rat).

Methods.—The tumor-bearing animals were given 0.5, 1, 2, or 5 mg/kg RAD001 or placebo, then killed. Samples from these rats were analyzed, as were samples from healthy human volunteers, which were treated with RAD001 or placebo. Measures included tumor growth; eukaryotic initiation factor 4E-binding protein 1 (4E-BP1) and translational activator ribosomal protein S6 kinase 1 (S6K1) activity in tumor, skin, and peripheral blood mononuclear cells (PBMCs); and correlations between efficacy and prolonged effects of RAD001 on mammalian target of rapamycin (mTOR) effectors.

Results.—All of the animals receiving RAD001 had suppressed tumor growth equal to that noted with cytotoxic 5-fluorouracil. Compared with controls, rats receiving RAD001 treatment at 0.5 or 2.5 mg/kg per day 6 times a week had significant inhibition of tumor growth. With 5 mg/kg of RAD001 given twice a week or once a week, tumor growth suppression was also significant. RAD001 was well tolerated in the rats. On biochemical profiles of mTOR signaling in tumors, skin, and PBMCs, a single 5-mg/kg dose of RAD001 was able to block the phosphorylation of the translational repressor 4E-BP1. In addition, S6K1 was inactivated by RAD001. With an intermittent dosing schedule, S6K1 was inactivated for at least 72 hours in tumors and surrogate tissues. Antitumor efficacy and effects lasting 7 days or longer on PBMC-derived S6K1 activity were correlated. A concentration-dependent inactivation of S6K1 activity was also noted on human PBMCs. RAD001 treatment had no effect on the hypophosphorylated form of 4E-BP1.

Conclusions.—Because short-term exposure to rapamycin in vitro retained its antiproliferative effects on tumor cell lines, continuous and intermittent treatment schedules for RAD001 may be equally effective. The antitumor efficacy of RAD001 and prolonged S6K1 inactivation in PBMCs were correlated. RAD001 treatment schedules could be evaluated by studying the PBMC-derived S6K1 activity levels in patients with cancer.

▶ Targeted therapy has become an extremely exciting phenomenon in cancer therapy. The use of drugs such as imatinib in specific cases where diseases are "addicted" to specific activating mutations, such as is seen in chronic myeloid leukemia with regard to the *BCR-ABL* gene mutation. For diseases in which the target of treatment is not a mutated or constitutively activated receptor, it is difficult to know whether a specific agent has activity or, more importantly, whether the new agent is being used at an active dose and schedule. One example of new targeted therapies is the mTOR inhibitors, an example of which is the agent RAD001. This drug blocks the activity of mTOR, which is increased particularly in patients whose tumors have silencing of the *PTEN* tumor suppressor gene. As a result, patients who are *PTEN* deficient may be excellent candidates for mTOR-directed therapy. Because RAD001 is an oral agent, it is difficult to know if the dosage is optimized in all patients. The authors of this study assessed the value of measuring S6K1 protein phosphorylation in mice receiving RAD001 on an intermittent dosing regimen with chemotherapy. They were able to demonstrate that effective mTOR inhibition by RAD001 was associated with inhibition of S6 phosphorylation. S6 is a downstream regulator that is phosphorylated to the active moiety by mTOR and, in in vitro studies, its phosphorylation status is reduced by treatment with mTOR inhibitors. What is lacking in this report is a direct correlation between PBMC S6 status and the status of S6 in tumors treated at the same time. This correlation would aid in confirming that the mononuclear cells can serve as a useful surrogate. Further studies need to be performed clinically to verify this approach. The other interesting issue raised by this study is the ability to inhibit mTOR on a long-term basis with bolus intermittent dosing, suggesting that long-term dosing may not be necessary to achieve biologically relevant end points.

M. S. Gordon, MD

Stable Expression of Small Interfering RNA Sensitizes TEL-PDGFβR to Inhibition With Imatinib or Rapamycin

Chen J, Wall NR, Kocher K, et al (Harvard Med School, Boston; Novartis Pharma AG, Basel, Switzerland; Dana-Farber Cancer Inst, Boston)

J Clin Invest 113:1784-1791, 2004 16–3

Background.—The tyrosine kinase fusions, such as BCR-ABL and TEL-PDGFβR receptors, are proven targets in patients with leukemia. Small-molecule inhibitors, such as imatinib, are effective for BCR-ABL- and TEL-PDGFβR-mediated leukemias. The unique fusion junction of these molecules may be a good candidate for molecularly targeted therapy based on RNA interference (RNAi). The RNAi process is mediated by small interfering RNA (siRNA). A retroviral-based system was developed that results in the stable expression of siRNA directed to the unique junctional sequence of TEL-PDGFβR (TPsiRNA) in transformed hematopoietic cells and describes the effects of TPsiRNA, alone or in combination with imatinib, on TEL-PDGFβR expression.

Methods.—A 19-bp stem-loop structure was designed by cloning the human pol III promoter H1 from genomic DNA by polymerase chain reaction (PCR) and inserting it into pBluescript II to make pSUPER. Oligonucleotides encoding the TPsiRNA were annealed and subcloned downstream of the H1 promoter in pSUPER. H1-TPsiRNA was then subcloned into a self-inactivating retroviral vector (pQCXIP-H1-TPsiRNA). This vector was introduced into cultured Ba/F3 cells stably transduced with TEL-PDGFαR, and TEL-PDGFβR expression was examined by Western blotting and PCR. Ba/F3 cells stably expressing TEL-PDGFβR, with or without TPsiRNA, were also injected into athymic nude mice, and TEL-PDGFαR expression, tumor progression, and death were assessed. Additionally, a possible synergistic effect between TPsiRNA and imatinib, a small-molecule inhibitor of TEL-PDGFβR tyrosine kinase activity, on TEL-PDGFαR expression was also examined.

Results.—Introduction of pQCIP-H1-TPsiRNA into Ba/F3 cells suppressed TEL-PDGFβR expression in the cultured Ba/F3 cells by approximately 4000-fold. Stable expression of TPsiRNA was associated with an approximately 90% decrease in expression of TEL-PDGFβR and its downstream effectors, including mammalian target of rapamycin (mTOR). TPsiRNA significantly impaired the proliferation of TEL-PDGFβR-transformed Ba/F3 cells in vitro. In mice, tumor development and death occurred a median of 24 days after the injection of TEL-PDGFβR-transformed Ba/F3 cells. Disease latency and death were significantly prolonged (median latency, 41 days) after injection of TPsiRNA. Stable TPsiRNA expression sensitized TEL-PDGFβR to imatinib and to rapamycin; at high imatinib doses (>100 nmol/L), coexpression with TPsiRNA almost completely blocked the kinase activity of TEL-PDGFβR. A similar inhibitory effect was seen with TPsiRNA in combination with PKC412, another TEL-PDGFβR inhibitor.

Conclusion.—Delivery of the pQCXIP-H1-TPsiRNA vector to the unique fusion junction sequence of TEL-PDGFβR results in stable expression of TPsiRNA in hematopoietic cells. This approach resulted in significant inhibition of TEL-PDGFβR expression both in vitro and in vivo. Furthermore, in this mouse model, TPsiRNA was able to prolong tumor development and death and virtually reverse resistance to imatinib. Thus, small-molecule kinase inhibitors targeted at the unique fusion junction sequence of TEL-PDGFβR deserve further study as a potential treatment for hematologic malignancy.

▶ siRNA represents an increasingly valuable tool in the assessment of the biology of tumors. The idea of using this technology is increasingly being explored and initial focus is being placed on disease states in which the target protein is unique to the tumor, such as the BCR-ABL translocation in chronic myeloid leukemia or the recently recognized TEL-PDGFβR, which has been seen in acute leukemias associated with the 11q23 chromosomal abnormality. In this study, the investigators assessed the ability of an siRNA directed against this target to inhibit downstream effectors. The siRNA was able to block signaling through this activating mutation, although it was not sufficient to induce apoptosis of the target cells. Of note, however, was the fact that pretreatment with siRNA was able to induce increased sensitivity to the tyrosine kinase inhibitor imatinib and inhibited an imatinib-resistant cell line, suggesting that if the specifics of administration can be worked out, this therapy could be used as an adjunct to other targeted therapies.

M. S. Gordon, MD

A Fully Human Monoclonal Antibody to the Insulin-Like Growth Factor I Receptor Blocks Ligand-Dependent Signaling and Inhibits Human Tumor Growth In Vivo

Burtrum D, Zhu Z, Lu D, et al (ImClone Systems Incorporated, New York)

Cancer Res 63:8912-8921, 2003 16–4

Background.—Insulin-like growth factor I receptor (IGF-IR), a critical signaling molecule for tumor cell proliferation and survival, is overexpressed in many tumor types. Therefore, treatment strategies that target the IGF-IR may be effective broad-spectrum anticancer agents. The development of a fully human antibody (A12) that binds to the IGF-IR and inhibits ligand binding was reported.

Methods and Findings.—The antibody was generated through screening of a Fab phage display library. The antibody binds with high affinity to the IGF-IR, inhibiting ligand binding with an IC_{50} of 0.6 to 1 nmol. In MCF7 human breast cancer cells, antibody-mediated blockade of ligand binding to the IGF-IR inhibited downstream signaling of mitogen-activated protein kinase and phosphatidylinositol 3'-kinase/Akt, the 2 major IGF pathways. This significantly decreased the mitogenic and proliferative potential of IGF-I and IGF-II. A12 did not block insulin binding to the insulin receptor, yet it did block binding to atypical IGF-IR in these cells. Also, A12 induced IGF-IR internalization and degradation on specific binding to tumor cells, which significantly decreased cell surface receptor density. In xenograft tumor models in vivo, A12-induced IGF-IR blockade occurred rapidly, leading to significant growth inhibition of breast, renal, and pancreatic tumors. Histologic analysis of tumor sections showed a substantial increase in apoptotic tumor cells in antibody-treated animals.

Conclusions.—This antibody has strong antitumor activity in vitro and in vivo. Thus, A12 may be an effective candidate for treating cancers dependent on IGF-IR signaling for growth and survival.

► The IGF-IR axis has become an extensively studied target for anticancer therapy. Preclinical studies have demonstrated that the stimulation of the IGF-IR system may play a role in the resistance of tumors to other targeted therapies such as those directed at the epidermal growth factor (EGF) receptor and other HER family members. In addition, resistance to antiestrogen therapy in hormone-sensitive tumors such as prostate cancer and breast cancer may be mediated by changes in this receptor system. Attempts to target the postreceptor signaling pathway have been complicated by the cross-sensitivity of the insulin receptor to these agents and a resultant disruption of glucose metabolism that would be potentially difficult to manage in the clinical setting. This study identified a human antibody to the IGF-IR that binds the receptors thereby blocking ligand-induced activation of the receptor. In contrast to the recent studied with the EGF receptor and the earlier studied of c-kit in gastrointestinal stromal tumors, there have not been definable activating mutations in the IGF-IR receptor and hence, a blocking antibody would be expected to have similar activity compared with a small molecule inhibitor. The use of this antibody in MCF7 breast cancer cells was associated with the predicted effect of down-regulating the activation of the Akt pathway. IGF-IR blockade was associated with significant growth inhibition of a variety of tumor types as well as the induction of apoptosis. No effects on the insulin receptor were identified. This study recognizes the potential value of a novel antitumor strategy by targeting the IGF-IR pathway with a monoclonal antibody and it is expected that this therapy will move aggressively into the clinical arena.

M. S. Gordon, MD

17 Supportive Care

Human Recombinant Erythropoietin Significantly Improves Tumor Oxygenation Independent of Its Effects on Hemoglobin

Blackwell KL, Kirkpatrick JP, Snyder SA, et al (Duke Univ, Durham, NC; Johnson Pharmaceutical Research and Development, Raritan, NJ)

Cancer Res 63:6162-6165, 2003 17–1

Background.—Tumor oxygenation has been shown to be an important prognostic marker in a variety of tumors. Many interactions influence tumor oxygenation, including oxygen delivery and consumption. The current study determined the effects of erythropoietin (EPO) treatment on the oxygenation of breast carcinoma in a nonanemic, clinically relevant animal model.

Methods.—Thirty nonanemic, female Fischer 344 rats were assigned randomly to 1 of 3 groups: placebo, EPO after tumor implantation, or EPO before tumor implantation. Tumors were implanted in the hindflank. In vivo oxygenation was assessed at day 22 after implantation. A mean 180 measures per animal were obtained.

Findings.—The median tumor volume was 399 mm^3 on day 22. There were no differences in tumor volume between treatment groups. The average hematocrit was equal among groups at initiation of treatment but was significantly greater in the 2 EPO groups on day 22. Tumors treated with EPO had significantly lower hypoxic measures compared with those in the placebo and EPO before implantation groups (Figs 1 and 2).

Conclusions.—In this rat model, administration of EPO improved tumor oxygenation. This improvement appeared to be independent of hemoglobin effects.

▶ This is an article from a very solid group of investigators at Duke. The point that they are establishing in rats is that recombinant erythropoietin improves tumor oxygenation even in non-anemic animals. Theoretically, this is good. However, the report[1] from Europe on erythropoietin in head and neck patients actually being associated with a worsening outcome despite improvements in tumor oxygenation is alarming. Presumably, these stimulating factors work in multiple ways, and some of those ways involve stimulation of tumor cells directly, outside the whole oxygen story. Time will tell if the article by Henke et al

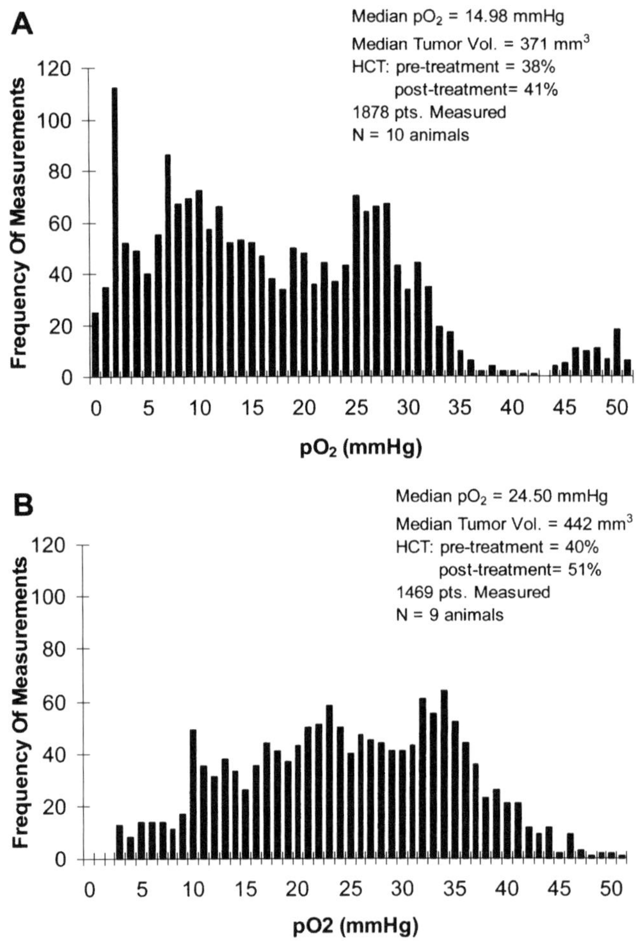

FIGURE 1.—Oxygen measurement histograms show reduction in hypoxia levels (<10 mm Hg) with the administration of EPO in a mammary carcinoma model (pooled data). **A**, group A (placebo); **B**, group B (EPO after tumor implantation). (Courtesy of Blackwell KL, Kirkpatrick JP, Snyder SA, et al: Human recombinant erythropoietin significantly improves tumor oxygenation independent of its effects on hemoglobin. *Cancer Res* 63:6162-6165, 2003.)

in *Lancet* is a fluke or if it really is a significant red flag over the casual administration of such agents.

E. Glatstein, MD

Reference

1. Henke M, Laszig R, Rube C, et al: Erythropoietin to treat head and neck cancer patients with anaemia undergoing radiotherapy: Randomised, double-blind, placebo-controlled trial. *Lancet* 362:1255-1260, 2003.

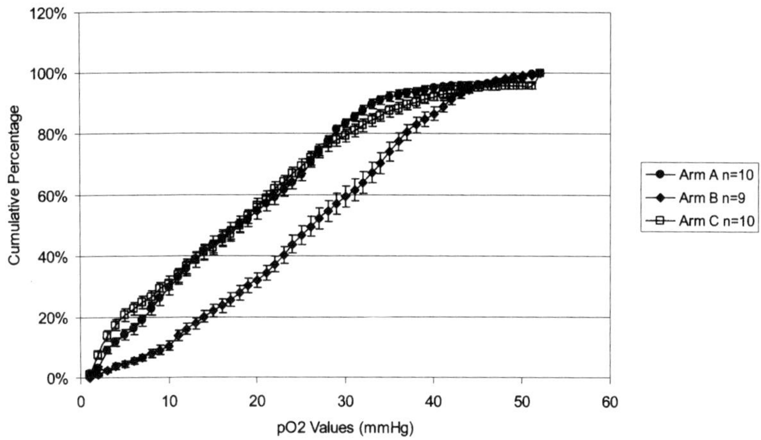

FIGURE 2.—EPO-treated tumors (Arm B) demonstrate significantly less pO_2 measurements < 10 mm Hg compared with saline-treated tumors (Arm A) or tumors pretreated with EPO (Arm C). There is no difference in tumor oxygenation measurements between saline-treated tumors and tumors pretreated with EPO. Error bars, SE. (Courtesy of Blackwell KL, Kirkpatrick JP, Snyder SA, et al: Human recombinant erythropoietin significantly improves tumor oxygenation independent of its effects on hemoglobin. *Cancer Res* 63:6162-6165, 2003.)

Focal Nodular Hyperplasia of the Hematopoietic Marrow Simulating Vertebral Metastasis on FDG Positron Emission Tomography

Bordalo-Rodrigues M, Galant C, Lonneux M, et al (Université Catholique de Louvain, Brussels, Belgium)
AJR 180:669-671, 2003 17–2

Introduction.—The case was reported of a patient with bronchioloalveolar carcinoma with focal nodular hyperplasia of the hematopoietic marrow in dorsal vertebral bodies identified on fluorodeoxyglucose (FDG) positron emission tomography (PET) and MR imaging.

Case Report.—Man, 77, was seen for a 1-month history of intermittent episodes of cough. He was a former smoker (60 packs/y; ceased smoking 10 years prior). A chest radiograph showed a spiculated pulmonary nodule in the right upper lobe. CT-guided transthoracic biopsy of the lesion identified bronchioloalveolar cell carcinoma. High uptake of the radiotracer was seen in the right upper lobe, corresponding to the primary tumor, and in the vertebral body of T-8.

Results of radiographs of the thoracic spine were normal. T1-weighted spin-echo MR images of the spine revealed a 2 × 2-cm focus of reduced signal intensity in the lateral aspect of the T-8 vertebral body and a 1 × 1-cm focus of reduced signal intensity in the lateral aspect of the T11 vertebral body. A CT-guided biopsy using a lateral scout image from S-3 to T-5 provided a lateral image of the

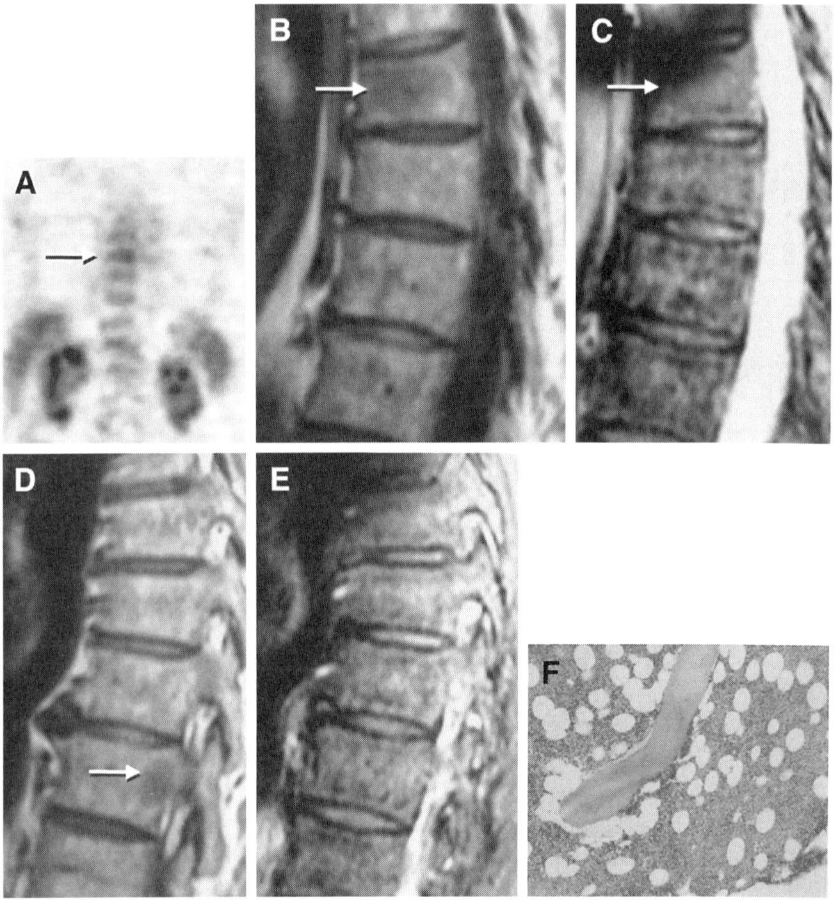

FIGURE 1.—A 77-year-old man with focal nodular hyperplasia of hematopoietic marrow. A, Posterior coronal fluorodeoxyglucose (FDG) positron emission tomography (PET) image obtained 60 minutes after injection of 370 MBq of FDG reveals hot spot (*arrow*) in lateral aspect of 1 vertebral body. Normal tracer uptake is seen in kidneys liver, and spleen. B, Sagittal T1- weighted spin-echo MR image of thoracic spine shows area of moderately decreased signal intensity (*arrow*) in vertebral body of T8. C, On sagittal fat-saturated T2-weighted MR image (corresponding to B), abnormality seen on T1-weighted image is not visible (*arrow*). Area of decreased signal intensity is artifact. *D*, Left parasagittal T1-weighted spin-echo MR image shows round area (*arrow*) of moderately decreased signal intensity in vertebral body of T11. E, On fat-saturated T2-weighted MR image, abnormality seen on T1-weighted image is not visible. The area was normal on FDG PET image (A). F, Low-power magnification photograph of biopsy specimen (hematoxylin-eosin; original magnification, ×80) of T8 abnormality shows hypercellullar marrow with reduced proportion of adipocytes. At higher power magnification (not shown), normal hematopoietic marrow devoid of neoplastic cells was found. (Courtesy of Bordalo-Rodrigues M, Galant C, Lonneux M, et al: Focal nodular hyperplasia of the hematopoietic marrow simulating vertebral metastasis of FDG positron emission tomography. *AJR* 180:669-671, 2003. Reprinted with permission from the *American Journal of Roentgenology*.)

spine to which the MR images of the thoracolumbar spine could be compared.

Histologic examination revealed hyperplastic hematopoietic bone marrow without neoplastic proliferation. Several islets of the various stem cell lines—including erythroid, myeloid, and lymphoid cells—

were present, along with megakaryocytes. The proportion of fat cells was substantially reduced with respect to the expressed proportion in normal bone marrow of a vertebral body (Fig 1). Normal immunohistochemical analysis using monoclonal antibodies raised against cytokeratins of low molecular weight demonstrated no carcinomatous cells, excluding the possibility of metastasis of the lung carcinoma. Because the T-8 vertebral lesion was a focal nodular hyperplasia of hematopoietic marrow, the pulmonary lesion was resected.

Conclusion.—In a case of focal nodular hyperplasia of hematopoietic marrow in dorsal vertebral bodies in a patient with bronchioloalveolar carcinoma, FDG PET and MRI produced findings that resembled bone metastases.

▶ Generally, I will not include a case report. However, this particular case report illustrates a really essential point and that is that everything that turns out to be abnormal in a patient who has cancer is not always due to cancer. Specifically, PET scanning has an incredible reputation for low false-negative and low false-positive.

This case report deals with a patient who had bronchioloalveolar carcinoma of the lung and a positive PET scan in the spine that turned out to be focal nodular hyperplasia of bone marrow. I have had the occasion of seeing several PET scans after treatment that were called positive but lacked corroboration on other imaging studies. I have simply watched those patients and repeated the scan a couple of months later and the scan was then negative.

I had 1 remarkable patient whom I had treated for relapse of her Hodgkin's disease following initial multi-agent chemotherapy. She later relapsed after radiation and underwent a bone marrow transplant. About 8 months later, she had what appeared to be a mass in her mediastinum and an enlarging spleen. A PET scan was done, and both of these areas lit up with very avid uptake of the FDG. We removed the mediastinal mass, which turned out to be thymic rebound without tumor; and because her spleen was still strongly positive by PET, we subjected her to a splenectomy, which also failed to show any evidence of tumor, even though it was bread loafed. The patient seemed thrilled with the news and felt that losing her spleen was relatively trivial.

I am not sure all the physicians agreed with that, but it turned out to be a good move. I should add that we did immunize her against pneumococcus, *Hemophilus*, and *Neisseria* about 10 days prior to her splenectomy, since the spleen is essential for opsonization of those antigens.

E. Glatstein, MD

The Oral Neurokinin-1 Antagonist Aprepitant for the Prevention of Chemotherapy-Induced Nausea and Vomiting: A Multinational, Randomized, Double-blind, Placebo-controlled Trial in Patients Receiving High-Dose Cisplatin: The Aprepitant Protocol 052 Study Group

Hesketh PJ, Grunberg SM, Gralla RJ, et al (Caritas St Elizabeth's Med Ctr, Brighton, Mass; Univ of Vermont, Burlington; New York Lung Cancer Alliance; et al)

J Clin Oncol 21:4112-4119, 2003 17–3

Background.—Patients dread the development of chemotherapy-induced nausea and vomiting (CINV), but selective type-three 5-hydroxytryptamine (5-HT_3) receptor antagonists (RAs) have provided a degree of control over CINV. Because the control remains suboptimal, new and more effective antiemetic agents are still being sought. Aprepitant is a potent selective CNS penetrating oral nonpeptide antagonist of the neurokinin-1 (NK_1) receptor. Other NK_1 RAs have proved efficacious against early and delayed emesis and with various emetic stimuli. Aprepitant has protected against acute emesis when used in combination with a 5-HT_3 RA and dexamethasone. Delayed emesis was prevented more effectively by a combination of aprepitant and dexamethasone than by dexamethasone alone. A phase III study was undertaken to establish the efficacy of aprepitant compared with standard therapy in preventing CINV.

Methods.—Five hundred twenty-one patients who were receiving cisplatin ($\geq$70 mg/m^2) for the first time were randomly assigned to receive either standard therapy (n = 260) or an aprepitant regimen (n = 261). The standard therapy consisted of ondansetron plus dexamethasone on day 1, and dexamethasone on days 2 to 4. The aprepitant regimen consisted of aprepitant plus ondansetron and dexamethasone on day 1, aprepitant plus dexamethasone on days 2 and 3, and dexamethasone only on day 4. A diary was kept to document episodes of nausea and vomiting. Complete response was defined as no emesis and no rescue therapy 1 to 5 days after receiving cisplatin. Adverse events and the results of physical and laboratory assessments were also noted.

Results.—The efficacy of the aprepitant regimen was superior to that of the standard regimen overall, with a 72.7% efficacy compared with a 52.3% efficacy. In addition, the aprepitant regimen had an 89.2% efficacy against acute CINV and a 75.4% efficacy against delayed CINV. These values were 78.1% and 55.8%, respectively, for the standard regimen. The percentages of men and women who had a complete response overall were similar (77.6% and 69.8%). For the standard regimen, the complete response rate for women was 38.8% and that for men was 60.5%. The comparisons for total control, no nausea, and no significant nausea also consistently favored the aprepitant regimen. The 2 treatment groups had similar overall incidences of clinical adverse events, drug-related adverse events, serious clinical adverse events, laboratory adverse events, drug-related laboratory events, and discontinuations because of adverse events. Seven patients (2.7%) in the aprepitant group and 9 (3.4%) in the standard therapy group died.

Conclusions.—Adding aprepitant to the ondansetron plus dexamethasone regimen achieved better control of CINV for patients taking highly emetogenic chemotherapy. The improved control included both acute and delayed CINV. The occurrence of adverse events was similar between the 2 regimens. Thus, the addition of aprepitant provided superior protection against CINV for patients who were receiving cisplatin-based chemotherapy.

Addition of the Oral NK_1 Antagonist Aprepitant to Standard Antiemetics Provides Protection Against Nausea and Vomiting During Multiple Cycles of Cisplatin-Based Chemotherapy

de Wit R, Herrstedt J, Rapoport B, et al (Rotterdam Cancer Inst, The Netherlands; Copenhagen Univ Hosp; Med Oncology Centre of Rosebank, Johannesburg, South Africa; et al)

J Clin Oncol 21:4105-4111, 2003 17–4

Background.—In 70% to 80% of cases of chemotherapy-induced nausea and vomiting (CINV), acute emesis is prevented with the use of a selective type-three 5-hydroxytryptamine (HT_3) receptor antagonist and a corticosteroid such as dexamethasone. However, 25% to 40% of patients still have delayed CINV, occurring 2 to 5 days into their first cycle of high-dose cisplatin therapy. When the neurokinin-1 receptor antagonist aprepitant is added to the standard regimen, both the acute and the delayed phases of CINV were handled better. Whether this effect is sustained for up to 6 cycles of cisplatin therapy was explored.

Methods.—Two hundred two patients receiving cisplatin ($\geq$70 mg/m^2) participated in the first cycle, 141 in the second cycle, and similar numbers through multiple cycles. In addition to the administration of ondansetron 32 mg and dexamethasone 20 mg before cisplatin, and dexamethasone 8 mg on days 2 to 5, patients were randomly assigned to receive 1 of the following 3 regimens: (1) aprepitant 375 mg 1 hour before cisplatin on day 1, and aprepitant 250 mg on days 2 to 5 (35 patients); (2) aprepitant 125 mg given before cisplatin, and aprepitant 80 mg on days 2 to 5 (81 patients); or (3) placebo before cisplatin on days 2 to 5 (86 patients). Complete response was defined as no emesis and no rescue therapy over 5 days after receiving cisplatin for up to 6 cycles.

Results.—In light of new pharmacokinetic data, the regimen of 375/250 mg of aprepitant was discontinued early. Among those receiving aprepitant 125/80 mg, all the patients with complete responses in the fifth and sixth cycles had complete responses consistently through all cycles. Higher and better sustained responses were found with aprepitant compared with standard therapy, with complete response rates of 64% in cycle 1 and 59% in cycle 6, compared with response rates of 49% and 34%, respectively, for the standard therapy group. The differences in response rate between the 2 groups at each cycle were also significant. More than 50% of the patients receiving standard therapy were treatment failures, but only 36.3% of those receiving aprepitant failed therapy. Nearly 75% of the 145 patients who completed the prestudy visit for cycle 2 had adverse clinical events in cycles 2 to 6, and 29 were serious. None of the serious events were linked to the drugs being taken. Laboratory adverse events occurred at comparable rates in the study groups.

Conclusions.—Protection against CINV was extended to multiple cycles of cisplatin therapy by using aprepitant along with standard antiemetic therapy. Patients had a nearly 2-fold greater chance of remaining emesis-free and not needing rescue medication when aprepitant was given in the 125/80-mg regimen compared with receiving standard therapy only.

▶ Aprepitant is an oral neurokinin-1 antagonist now available for use in preventing CINV. These 2 studies (Abstracts 17–3 and 17–4) evaluate its use in combination with standard antiemetic regimens. Both trials show that the addition of aprepitant to an antiemetic regimen that contains ondansetron and dexamethasone provides better and more sustained protection than the same regimen without aprepitant. These 2 studies provide a strong argument for the inclusion of aprepitant in the standard antiemetic regimen for patients receiving emetogenic chemotherapy.

J. T. Thigpen, MD

A Randomized Trial of Multivitamin Supplements and HIV Disease Progression and Mortality

Fawzi WW, Msamanga GI, Spiegelman D, et al (Harvard Univ, Boston; Muhimbili Univ, Dar es Salaam, Tanzania)
N Engl J Med 351:23-32, 2004 17–5

Background.—Observational studies suggest micronutrient supplements may slow disease progression in patients with HIV infection. Thus, the effects of micronutrient supplementation on virologic and immunologic variables in HIV-infected pregnant women were prospectively studied.

Methods.—The research subjects were 1078 pregnant women with HIV (mean age, about 24.7 years) living in Dar es Salaam, Tanzania. Patients were randomly assigned to 4 groups to receive daily supplements of either vitamin A alone (preformed vitamin A and beta carotene), multivitamins alone (vitamins B complex, C, and E), vitamin A plus multivitamins, or placebo. Patients were followed up for a median of 71 months to determine a combined end point of HIV disease progression (ie, World Health Organization [WHO] stage 4 disease) or death; CD4+ cell counts and viral loads were also examined according to treatment.

Results.—Vitamin A supplementation alone was not significantly more effective than placebo in improving clinical, virologic, and immunologic variables (Table 4). With multivitamin monotherapy, however, significantly fewer patients met the combined end point (24.7% vs 31.1% in the placebo group; relative risk [RR], 0.71). Specifically, multivitamins significantly decreased the risks of progression to WHO stage 4 disease (RR, 0.50), death

TABLE 4.—Effects of 3 Vitamin Regimens on T-Cell Counts and Viral Loads Compared With the Effects of Placebo

End Point	Mean Value in Placebo Group*	Multivitamins		Multivitamins + Vitamin A		Vitamin A Alone	
		Mean Difference (95% CI)†	*P* Value	Mean Difference (95% CI)†	*P* Value	Mean Difference (95% CI)†	*P* Value
Whole period							
CD4+ cell count/mm^3	449±255	48 (10 to 85)	0.01	41 (4 to 77)	0.03	−15 (−45 to 14)	0.30
CD8+ cell count/mm^3	968±479	43 (−15 to 101)	0.15	12 (−44 to 69)	0.67	−48 (−100 to 4)	0.07
CD3+ cell count/mm^3	1497±615	38 (14 to 161)	0.02	47 (−27 to 120)	0.21	−72 (−141 to −3)	0.04
Viral load (log)‡	4.67±0.86	−0.18 (−0.32 to −0.03)	0.02	−0.07 (−0.21 to 0.09)	0.40	−0.03 (−0.17 to 0.11)	0.68
First 2 years							
CD4+ cell count/mm^3	494±257	48 (18 to 79)	0.002	21 (−11 to 53)	0.20	−16 (−44 to 13)	0.28
CD8+ cell count/mm^3	973±425	56 (1 to 110)	0.05	40 (−18 to 97)	0.17	−36 (−89 to 17)	0.19
CD3+ cell count/mm^3	1544±587	109 (32 to 185)	0.006	64 (−15 to 143)	0.11	−59 (−132 to 15)	0.12
Viral load (log)‡	4.59±0.86	−0.18 (−0.34 to −0.03)	0.02	−0.11 (−0.27 to 0.05)	0.17	−0.07 (−0.23 to 0.08)	0.35
First 4 years							
CD4+ cell count/mm^3	470±254	38 (8 to 68)	0.01	19 (−12 to 50)	0.22	−18 (−46 to 11)	0.22
CD8+ cell count/mm^3	959±438	56 (2 to 111)	0.04	31 (−26 to 87)	0.29	−53 (−105 to −1)	0.05
CD3+ cell count/mm^3	1506±584	98 (25 to 171)	0.009	59 (−16 to 133)	0.12	−71 (−140 to −1)	0.05
Viral load (log)‡	4.65±0.86	−0.13 (−0.33 to −0.04)	0.01	−0.09 (−0.24 to 0.06)	0.24	−0.04 (−0.18 to 0.10)	0.57

*± Values are means ± SD. Baseline measurement was excluded.

†Values are mean difference between this group and placebo group. Mean differences, 95% confidence intervals (*Cis*), and corresponding *P* values were estimated from generalized estimating equations, after adjustment for baseline measurements.

‡Base-10 scale was used.

(Reprinted by permission of *The New England Journal of Medicine* from Fawzi WW, Msamanga GI, Spiegelman D, et al: A randomized trial of multivitamin supplements and HIV disease progression and mortality. *N Engl J Med* 351:23-32, 2004.)

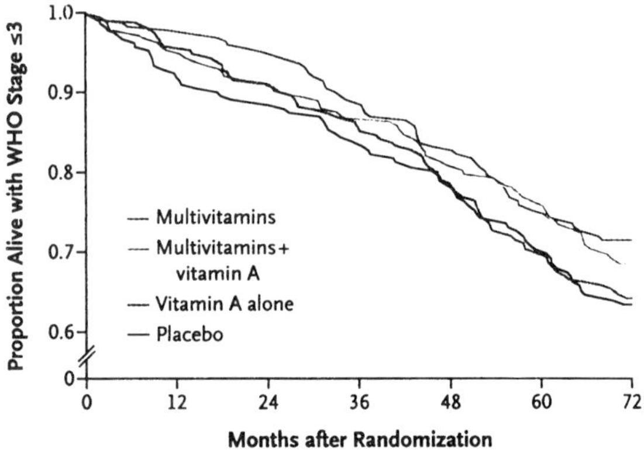

No. at Risk	0	24	48	72
Multivitamins	271	195	157	119
Multivitamins+ vitamin A	267	181	143	102
Vitamin A alone	272	190	147	104
Placebo	267	173	145	101

FIGURE 1.—Kaplan-Meier estimates of proportion of women alive with disease at WHO stage 3 or lower. (Reprinted by permission of *The New England Journal of Medicine* from Fawzi WW, Msamanga GI, Spiegelman D, et al: A randomized trial of multivitamin supplements and HIV disease progression and mortality. *N Engl J Med* 351:23-32, 2004.)

from AIDS-related causes (0.73), and progression to WHO stage 3 or higher disease (RR, 0.72) (Fig 1). These risk reductions were stronger during the first 2 years of therapy, but benefits were still significant at 4 years. Multivitamins were also associated with significant improvements in CD4+ cell counts (increase of 48 cells per cubic millimeter), CD8+ cell counts (increase of 43 cells per cubic millimeter), and viral load (decrease of 0.18 $\log_{10}$ units) compared with placebo. Oral and gastrointestinal manifestations of HIV disease were also significantly reduced by multivitamin use. Adding vitamin A to multivitamin therapy actually decreased some of the benefits seen with multivitamins alone.

Conclusion.—Among these HIV-infected pregnant women, supplementation with vitamin B complex and vitamins C and E significantly lowered the risk of HIV disease progression compared with placebo. Multivitamins also had positive effects on virologic and immune variables. These results suggest that daily multivitamins may be a low-cost approach to delaying the need for antiretroviral therapy in HIV-infected pregnant women.

▶ Although not directly cancer-related, this study does have oncologic relevance. This is a simple randomized trial, which demonstrates that a multivitamin (with or without vitamin A) was associated with higher CD4 and CD8+ cells and improved outcome compared with vitamin A alone in patients with HIV infections. Similar adverse outcome with vitamin A therapy has previously been reported in smokers with head and neck cancer. However, the impact of a relatively simple multivitamin on survival is an important observation and should be looked at in other scenarios, especially in those who are immunocompromised.

P. J. Loehrer, Sr, MD

Hormone Replacement Therapy and Life Expectancy After Prophylactic Oophorectomy in Women With *BRCA1/2* Mutations: A Decision Analysis

Armstrong K, Schwartz JS, Randall T, et al (Univ of Pennsylvania, Philadelphia)

J Clin Oncol 22:1045-1054, 2004 17–6

Background.—Prophylactic oophorectomy significantly reduces the risk of ovarian and breast cancer in premenopausal women with *BRCA1/2* mutations, but concerns about hormone replacement therapy (HRT) cause some women concern about this surgery. A decision analysis was performed to evaluate expected outcome of prophylactic oophorectomy and HRT in women with *BRCA1/2* mutations.

Study Design.—A Markov decision analytic model was developed to represent the impact of prophylactic oophorectomy and HRT on breast cancer, ovarian cancer, coronary heart disease, osteoporosis, and venous thrombosis. The health outcomes of each management strategy were estimated by simulating the life span of a hypothetical cohort of women at age 30, 40, and 50 years by using published studies as the source of epidemiologic data.

Findings.—The model demonstrated that prophylactic oophorectomy lengthened life expectancy for women with *BRCA1/2* mutations whether or not HRT was used after surgery. Use of HRT after surgery was associated with small decrements in life expectancy (<1 year) when HRT was discontinued by age 50 years but larger decrements when HRT was continued for life. HRT was associated with a gain in life expectancy of 0.39 to 0.79 years for those who had both prophylactic oophorectomy and mastectomy.

Conclusions.—This decision analysis found that for women with *BRCA1/2* mutations, premenopausal oophorectomy was associated with increase in life expectancy. The risks and benefit of postsurgery HRT were closely balanced, so women should make a decision on use up to age 50 years based on quality of life issues. If they choose to take HRT, they should plan to discontinue its use by the time of expected natural menopause.

Bilateral Prophylactic Mastectomy Reduces Breast Cancer Risk in BRCA1 and BRCA2 Mutation Carriers: The PROSE Study Group

Rebbeck TR, Friebel T, Lynch HT, et al (Univ of Pennsylvania; Fox Chase Cancer Ctr, Philadelphia; Creighton Univ, Omaha, Neb; et al)

J Clin Oncol 22:1055-1062, 2004 17–7

Background.—Women with *BRCA1* or *BRCA2* (*BRCA1/2*) germline mutations are at increased risk of developing breast cancer, and many of these women choose to undergo bilateral prophylactic mastectomy to reduce this risk. But does this strategy work? The purpose of this prospective case-control study was to assess degree of reduction in breast cancer risk after bilateral prophylactic mastectomy in *BRCA1/2* carriers.

Methods.—The subjects were 483 women (aged 20-63 years) with disease-associated *BRCA1/2* germline mutations without breast cancer identified from 11 North American and European institutions. The cases were 105 women who underwent bilateral prophylactic mastectomy; these women were followed prospectively. Control subjects were 378 women matched for type of mutation, treatment center, and age but who did not undergo prophylactic mastectomy. The mean follow-up to data censoring for cases was 5.3 years (range, 0-31.1 years) and that for the controls was 7.5 years (range, 0.02-33.8 years).

Findings.—The incidence of breast cancer was much lower among the cases (2 of 105, or 2%) than in the controls (184 of 378, or 49%); mean time to diagnosis was no different between the groups (5.7 years for cases vs 6.0 years for controls). In Cox proportional hazards modeling, bilateral prophylactic mastectomy markedly reduced the risk of breast cancer in women with intact ovaries (hazard ratio [HR], 0.09; 95% confidence interval [CI] 0.02-0.38) and in women with prior or concurrent prophylactic bilateral oophorectomy (HR, 0.05; 95% CI, 0.01-0.22). Too few breast cancers occurred after bilateral prophylactic mastectomy to determine the extent of reduction in risk.

Conclusions.—For women with *BRCA1/2* germline mutations, bilateral prophylactic mastectomy reduced the risk of breast cancer by more than 90%. Undergoing bilateral prophylactic mastectomy can effectively prevent breast cancer in *BRCA1/2* germline mutation carriers.

► The potential roles of prophylactic mastectomy and oophorectomy and the potential role of hormone replacement therapy in women with *BRCA1* or *BRCA2* mutations have posed difficult questions for physicians who deal with patients with these mutations. These 2 articles (Abstracts 17–6 and 17–7) provide some insight and help into the management of such patients, at least at the present time. Armstrong et al (Abstract 17–6) examine prophylactic oophorectomy and hormone replacement therapy in such patients. Their approach is based on a decision-analysis model and concludes that women with these mutations should undergo prophylactic oophorectomy on completion of childbearing based on a survival gain of 3.34 to 4.65 years. Their analysis suggests that hormone replacement therapy contributes only a small gain in survival (0.39-0.79 years) and should be used on a short-term basis (until the expected time of a natural menopause) for control of vasomotor symptoms. The major concern for hormone replacement therapy use is the breast cancer risk, which is perhaps a greater concern for *BRCA2* mutations (associated with hormone receptor–positive cancers) than for *BRCA1* mutations, which are associated with predominantly receptor-negative cancers. Rebbeck et al (Abstract 17–7) report a case-control study of the impact of bilateral prophylactic mastectomies on breast cancer risk in *BRCA1/BRCA2* patients and find a 90% reduction in breast cancer risk with bilateral mastectomies. For those willing to undergo bilateral mastectomies, the reduction in breast cancer risk addresses the concern about increased breast cancer risk in those who undergo prophylactic oophorectomy and subsequently wish to take hormone replacement therapy.

While these 2 studies certainly do not provide definitive answers because of the nature of the study methodology used by each, they do provide additional information on which to base decisions at the present time.

J. T. Thigpen, MD

Itraconazole Prevents Invasive Fungal Infections in Neutropenic Patients Treated for Hematologic Malignancies: Evidence From a Meta-analysis of 3,597 Patients

Glasmacher A, Prentice A, Gorschlüter M, et al (Univ of Bonn, Germany; Derriford Hosp, Plymouth, United Kingdom; Univ of South Florida, Tampa)
J Clin Oncol 21:4615-4626, 2003 17–8

Background.—Many studies of various antifungal agents to date have not proved the efficacy of antifungal prophylaxis. However, new evidence and the anti-*Aspergillus* efficacy of itraconazole prompted a review of the data on preventing invasive fungal infections.

Methods.—A literature review was performed to identify randomized, controlled studies of itraconazole for antifungal prophylaxis in neutropenic patients with hematologic malignancies. Thirteen studies involving a total of 3597 patients evaluable for invasive fungal infections were analyzed.

Findings.—Itraconazole decreased the incidence of invasive fungal infection by a mean of 40%. In addition, it reduced the mean incidence of invasive yeast infections by 53%. Mortality from invasive fungal infections declined by a mean 35%. All of these reductions were significant. The incidence of invasive *Aspergillus* infections declined only in studies of the itraconazole cyclodextrine solution and not the itraconazole capsules. The overall mortality rate did not change. Adverse effects were rare. Hypokalemia was reported in 3 studies. Trials comparing itraconazole cyclodextrine solution with a no-cyclodextrine control reported a higher rate of drug discontinuation. The effect of prophylaxis clearly correlated with a greater bioavailable dose of itraconazole.

Conclusions.—Antifungal prophylaxis with itraconazole is effective in preventing proved invasive fungal infections in neutropenic patients with hematologic malignancies. For the first time, this analysis shows that itraconazole prophylaxis reduces mortality from these infections as well as the rate of invasive *Aspergillus* infections in this patient population. The efficacy of this prophylaxis relies on sufficient doses of oral cyclodextrine solution (at least 400 mg/d) or IV formulations (200 mg/d).

► Patients who are severely neutropenic have various infectious complications including bacterial and fungal infection. Early studies in severely neutropenic patients have demonstrated that the longer and more profound the neutropenic period, the higher the likelihood of serious infectious complications. The treatment of hematologic malignancies such as the acute leukemias is often associated with periods of severe neutropenia in excess of 2 to 3 weeks with an associated risk of fungal infections, particularly after antibacterial therapy has been used. In this article, a meta-analysis was performed of all randomized controlled trials wherein 1 arm used itraconazole as fungal prophylaxis compared with either placebo or standard antifungal prophylaxis. Thirteen randomized trials were reviewed representing level I evidence for the assessment of this end point. The patient population in question was predominantly those with underlying hematologic malignancies because these are the patients who tend to have prolonged neutropenia, the major risk factor for the development of invasive fungal infections. The use of itraconazole solution was associated with a statistically significant decrease in the incidence of invasive fungal infections, particularly of invasive *Aspergillus* and as would be expected, this reduced incidence was accompanied with a decreased mortality associated with the invasive fungal infections. Importantly, this effect was most significantly seen in patients who were treated with itraconazole solution and not with itraconazole capsules suggesting that bioavailability, improved with the solution, may be a critical determinant of benefit and highlighting the fact that if such prophylaxis is to be administered, the intraconazole solution should be used.

M. S. Gordon, MD

18 Late Effects of Therapy

Radiation Exposure at Chest CT: A Statement of the Fleischner Society

Mayo JR, Aldrich J, Müller NL (Vancouver Gen Hosp, BC, Canada)

Radiology 228:15-21, 2003 18–1

Background.—With the increase in clinical indications for CT, CT studies now account for more than one half of the radiation dose resulting from medical procedures in the North American population. The level of CT radiation dose, especially in children, is a concern. The radiation dose from chest CT is presented.

Discussion.—The introduction of helical and multi-detector row scanners has increased the number of indications for, and diagnostic accuracy of CT. Thus, the current level of radiation exposure from CT is high. Surveys of radiation dose show a large variation in technical factors (Table 1). Therefore, there is a large variation in radiation doses to patients. Reference dose values for chest CT have been published (Table 3). Radiologic societies should consider the benefits of adopting such standards. More research on the complex relationship among radiation exposure, image noise, and diagnostic accuracy is needed to scientifically determine the minimum radiation doses that will provide adequate diagnostic information for standard clinical questions. With minimum levels of image quality validated, automatic exposure controls for CT scanners need to be developed to ensure that all

TABLE 1.—Methods of Quantifying Ionizing Radiation

Method	Conventional Units	International System of Units, or SI
Radiation exposure	roentgens (R)	coulombs per kilogram (C/kg)
Absorbed dose	rads (rad)	grays (Gy)
Equivalent dose	rems	sieverts (Sv)†
Effective dose	Effective dose equivalent (Sv)*	sieverts (Sv)‡

Note: Abbreviations of the units of measure are in parentheses.
*1977 tissue-weighting factors.
†D multiplied by ICRP radiation weighting factor w_R. The w_R for X-rays is 1.
‡1990 tissue-weighting factors.
(Courtesy of Mayo JR, Aldrich J, Müller NL: Radiation exposure at chest CT: A statement of the Fleischner Society. *Radiology* 228:15-21, 2003. Radiological Society of North America.)

TABLE 3.—Proposed Reference Dose Values for Routine CT Examinations on the Basis of Absorbed Dose to Air

Examination	Reference Dose Value CTDI$_w$ (mGy)	DLP (mGy · cm)
Routine head*	60	1,050
Face and sinuses*	35	360
Vertebral trauma†	70	460
Routine chest†	30	650
High-resolution CT of lung†	35	280
Routine abdomen†	35	780
Liver and spleen†	35	900
Routine pelvis†	35	570
Osseous pelvis†	25	520

*Data relate to head phantom (polymethylmethacrylate, 16 cm diameter).
†Data relate to body phantom (polymethylmethacrylate, 32 cm diameter).
(Courtesy of Mayo JR, Aldrich J, Müller NL: Radiation exposure at chest CT: A statement of the Fleischner Society. *Radiology* 228:15-21, 2003. Radiological Society of North America.)

patients undergo CT with methods conforming to the principle of "as low as reasonably achievable" (ALARA) (Table 4). Because children have an increased radiation sensitivity, initial efforts to reduce dose should be focused on children. Recently, the Society for Pediatric Radiology has published their recommendations. To successfully decrease radiation dose but still maintain diagnostic accuracy, radiologists and medical physicits need to collaborate closely.

► Most of us are concerned about the issues of radiation exposure that a patient receives diagnostically. Certainly, patients who do not have a diagnosis of malignant disease need to have their exposures minimized. For patients who have a diagnosis of malignancy, the information to be gained in that particular individual is presumably high enough that it merits the kind of exposures that we subject patients to. This analysis from Canada looks at the determinants of

TABLE 4.—Comparison of Effective Doses

Procedure	Effective Dose (mSv)
Posteroanterior chest radiograph	0.05
Conventional CT	7.0
Spiral CT pitch 1	7.0
Spiral CT pitch 2	3.5
High-resolution CT with 10-mm intersection gap	0.7
High-resolution CT with 20-mm intersection gap	0.35
Thin-section low-dose high-resolution CT	0.02
Conventional pulmonary angiography	9.0
Digital pulmonary angiography	6.0
Conventional bronchography	3.0*
Annual natural background radiation	2.5

*Bronchography performed with the assumption of 2 minutes of fluoroscopy and 6 posteroanterior and 6 lateral views.
(Courtesy of Mayo JR, Aldrich J, Müller NL: Radiation exposure at chest CT: A statement of the Fleischner Society. *Radiology* 228:15-21, 2003. Radiological Society of North America.)

radiation dose for thoracic CT, and discusses the interactions between the dose, and the quality of the image.

I think this is an area that most oncologists are not particularly knowledgeable about. The thing to understand is that the radiation dose associated with a CT is relatively high compared to other diagnostic studies. This article is jammed with information that I think is relevant and thus worth the reader's time.

E. Glatstein, MD

Risk of Cancer From Diagnostic X-rays: Estimates for the UK and 14 Other Countries

de González AB, Darby S (Univ of Oxford, England)
Lancet 363:345-351, 2004 18–2

Introduction.—Diagnostic radiographs are the greatest man-made source of radiation exposure to the general population. This modality contributes

TABLE 1.—Estimated Organ-specific Radiation Doses (mGy) by Type of Diagnostic X-ray

	Organ								
	Bladder	Breast	Colon	Liver	Lung	Oesophagus*	RBM	Stomach	Thyroid
X-ray type									
Abdomen	1·14	0·05	1·63	1·10	0·27	0·03	0·37	1·64	0·03
Coronary angiography	0·23	0·42	0·51	1·54	37·69	13·79	7·39	0·67	1·08
Cerebral angiography	0·00	0·02	0·00	0·01	1·14	1·98	9·27	0·01	25·06
Barium meal	0·28	0·62	1·82	9·48	1·23	0·54	1·69	8·24	0·22
Barium enema	14·45	0·14	21·51	3·55	0·39	0·06	7·49	4·98	0·01
Cardiac catheterisation	0·23	0·42	0·51	1·54	37·69	13·79	7·39	0·67	1·08
Cervical spine	0·00	0·00	0·00	0·00	0·07	0·12	0·07	0·00	0·84
Chest	0·00	0·01	0·00	0·03	0·07	0·04	0·02	0·02	0·01
Hip	1·16	0·00	0·71	0·01	0·00	0·00	0·12	0 02	0·00
Hysterosalpingography	4·67	0·00	2·82	0·01	0·00	0·00	0·81	0·03	0·00
Intravenous urogram (IVU)	4·42	0·20	5·10	3·49	0·42	0·03	0·83	6·04	0·00
Lumbar myelography	7·90	0·01	10·85	1·30	0·04	0·01	4·06	1·62	0·00
Lumbar spine	2·49	0·03	2·40	2·16	0·15	0·02	0·68	1·51	0·00
Mammography (1-view screen)	0·00	2·00	0·00	0·00	0·00	0·00	0·00	0·00	0·00
Pelvis	2·13	0·01	1·85	0·13	0·01	0·00	0·25	0·29	0·00
Skull	0·00	0·00	0·00	0·00	0·01	0·02	0·12	0·00	0·14
Thoracic spine	0·00	0·47	0·00	0·57	2·25	1·15	0·55	0·25	2·97
CT: abdomen	5·07	0·72	6·60	0·05	2·70	0·56	5·58	22·20	0·05
CT: chest	0·02	21·40	0·07	5·64	22·40	28·30	5·94	4·06	2·25
CT: head	0·00	0·03	0·00	0·01	0·09	0·07	2·67	0·00	1·85
CT: internal auditory meatus	0·00	0·02	0·00	0·01	0·08	0·07	0·83	0·00	2·03
CT: orbits	0·00	0·01	0·00	0·00	0·04	0·03	1·05	0·00	0·87
CT: pituitary	0·00	0·01	0·00	0·00	0·04	0·03	0·96	0·00	0·77
CT: pelvis	23·20	0·03	15·10	0·68	0·05	0·01	5·62	1·06	0·00
CT: cervical spine	0·00	0·09	0·00	0·03	0·58	0·51	1·12	0·02	43·90
CT: thoracic spine	0·00	27·70	0·02	1·48	13·40	15·70	2·92	0·98	0·46
CT: lumbar spine	0·67	0·13	3·30	6·88	0·34	0·08	2·52	10·50	0·01

*CT scan doses not available and assumed equal to thymus dose.

Abbreviation: RBM, Red bone marrow.

(Courtesy of de González AB, Darby S: Risk of cancer from diagnostic X-rays: Estimates for the UK and 14 other countries. *Lancet* 363:345-351, 2004. Reprinted with permission from Elsevier.)

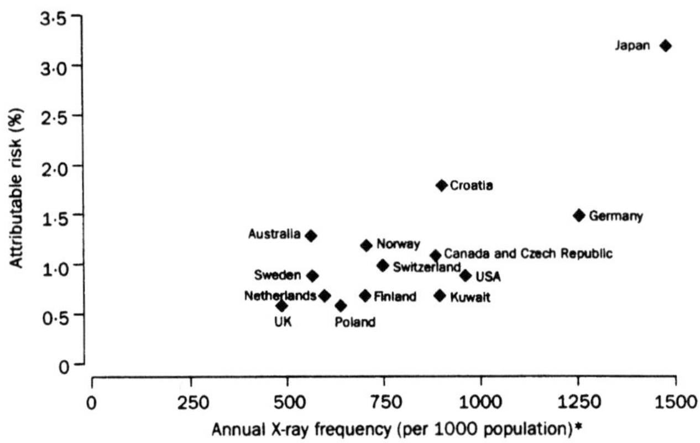

FIGURE 3.—Risk of cancer attributable to diagnostic X-ray exposures versus annual X-ray frequency. *Taken from worldwide survey. (Courtesy of de González AB, Darby S: Risk of cancer from diagnostic X-rays: Estimates for the UK and 14 other countries. *Lancet* 363:345-351, 2004. Reprinted with permission from Elsevier.)

about 14% of the total annual exposure worldwide from all sources. Diagnostic radiographs provide great benefits. Their use involves some small risk of development of cancer, which is generally accepted. The extent of this risk on the basis of the annual number of diagnostic radiographs performed in the United Kingdom and 14 other developed countries was assessed.

Methods.—Data were combined concerning the frequency of diagnostic radiography use, estimated radiation doses from radiographs to individual body organs, and risk models, based primarily on the Japanese atomic bomb survivors (Table 1 and Fig 3). Population-based cancer incidence rates and mortality rates for all causes of death were determined by life table methods.

Results.—In the United Kingdom, about 0.6% of the cumulative risk of cancer to age 75 years could be attributable to diagnostic radiographs of specific cancer sites or diagnostic procedures (Fig 2 and Table 3). This incidence is equivalent to about 700 cases of radiation-induced cancer per year. In 13 other developed countries, estimates of the attributable risk ranged from 0.6% to 1.8%. In Japan, which had the highest estimated annual exposure frequency in the world, the rate was over 3%.

Conclusion.—The calculations for estimates of cancer risk from diagnostic radiographs involved several assumptions and thus are inevitably subject to considerable uncertainty. The possibility that the risk was overestimated cannot be excluded; it is not likely that it has been overestimated substantially.

▶ These British epidemiologists have used the doses from radiologic procedures to individual body organs in order to estimate the subsequent risk of developing cancer. Obviously they have made a number of assumptions to permit this estimate, the most important of which is assuming a linear model. In addition, the estimates of cancer have been based on the survivors of atomic bomb survivors in Japan.

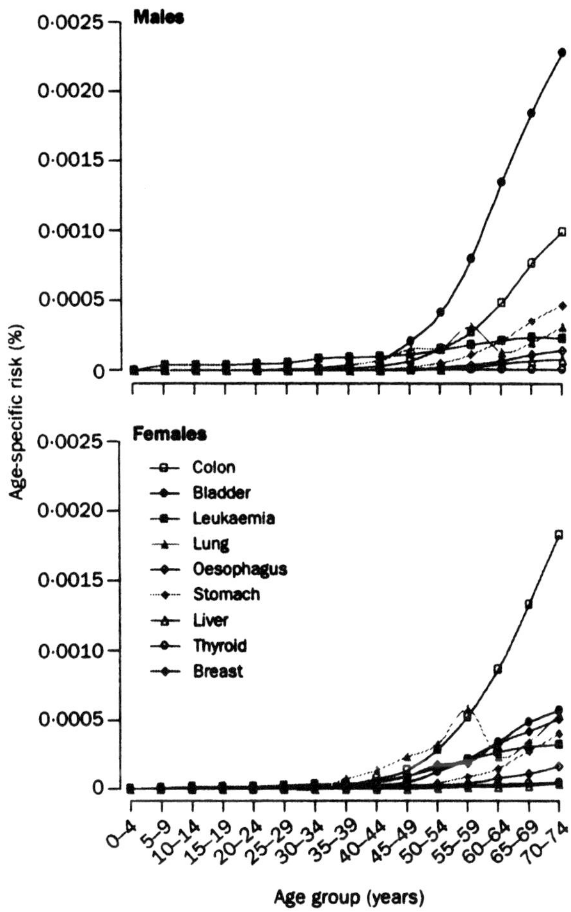

FIGURE 2.—Estimated annual risk of radiation-induced cancer from diagnostic X-rays in 5-year age groups in the United Kingdom population. (Courtesy of de González AB, Darby S: Risk of cancer from diagnostic X-rays: Estimates for the UK and 14 other countries. *Lancet* 363:345-351, 2004. Reprinted with permission from Elsevier.)

The radiation from the atomic bomb explosions in Japan is considerably different than a diagnostic X-ray. Not only is there an immediate photon exposure, but also there is beta and alpha emission from a variety of particles that were contaminated at the time of the explosion and which add to an internal dose of considerable but variable amounts. It is also true that the dose is fundamentally a "guesstimate," based on the distance that the survivor was thought to be from the epicenter of the explosion when it occurred. This does not take into account any type of structural protection that might have been situated between the survivor and the explosion. Thus, the doses from the Japanese explosions are extremely crude. Nonetheless, I think this is worth the reader's attention, largely because of (1) the consistent increase in diagnostic X-rays going on throughout this country and most of the other devel-

TABLE 3.—Estimated Number of Radiation-induced Cases of Cancer per Year in the UK by Type of X-ray

	Cases of Radiation-Induced Cancer Per Year*			Cases Per Million Examinations*
	Males	Females	Total	
X-ray type				
Abdomen	16	15	31	30
Barium meal	5	6	11	40
Barium enema	27	28	55	170
Chest	1	3	4	1
Coronary angiography	13	28	41	280
CT scan	31	39	70	60
Cerebral angiography	1	1	2	180
Hip or pelvis	28	24	52	30
Lumbar spine	23	16	39	40
Screening mammography	..	8	8	8
Thoracic spine	2	4	6	20
Each other type	<10	<10	<20	..

*Includes only the following 9 cancer sites: esophagus, stomach, colon, liver, lung, breast, bladder, thyroid, blood (leukemia). Detailed estimation of number of radiation-induced cases for all cancers is not possible, since estimates of organ-specific doses are not available for other cancers.

(Courtesy of de González AB, Darby S: Risk of cancer from diagnostic X-rays: Estimates for the UK and 14 other countries. *Lancet* 363:345-351, 2004. Reprinted with permission from Elsevier.)

oped countries in the world; and (2) because I think their Table 1 is extremely valuable in terms of giving the reader an estimate of doses in milligray according to individual radiologic studies. That information is not easy to come by, and the point is not in the absolute values, but in the relative values that are quoted for organs, particularly the lung, esophagus, colon, breast and bladder. CTs make an enormous contribution that needs to be recognized by the physicians who order these exams.

The numbers of cancers that are estimated will probably be reduced by new developments on the horizon, such as digital luminescent radiography, suggesting a substantial decrease in the radiation exposure. Nonetheless, the cancers will not be eliminated. One could argue not to do diagnostic imaging studies, but obviously the benefit derived from those studies is clearly important to the individual patient with a malignant diagnosis. The physician has to be aware of when the study really needs to be done and when he can afford not to do it.

E. Glatstein, MD

Second Malignancies After Chemotherapy and Radiotherapy for Hodgkin Disease

Chronowski GM, Wilder RB, Lovy LB, et al (Univ of Texas, Houston)
Am J Clin Oncol 27:73-80, 2004 18–3

Background.—Radiotherapy techniques have been used to cure early stage Hodgkin's disease, yet patients who are cured remain at increased risk for developing second malignancies. To improve the relapse-free survival time of Hodgkin's disease, treatment has evolved to induction chemotherapy followed by radiotherapy, but this approach also has led to an increased risk of solid tumors in survivors of Hodgkin's disease. The incidence of second malignancies among adults with early stage Hodgkin's disease who received chemotherapy followed by radiotherapy was explored. The risk accompanying the use of mitoxantrone, vincristine, vinblastine, and prednisone (NOVP) chemotherapy was compared with that seen when chemotherapeutic regimens containing alkylating agents were used. The frequency with which solid tumors developed in radiotherapy fields and the incidence of second malignancies when consolidative radiotherapy to both sides of the diaphragm was used were also explored.

Methods.—A retrospective analysis of the medical records of 286 patients with stage I or II Hodgkin's disease was conducted. Patients ranged in age from 16 to 88 years and received chemotherapy followed in 3 to 4 weeks by radiotherapy. A median of 3 cycles of induction chemotherapy were given. One hundred sixty-one patients received NOVP; 67 received nitrogen mustard, vincristine, procarbazine, and prednisone (MOPP); 19 received doxorubicin, bleomycin, vinblastine, and dacarbazine (ABVD); 18 received lomustine, vinblastine, procarbazine, and prednisone alternating with

TABLE 3.—Relative and Absolute Excess Risks of Second Malignancies in 286 Patients With Hodgkin Disease Treated With Alkylating-Agent (n = 125) vs NOVP (n = 161) Chemotherapy Followed by Radiotherapy

Second Malignancy (SEER Category)	Observed No. of Cases	Expected No. of Cases	RR	95% CI	AER
Acute myeloid leukemia (all cases)	3	0.04	69.3	14.3-202.6	13.3
Treated with an alkylating agent	1	0.02	41.0	1.2-228.4	8.4
Treated with NOVP	2	0.02	105.9	12.9-382.4	18.6
Non-Hodgkin lymphoma	1	0.30	3.4	0.1-18.8	3.2
All solid tumors (not leukemia or non-Hodgkin lymphoma)	17	7.52	2.4	1.3-3.6	42.5
Treated with alkylating agent	6	4.38	1.4	0.5-3.0	13.9
Treated with NOVP	11	3.14	3.5	1.8-6.3	74.0
Treated with RT to 1 side of diaphragm	5	4.43	1.1	0.4-2.6	6.5
Treated with RT to both sides of diaphragm	12	3.09	3.9	2.0-6.8	65.7
Basal cell carcinoma, NOS	4	—	—	—	—
Melanoma (skin)	3	0.41	7.3	1.5-21.3	11.6
Female genital system	2	1.71	1.2	0.1-4.2	1.3
Male genital system	1	1.12	0.9	0.0-5.0	−0.5
Urinary system	1	0.40	2.5	0.1-13.9	2.7
Lung and bronchus	1	0.78	1.3	0.0-7.2	1.0
Breast	1	0.96	1.0	0.0-5.8	0.2
Digestive system	1	0.42	2.4	0.1-13.3	2.6
Endocrine system	1	0.16	6.3	0.2-34.9	3.8
Brain	1	0.11	9.4	0.3-52.4	4.0
Soft tissue	1	0.05	21.5	0.6-119.9	4.3
All second malignancies	21	7.97	2.6	1.6-4.0	58.4

Abbreviations: AER, Absolute excess risk; *CI*, confidence interval; *NOS*, not otherwise specified; *NOVP*, mitoxantrone, vincristine, vinblastine, and prednisone; *RR*, relative risk; *RT*, radiotherapy; *SEER*, surveillance, epidemiology, and end results.

(Courtesy of Chronowski GM, Wilder RB, Levy LB, et al: Second malignancies after chemotherapy and radiotherapy for Hodgkin disease. *Am J Clin Oncol* 27:73-80, 2004.)

doxorubicin, bleomycin, dacarbazine, and lomustine; and 21 had various other combinations. Eighty-five patients were given involved-field (IF) radiotherapy, and 201 received extended-field radiotherapy. The median follow-up for survivors was 7.4 years.

Results.—In the 2230 patient-years of observation, the 5-year relapse-free survival rate was 88%, and the overall survival rate was 93%. Twenty-one second malignancies were found, compared with 7.97 events expected on the basis of incidence in the general population (Table 3). No leukemias developed more than 5.2 years after treatment, but the incidence of solid tumors rose with longer follow-up (Fig 1). At 5 years, the solid tumor risk was 1.9%; at 10 years, 9.3%; and at 15 years, 16.8%. Thirteen of the 17 solid tumors developed in the radiotherapy fields. Acute myeloid leukemia and melanoma also had significantly increased relative risk values of 69.3 and 7.3, respectively. No lower actuarial risk of leukemia attended the use of NOVP, and no higher actuarial risk of leukemia was associated with extended radiotherapy fields. Extended fields showed a trend toward a greater risk of solid tumors in comparison with the use of IF or regional fields. The cumulative risk of solid tumors with extended-field radiotherapy at 5 years was 2.7%; at 10 years, 11.1%; and at 15 years, 28.7% (Fig 2). These values were 0.0%, 6.9%, and 11.4% with consolidation IF or regional radiotherapy.

Conclusions.—Patients with Hodgkin disease carry a higher risk of having solid tumors develop, specifically melanoma. Because alkylating agents may contribute to this higher risk, it is recommended that nitrogen mustard and procarbazine be discontinued for these patients, as well as elective para-aortic and splenic radiotherapy after chemotherapy.

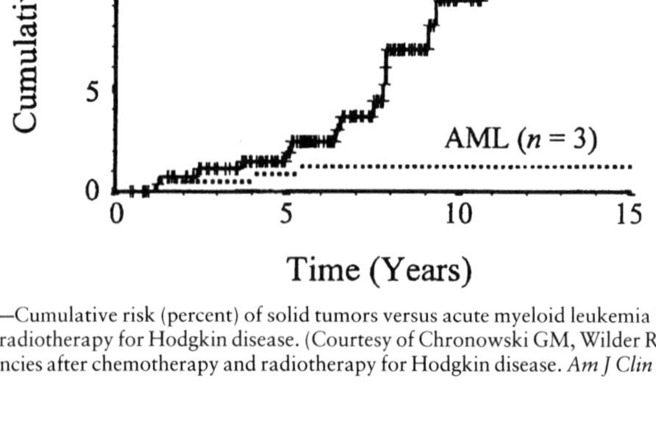

FIGURE 1.—Cumulative risk (percent) of solid tumors versus acute myeloid leukemia (*AML*) after chemotherapy and radiotherapy for Hodgkin disease. (Courtesy of Chronowski GM, Wilder RB, Levy LB, et al: Second malignancies after chemotherapy and radiotherapy for Hodgkin disease. *Am J Clin Oncol* 27:73-80, 2004.)

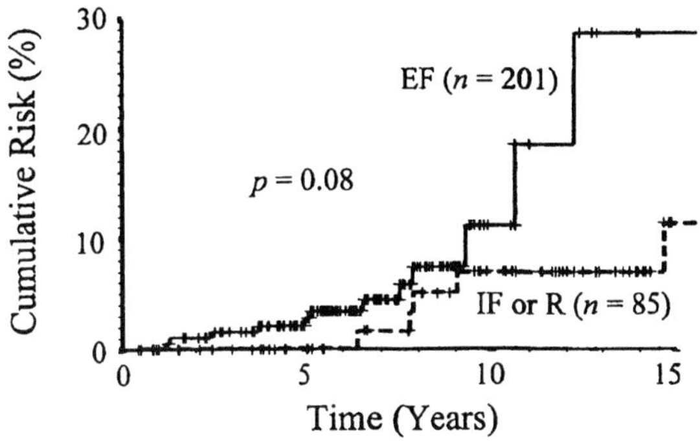

Field Size	Cumulative Incidence of Solid Tumors			
IF or R	0	0	4	5
EF	0	5	10	12

FIGURE 2.—Cumulative risk (percent) of solid tumors in terms of whether extended-field (*EF*) radiotherapy was delivered as opposed to involved-field (*IF*) or regional (*R*) radiotherapy after induction chemotherapy. (Courtesy of Chronowski GM, Wilder RB, Levy LB, et al: Second malignancies after chemotherapy and radiotherapy for Hodgkin disease. *Am J Clin Oncol* 27:73-80, 2004.)

▶ This article from the M. D. Anderson Cancer Center looks at the issue of second malignancy after combined-modality treatment for Hodgkin's disease. Certainly, increased risks were seen for acute myeloid leukemia and for melanoma. The authors say that to address this problem, they have stopped using regimens that use alkylating agents (nitrogen mustard and procarbazine), and they have stopped using elective irradiation to uninvolved nodes.

Currently, most people point the finger at radiation and chemotherapy as the critical issues in the second malignancy story in Hodgkin's patients. The fact remains that these patients have abnormal cell-mediated immunity, and those deficits persist even when patients are cured. It is hard for me to believe that this is not a factor in this phenomenon, simply because what we see in this group of patients seems disproportionate to all other groups of patients that we follow. In today's world where patients receive chemotherapy first, I virtually never treat the axilla anymore so that the mantle has undergone a major modification. This not only keeps the lateral breast out of the field of treatment (and in my experience that is where most of the second malignancies of breast have occurred among female patients), but it also markedly reduces the dose to the lungs. The scatter dose under the blocks can be enormous, depending upon the ratio of the mediastinal cutout to the transverse diameter of the chest. Particularly when patients receive ABVD, I try very hard to keep that scatter dose to a minimum, and omitting the axilla is an important step in that direction.

E. Glatstein, MD

Long-term Outcome for Patients With Non-metastatic Ewing's Sarcoma Treated With Adjuvant and Neoadjuvant Chemotherapies. 402 Patients Treated at Rizzoli Between 1972 and 1992

Bacci G, Forni C, Longhi A, et al (Istituto Ortopedico Rizzoli, Bologna, Italy)
Eur J Cancer 40:73-83, 2004 18–4

Background.—The prognosis of patients with nonmetastatic Ewing's sarcoma (ES) of bone is improved dramatically by current adjuvant and neoadjuvant chemotherapies. Long-term survival increases from between 10% and 15% to between 60% and 70%. Long-term follow-up data for patients with ES were obtained.

Methods.—Over 20 years, 402 patients with nonmetastatic ES of bone received adjuvant and neoadjuvant chemotherapy (Table 1). Follow-up lasted a mean of 17.7 years (range, 10-30 years).

Results.—Local treatment consisted of radiotherapy in 46.3% of patients, surgery in 25.4%, and surgery plus radiotherapy in 28.1% of patients. One patient had no local treatment. Surgery was used increasingly, rising from 32.9% to 64.1%. Event-free survival (EFS) was 44.0%. Relapse occurred in 53.5% of patients, a second neoplasm developed in 2.0%, and 2 patients died of cardiotoxicity related to doxorubicin. For 85.7% of patients, the adverse events were early; for 14.3% they were late. At 10 years, the EFS was 45.4% and the overall survival (OS) was 48.9%. Better OS was noted in women, persons younger than 14 years, those with tumors in the extremities, and with normal serum lactate dehydrogenase (LDH) levels at presentation. Surgery had an OS of 64.7% and radiotherapy an OS of 36.6%; the combination had an OS of 56.6%. Site and treatment period (1972-1990 vs 1991-1992) also influenced outcome. The 10-year survival of good responders (80.1%) was significantly better than that of poor responders (31.3%). Multivariate analysis showed only serum LDH level and gender were significantly independently related to increased survival (Table 3). Local recurrence developed in 18% of cases and metastases in 52%. Patients who had only radiotherapy had local relapse at a significantly higher rate than those treated surgically or with surgery plus radiotherapy. Seventy patients had local recurrence and metastases. Sites of recurrence included the lung, bone, or both. Relapse developed in a mean of 28.1 months, with 87% of cases found in the first 5 years after treatment. Late relapse occurred significantly less often in patients given radiotherapy only. Good responders had a higher late relapse rate than poor responders. Serum LDH levels, type of local treatment, and histologic response to chemotherapy were significantly related to time to relapse. Treatment of relapse was individualized. Of 215 patients who relapsed, 14 are alive and free of disease, 200 died of the tumor, and 1 is alive with uncontrolled disease. OS rates plateaued at 57.2% at 5 years and then declined to 38.4% at 20 years. Of 8 patients with a second malignancy (Table 7), 7 involved extremities and 1 the scapula. Radiotherapy was used in all cases; 2 also had surgery. The second malignancies developed 4 to 20 years after the first tumor. One patient had severe doxorubicin-linked cardiotoxicity develop 8 years after chemotherapy con-

TABLE 1.—Event-Free Survival and 10-Year Overall Survival According to Several Variables

	No. Cases	% EFS	*P* Value	% OS	*P* Value
All cases	402	44.5		49.3	
Gender					
Male	257	40.1		44.4	
			0.01		<0.01
Female	145	52.4		55.6	
Age					
≤14 yr	190	51.6		55.3	
			0.01		<0.02
>14 yr	212	38.2		44.7	
Site					
Extremity	253	49.8		55.3	
			0.01		<0.004
Other sites	149	35.6		45.1	
Serum LDH					
Normal	248	54.4		60.5	
			0.0001		<0.0001
Elevated	144	26.4		39.5	
Tumour volume (ml)					
≤150 ml	228	46.9		52.2	
		0.22		0.09	
>150 ml	147	38.9		47.8	
Local treatment[a]					
Radiotherapy	186	32.8		36.6	
Surgery	102	59.8	0.0007	64.7	<0.0001
Surgery + radiotherapy	113	50.4		56.6	
Histological response to chemotherapy[a]					
Poor	67	26.8		31.3	
			0.0001		<0.0001
Good	83	74.6		80.1	
Protocol of chemotherapy					
Three-drug regimen	86	26.7		34.8	
Four-drug regimen	168	44.0	0.001	50.0	<0.005
Six drug regimen	148	55.4		56.8	
Protocol of chemotherapy					
REA-1	86	26.7		34.9	
REA-2	59	50.8		57.6	
REN-1	109	40.4	0.002	45.9	<0.002
REN-2	81	49.4		50.6	
REN-3	67	62.7		64.2	

[a]Some of the data are missing in these subgroups.

Abbreviations: LDH, Lactate dehydrogenase; *EFS*, event-free survival; *OS*, overall survival; *REA-1*, 86 patients were treated for 24 months with a 3-drug regimen (cyclophosphamide [CP], doxorubicin [DX], and vincristine [VC]); *REA-2*, 59 patients were treated for 45 weeks with a 4-drug regimen (VC, dactinomycin [DT], CP, and DX); *REN-1*, 109 patients received 2 months of induction chemotherapy with 3 cycles of VC, DX, CP (VAC regimen), and maintenance chemotherapy with 5 cycles of VC/DX, 6 cycles of VC/DT, and 6 cycles of VC/CP; *REN-2*, 81 patients received 2 cycles of VAC regimen as induction chemotherapy, and 4 cycles of the same regimen were administered in maintenance chemotherapy, intercalated with 3 cycles of VC/ifosfamide (IF)/DT, followed by 3 cycles of etoposide (ET)/IF and 2 cycles of VC/DC/CP; *REN-3*, 67 patients received induction chemotherapy consisting of 2 cycles of VAC intercalated with 1 cycle of VC/IF/DT, with maintenance chemotherapy the same as that used in the REN-2 protocol.

(Reprinted from Bacci G, Forni C, Longhi A, et al: Long-term outcome for patients with non-metastatic Ewing's sarcoma treated with adjuvant and neoadjuvant chemotherapies. 402 patients treated at Rizzoli between 1972 and 1992. *Eur J Cancer* 40:73-83, 2004. Copyright 2004, with permission from Elsevier Science.)

TABLE 3.—Multivariate Analyses of the Variables Significant at the Univariate Examination

Variable	Odds Ratio	95% CI	*P* Value
Gender			
Female	1		
Male	1.23	1.02-1.45	<0.03
Site			
Other sites	1		
Extremities	0.86	0.72-1.03	<0.09
Age (years)			
>14	1		
≥14	0.84	0.70-0.99	<0.04
Local treatment			
Surgery alone or + radiotherapy	1		
Radiotherapy	1.17	0.97-1.40	<0.09
Serum LDH			
Elevated	1		
Normal	0.64	0.54-0.76	<0.0001

Abbreviations: 95% CI, 95% confidence interval; *LDH*, lactate dehydrogenase.

(Reprinted from Bacci G, Forni C, Longhi A, et al: Long-term outcome for patients with non-metastatic Ewing's sarcoma treated with adjuvant and neoadjuvant chemotherapies. 402 patients treated at Rizzoli between 1972 and 1992. *Eur J Cancer* 40:73-83, 2004. Copyright 2004, with permission from Elsevier Science.)

cluded, and 6 had azoospermia 5 to 8 years after treatment. All had chemotherapy after puberty. The 17 women who desired a pregnancy succeeded, with 2 early spontaneous abortions and 15 healthy newborns.

Conclusions.—Patients with ES with no evidence of disease 5 years after starting therapy are expected to live as long as persons without cancer. Of 231 patients alive after 5 years, 35 died (15.2%) and 10 of 197 patients (5.1%) alive after 10 years died of relapse or second tumors. Even with successful treatment, patients with ES of bone require careful follow-up to identify late relapses, complications of treatment, and second neoplasms.

► This is a very thorough review from the Rizzoli Institute in Bologna, Italy, on patients with nonmetastatic ES seen over a 20-year period. These patients were on a variety of studies that are detailed, and 402 patients are analyzed. There are not many real surprises here; elevated LDH was probably the most important prognostic variable. The differences in outcome according to local treatment presumably reflect patient selection for surgery. With a cure rate of 44%, and 2 patients dying of doxorubicin cardiotoxicity and another 8 developing second neoplasms, predominantly bony, it is a sobering experience that should give most of us a lot to shoot for in the future. The analysis would have been helped with some overall survival and relapse-free survival curves.

E. Glatstein, MD

TABLE 7.—Secondary Malignancies: Clinical Characteristics, Treatment and Outcome

Patient	Gender/Age (Years)	Protocol of Chemotherapy	Local Treatment	Second Neoplasm	Latency Time (Months)	Treatment	Outcome (m = months, y = years)
1	M/20	REA-1	RxT (60 Gy)	Radio-induced	48	Amputation	Dead after 12 m
2	F/10	REA-1	RxT (50 Gy)	ALL	10	Chemotherapy	Dead after 13 m
3	F/6	REN-1	Surgery + RxT (40 Gy)	Radio-induced osteosarcoma	48	Amputation + chemotherapy	Dead after 18 m
4	M/9	REA-1	RxT (60 Gy)	Radio-induced osteosarcoma	86	Limb salvage	NED at 20 y
5	M/17	REA-1	RxT (60 Gy)	Radio-induced MFH of bone	93	Amputation	NED at 22 y
6	M/10	REN-1	RxT (60 Gy)	Radio-induced osteosarcoma	120	Limb salvage + chemotherapy	Dead after 48 m
7	F/14	REA-2	RxT (56 Gy)	ALL	32	Chemotherapy	Dead after 6 m
8	F/17	REA-2	Surgery + RxT (44 Gy)	Radio-induced osteosarcoma	240	Limb salvage + chemotherapy	NED at 5 y

Abbreviations: M, Male; *F*, female; *RxT*, radiotherapy; *NED*, no evidence of disease; *MFH*, malignant fibrous histiocytoma; *ALL*, acute lymphoblastic leukemia.

(Reprinted from Bacci G, Forni C, Longhi A, et al: Long-term outcome for patients with non-metastatic Ewing's sarcoma treated with adjuvant and neoadjuvant chemotherapies. 402 patients treated at Rizzoli between 1972 and 1992. *Eur J Cancer* 40:73-83, 2004. Copyright 2004, with permission from Elsevier Science.)

Risk of Malignant Mixed Mullerian Tumors After Tamoxifen Therapy for Breast Cancer

Curtis RE, Freedman DM, Sherman ME, et al (NIH, Bethesda, Md)

J Natl Cancer Inst 96:70-74, 2004 18–5

Background.—Tamoxifen is used to improve survival in women with breast cancer and to reduce the risk of estrogen receptor–positive breast cancer in high-risk populations. However, its weakly estrogenic properties can lead to endometrial cell proliferation and a 2- to 3-fold increased risk of endometrial cancer. A substantially higher risk for rare, aggressive forms of uterine tumors, particularly malignant mixed mullerian tumors (MMMTs) and uterine sarcomas, also accompanies tamoxifen use. The relative and absolute risks of subsequent malignant uterine tumors were estimated by histologic type for women taking tamoxifen for breast cancer.

Methods.—The data from 39,451 breast cancer patients who received tamoxifen for initial treatment were evaluated. All had survived at least 1 year and were included in a population-based cancer registry in the Surveillance, Epidemiology, and End Results (SEER) program.

Results.—A more than 2-fold increased risk of developing a subsequent uterine cancer was found in these women in comparison with the SEER general population. The relative risk was substantially higher for subsequent MMMTs than for endometrial adenocarcinomas. Tamoxifen users who survived 5 years or longer had an 8-fold greater risk of MMMTs compared with a 2.3-fold greater risk for endometrial adenocarcinomas. MMMTs were diagnosed a median of 7.5 years after the initial tumor, whereas adenocarcinomas were diagnosed a median of 4.5 years later. For non–tamoxifen users, there was no increased risk for uterine corpus cancer overall or for endometrial adenocarcinomas (Table 1). A statistically nonsignificant increased risk of MMMTs was noted in non–tamoxifen users treated between 1973 and 1984. Age at diagnosis and stage of initial breast cancer did not influence endometrial adenocarcinoma or MMMT risk appreciably. The highest risk of MMMTs was noted in women aged 60 to 69 years when they received their initial treatment (Table 2). A very low cumulative mortality from uterine corpus cancer was found among tamoxifen users 15 years after their initial treatment. However, 25 of the 34 women who developed MMMTs died, with at least 15 of these deaths linked to uterine cancer or sarcoma. Death related to MMMTs among tamoxifen users was rare, with an estimated 0.8 deaths per 10,000 woman-years-at-risk, or about 11 or 12 deaths among 10,000 breast cancer patients followed up for 15 years.

Conclusions.—Tamoxifen users have about a 4-fold greater risk of having MMMTs develop than does the general population. For long-term breast cancer survivors who have received tamoxifen, the relative risk of an MMMT developing was 8-fold, compared with a 2-fold risk for endometrial adenocarcinoma. MMMTs have a poor prognosis, but the tumors are rare,

TABLE 1.—Risk of Uterine Corpus Cancer After Breast Cancer, by Type of Initial Therapy, Histologic Type of Uterine Cancer, and Time Since Breast Cancer Diagnosis*

	Time Since Breast Cancer Diagnosis									
	1-4 y		5-9 y		≥10 y		Total ≥1 y			
No. of patients entering interval*										
Tamoxifen†	39 451		20 053		5522		39 451			
No tamoxifen‡	67 190		51 918		39 050		67 190			
Woman-years at risk										
Tamoxifen	116 191		60 454		11 926		188 571			
No tamoxifen	236 596		224 642		336 526		797 764			
Second Uterine Cancer/Therapy	**O**	**O/E**	**O**	**O/E**	**O**	**O/E**	**O**	**O/E**	**95% CI**	**EAR**
All uterine corpus cancers										
Tamoxifen†	193	1.95§	132	2.49§	29	2.72§	354	2.17§	195 to 2.41	10.14
No tamoxifen‡	185	0.98	189	1.05	274	0.95	648	0.99	0.91 to 1.06	−0.12
Group I. Adenocarcinoma‖										
Tamoxifen¶	176	1.96§	109	2.27§	21	2.19§	306	2.07§	1.85 to 2.32	8.40
No tamoxifen	168	0.97	173	1.06	241	0.92	582	0.97	0.90 to 1.06	−0.21
Group II. Malignant mixed mullerian tumors (MMMTs)‖										
Tamoxifen**	10	2.29§	18	7.32§	6	11.52§	34	4.62§	3.20 to 6.46	1.41
No tamoxifen	9	1.45	8	1.14	19	1.48	36	1.38	0.97 to 1.91	0.12
Group III. Leiomyosarcomas‖										
Tamoxifen	0	(0.83)††	0	(0.39)††	0	(0.07)††	0	(1.29)††	0.00 to 2.85	−0.07
No tamoxifen	1	0.44	2	1.10	1	0.44	4	0.63	0.17 to 1.61	−0.03

(Continued)

TABLE 1. (cont.)

Second Uterine Cancer/Therapy	O	O/E	O	O/E	O	O/E	O	O/E	95% CI	EAR
Group IV. Endometria stromal, adenosarcoma‖										
Tamoxifen	2	1.90	1	1.82	1	9.57	4	2.34	0.63 to 5.99	0.12
No tamoxifen	0	(1.26)††	1	0.67	3	1.05	4	0.71	0.19 to 1.82	−0.02
Group V. Other uterine corpus cancers‖										
Tamoxifen	5	1.76	4	2.51	1	2.88	10	2.09§	1.00 to 3.84	0.28
No tamoxifen	7	1.08	5	0.84	10	1.12	22	1.03	0.65 to 1.56	0.01

*All patients survived or more years following an invasive breast cancer identified through the Surveillance, Epidemiology, and End Results (SEER) Program population registries. Patients who received initial therapy with chemotherapy, endocrine surgery, or endocrine radiation therapy were excluded from the analysis.

†Patients included in the tamoxifen group were diagnosed from 1980 through 2000.

‡Patients included in the no-tamoxifen group were diagnosed from 1973 through 1979 (women with all stages of disease) or from 1980 through 1984 (women with localized stage breast cancer only).

§Statistically significant when 95% CI excludes 1.0.

‖International Classification of Diseases for Oncology (2nd ed.) histologic type (morphology) groupings of uterine corpus cancers: Group I. Adenocarcinoma, type 1: 8050, 8140-8141, 8143, 8210-8211, 8260-8263, 8323, 8340, 8380-8381, 8440, 8470-8471, 8480-8481, 8490, 8550, 8560, 8570-8573; adenocarcinoma, type II: 8310 clear-cell adenocarcinoma, 8441 serous cystadenocarcinoma, not otherwise specified, 8460-8462 papillary serous cystadenocarcinoma. Group II. Malignant mixed mullerian tumors (MMMT): 8950 mullerian mixed tumor, 8951 mesodermal mixed tumor, 8980 carcinosarcoma, not otherwise specified, 8981 carcinosarcoma, embryonal type. Group III. Leiomyosarcomas 8890-8891, 8896. Group IV. Endometrial stromal, adenosarcoma: 8910 embryonal rhabdomyosarcoma, 8930 endometrial stromal sarcoma, 8933 adenosarcoma. Group V. Other uterine corpus cancers include all other histologic types not included in groups I-IV.

¶Adenocarcinoma tamoxifen group includes one patient with a second papillary serous cystadenocarcinoma and a third endometrioid carcinoma and one patient with a second MMMT (second cancer counted in the MMMT group) and a third serous surface papillary carcinoma (third cancer was counted in the adenocarcinoma group).

**MMMT tamoxifen group includes one patient with a second MMMT (second cancer counted in the MMMT group) and a third serous surface papillary carcinoma (third cancer was counted in the adenocarcinoma group).

††Numbers in parentheses are expected numbers of cancers.

Abbreviations: O, Observed number of subsequent (ie, second and third) cancers; *E*, expected number of subsequent cancers; *O/E*, observed-to-expected ratio; *tamoxifen group*, patients who received hormones as their initial therapy; *no-tamoxifen group*, patients who did not receive hormones as their initial therapy; *CI*, confidence interval; *EAR*, excess absolute risk per 10,000 women-years-at-risk, ([O − E]/women-years-at-risk) × 10,000.

(Courtesy of Curtis RE, Freedman DM, Sherman ME, et al: Risk of malignant mixed mullerian tumors after tamoxifen therapy for breast cancer. *J Natl Cancer Inst* 96:70-74, 2004. By permission of Oxford University Press.)

TABLE 2.—Risk of Subsequent Uterine Corpus Cancer Following Tamoxifen Therapy, by Age, Stage, Race, and Histologic Type of Breast Cancer, and Vital Status Among Patients Developing Uterine Corpus Cancer*

		Adenocarcinoma			MMMT		
Characteristic	No. of Patients	O	O/E	95% CI	O	O/E	95% CI
Total uterine corpus cancers	39 451	306	2.07†	1.85 to 2.32	34	4.62†	3.20 to 6.46
Age at breast cancer diagnosis, y							
<50	3002	12	2.33†	1.20 to 4.06	0	(0.10)‡	0.00 to 36.11
50-59	7053	46	1.78†	1.30 to 2.37	3	3.57	0.72 to 10.43
60-69	11 553	118	2.07†	1.72 to 2.48	18	6.91†	4.09 to 10.91
≥70	17 843	130	2.18†	1.82 to 2.59	13	3.42†	1.82 to 5.84
Stage at breast cancer diagnosis							
Localized	25 142	178	1.97†	1.69 to 2.29	23	5.34†	3.38 to 8.01
Regional	11 045	110	2.21†	1.82 to 2.66	10	3.82†	1.83 to 7.02
Distant	2302	11	2.31†	1.15 to 4.14	1	3.98	0.05 to 2.22
Unstaged	962	7	2.41	0.97 to 4.97	0	(0.17)‡	0.00 to 21.05
Race							
White	34 702	275	2.00†	1.77 to 2.26	26	4.11†	2.68 to 6.02
Black	2273	9	1.83	0.83 to 3.47	7	8.55†	3.43 to 17.62
Other	2405	22	4.78†	3.00 to 7.24	1	5.14	0.07 to 28.59
		No.	%		No.	%	
Vital status§		305	100.0		34	100.0	
Total alive		174	57.1		9	26.5	
Total dead		131	42.9		25	73.5	
Uterine cancer deaths‖		29	9.5		15	44.1	

*All patients survived 1 or more years following invasive breast cancer diagnosed from 1980 through 2000. Patients who received hormonal therapy (tamoxifen) as their initial therapy. Patients who received initial therapy in the form or chemotherapy, endocrine surgery, or endocrine radiation therapy were excluded from the analyses. All patients were identified from the Surveillance, Epidemiology, and End Results (SEER) Program population registries.

†Statistically significant when 95% confidence interval excludes 1.0.

‡Numbers in parentheses are expected numbers of uterine corpus cancers.

§Vital status of breast cancer patients who developed uterine corpus cancer as their second cancer. Number of patients with uterine adenocarcinomas (n = 305) excludes one patient who had a second MMMT uterine tumor and a third uterine adenocarcinoma.

‖Includes deaths due to uterine cancer or sarcoma.

Abbreviations: MMMT, Malignant mixed mullerian tumor; *O*, observed number of subsequent (eg, second and third) cancers; *E*, expected number of subsequent cancers; *O/E*, observed-to-expected ratio.

(Courtesy of Curtis RE, Freedman DM, Sherman ME, et al: Risk of malignant mixed mullerian tumors after tamoxifen therapy for breast cancer. *J Natl Cancer Inst* 96:70-74, 2004. By permission of Oxford University Press.)

so the absolute risk of death is small. These results indicate that tamoxifen may produce delayed effects in some patients.

► This is an important epidemiologic study from the National Cancer Institute evaluating the risk of uterine cancer in patients receiving tamoxifen for breast cancer. The investigators evaluated data from almost 40,000 patients over a 20-year period. The increased risk of uterine cancer associated with the use of tamoxifen was more than double what was expected on the basis of the SEER population. A surprisingly higher risk was seen for MMMTs, which have a relatively unfavorable prognosis. These risks are probably justified in terms of the benefits of tamoxifen in the population of women with breast cancer, but it is important that physicians be aware that these benefits do have a price associated with them, and they need to inform patients about these small but finite risks.

E. Glatstein, MD

Long-term Risk of Second Malignant Neoplasms After Neuroblastoma in Childhood: Role of Treatment

Rubino C, Adjadj E, Guérin S, et al (Institut Gustave Roussy, Villejuif, France; Univ of Birmingham, England)
Int J Cancer 107:791-796, 2003 18–6

Background.—Neuroblastoma is one of the most common solid tumors in childhood. Surgery, radiation therapy, combination therapy, and in recent years, high-dose chemotherapy followed by bone marrow transplantation are integrated in the conventional treatment of neuroblastoma. The selection of treatment options is made on the basis of the age of the child, the location and biology of the tumor, and the stage of disease. As successful treatments of malignant diseases in childhood have advanced, the problem of long-term complications has become prominent. General evaluations of the long-term carcinogenic risks induced by radiotherapy, chemotherapy, and their association after treatment for childhood cancer have already been

TABLE 1.—General Characteristics of 544 Five-Year Survivors of a Neuroblastoma in Childhood According to the Type of Treatment

Treatment	Patients n	Sex (% Female)	Year of Treatment Median (min-max)	Age at Diagnosis in Months Median (min-max)	Follow-up in Years Median (min-max)
No Ct no Rt	72	47	1979 (1951-1985)	8 (0-154)	11 (5-38)
Rt no Ct	85	59	1965 (1948-1982)	9 (0-178)	22 (6-37)
Ct no Rt	173	51	1981 (1962-1986)	10 (0-177)	10 (5-38)
Rt & Ct	214	46	1975 (1955-1985)	13 (0-198)	15 (5-37)
All	544	50	1977 (1948-1986)	11 (0-198)	14 (5-38)

Abbreviations: Ct, Chemotherapy; *Rt*, radiotherapy.

(Courtesy of Rubino C, Adjadj E, Guérin S, et al: Long-term risk of second malignant neoplasms after neuroblastoma in childhood: Role of treatment. *Int J Cancer* 107:791-796, 2003.

TABLE 2.—Radiotherapy: Period of Treatment and Mean Radiation Dose to Selected Organs and Active Bone Marrow According to the Type of Machine, for 285 Children Treated by Radiotherapy Among the 544 5-Year Survivors of a Neuroblastoma

Type of Machine	Patients	Median Period of Treatment: (Range)	Mean Duration of Courses in Day	Mean Number of Fractions	Mean Dose in Gy			
					Breasts	Thyroid	Brain	Active Bone Marrow
Orthovoltage x-rays (200-250 KV)	65	1962 (1948-1974)	34	18	5.0	2.2	0.98	2.8
Cobalt 60 (γ-rays)	159	1976 (1952-1989)	28	18	5.3	4.9	3.2	5.1
Megavoltage x-rays (4-25 MV)	25	1973 (1961-1985)	21	12	2.7	0.33	2.1	2.1
Electrons (6-22 MV)	54	1974 (1965-1985)	21	10	6.3	1.6	0.006	2.5
All types*	285	1972 (1948-1989)	29	17	5.5	3.4	2.2	4.1

*15 children were treated with more than one type of machine.

(Courtesy of Rubino C, Adjadj E, Guérin S, et al: Long-term risk of second malignant neoplasms after neuroblastoma in childhood: Role of treatment. *Int J Cancer* 107:791-796, 2003. Copyright 2003. Reprinted by permission of Wiley-Liss, Inc, a subsidiary of John Wiley & Sons, Inc.)

TABLE 4.—Characteristics of 13 Second Malignant Neoplasms (Smn) Developed in 12 of 544 Neuroblastoma 5-Year Survivors

	Neuroblastoma Treatment								
Site of the SMN (Sex)	Year	Age in Months	Tumor Site	Chemotherapy	Radiotherapy	Year	Age in Year	SMN Within the Irradiation Field	Radiation Dose at SMN (Gy)
Thyroid									
Papillary carcinoma (M)	1950	8	Thorax	No	Orthovoltage	1976	27	Yes	17.9
Papillary carcinoma (M)	1953	15	Pelvis	No	Orthovoltage	1975	23	No	0.7
Carcinoma (F)	1963	35	Abdomen	No	Orthovoltage	1981	20	No	0.4
Papillary carcinoma (F)	1968	26	Abdomen	No	Orthovoltage	1988	22	Yes	13.8
Well differentiated vesicular carcinoma (F)	1968	7	NA	No	Cobalt-60	1987	19	No	0.9
Breast									
Invasive ductal carcinoma (F)	1954	19	Abdomen	No	Orthovoltage	1991	38	Yes	10.0
Carcinoma (F)	1956	7	Thorax	No	Orthovoltage	1983	27	No	1.0
Malignant phyllode tumour (F)*	1961	29	Abdomen	No	Orthovoltage	1975	16	Yes	12.9
Glioblastoma (F)	1958	8	Thorax	No	Orthovoltage	1988	30	No	0.02
Osteosarcoma-head (F)	1977	18	Pelvis	Adr Vcr Cpm	Cobalt-60	1983	7	No	1.2
Soft tissue sarcoma-abdomen (M)	1962	3	Pelvis	Act	Orthovoltage	1981	19	Yes	25.6
Acute myeloid leukaemia (F)*	1961	29	Abdomen	No	Orthovoltage	1991	32	—	3.1
Acute lymphoid leukaemia (F)	1979	29	Pelvis	Vm26 Adr Vcr Cpm Cddp	No	1984	7	—	—

Abbreviations: NA, Not available; *Adr*, adriamycin; *Vcr*, vincristine; *Cpm*, cyclophosphamide; *Act*, actinomycin; *Vm26*, teniposide; *Cddp*, cisplatinum.
*These 2 second malignancies occurred in the same patient.
(Courtesy of Rubino C, Adjadj E, Guérin S, et al: Long-term risk of second malignant neoplasms after neuroblastoma in childhood: Role of treatment. *Int J Cancer* 107:791-796, 2003.

published. However, few cohort studies have examined the very long-term incidence of second malignant neoplasms (SMNs) in children initially treated for a neuroblastoma. The risk of SMNs among long-term survivors of neuroblastomas was quantified, and the influence of treatment on this risk was examined.

Methods.—Data were obtained from 544 five-year survival patients who had neuroblastoma diagnosed before 16 years of age at 8 British and French treatment centers from 1948 to 1986 (Table 1).

Results.—After an average follow-up of 15 years (range, 5-38 years), 12 children had a total of 13 SMNs develop, whereas only 1.19 SMNs were expected from general population rates (Tables 2 and 4). Among these SMNs, there were 5 thyroid and 3 breast cancers. Increases in the risks of SMN were observed with time since neuroblastoma diagnosis (Fig 1) and attained age (Table 7). In a multivariate analysis, the relative risk of SMN occurring in

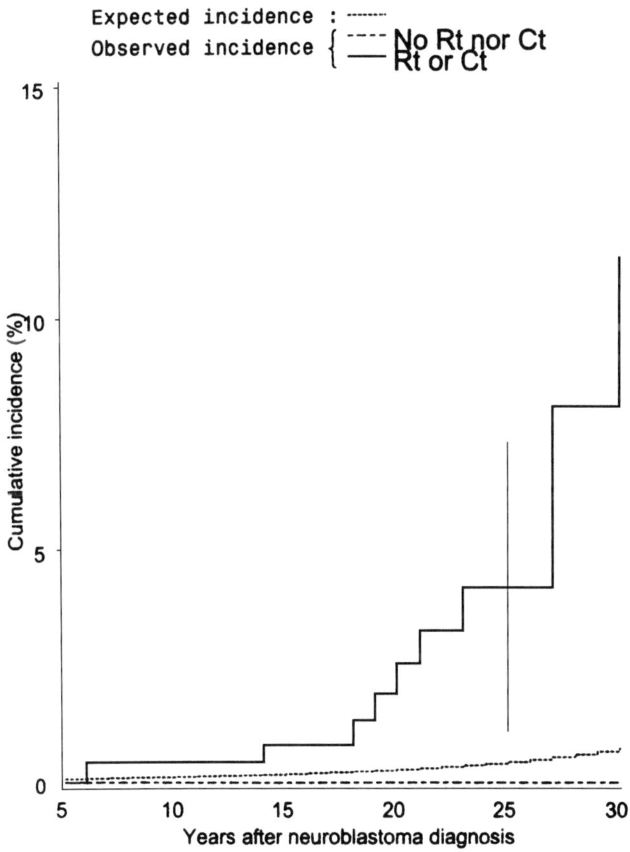

FIGURE 1.—Expected and cumulative incidence of second malignant neoplasm and 95% confidence interval. *Abbreviations: Rt,* Radiotherapy; *Ct,* chemotherapy. (Courtesy of Rubino C, Adjadj E, Guérin S, et al: Long-term risk of second malignant neoplasms after neuroblastoma in childhood: Role of treatment. *Int J Cancer* 107:791-796, 2003. Copyright 2003. Reprinted by permission of Wiley-Liss, Inc, a subsidiary of John Wiley & Sons, Inc.)

TABLE 7.—Occurrence of SMN in 544 Neuroblastoma 5-Year Survivors According to Attained Age

Attained Age	Number of PYR	Number of SMN: O	Number of SMN: E	Annual Incidence/10^5 persons (95% CI): Total	Excess (AER)	*P* for Trend	SIR (95% CI)	*P* for Trend
3-9	3242	2	0.32	61.7 (10.3-190.5)	54.4 (3.0-183.2)	Crude	6.3 (1.0-10.3)	Crude
10-19	3020	3	0.34	99.9 (24.7-257.6)	85.6 (11.1-243.8)	0.001	8.9 (2.2-23.0)	0.1
20-29	1104	5	0.30	453.0 (162.5-973.7)	424.1 (133.6-944.8)	Adjusted	16.6 (5.9-35.6)	Adjusted*
≥30	197	2	0.20	1016.5 (169.0-3137.9)	901.5 (56.0-3022.7)	0.2	10.0 (1.7-31.0)	0.5

Abbreviations: SMN, Second malignant neoplasm; *PYR*, person year at risk; *O*, observed number of SMN; *E*, expected number of SMN; *AER*, absolute excess risk; *SIR*, standardized incidence ratio; *95% CI*, 95% confidence interval.

*Stratified on period of treatment.

(Courtesy of Rubino C, Adjadj E, Guérin S, et al: Long-term risk of second malignant neoplasms after neuroblastoma in childhood: Role of treatment. *Int J Cancer* 107:791-796, 2003.

association with radiotherapy was 4.3, whereas no increased risk of SMN was associated with the administration of chemotherapy as a whole.

Conclusions.—Young children treated for a neuroblastoma have significantly increased risks of SMNs over 30 years of follow-up. Radiotherapy was found to be an important risk factor for the development of SMNs, although no similar effect of chemotherapy was observed. The importance of long-term surveillance of young children treated for neuroblastoma is underscored by these findings.

▶ This is an important article dealing with the risk of SMNs among survivors of neuroblastoma. The data come from a group of solid investigators from France and England. They had 544 patients who survived neuroblastoma for at least 5 years. There were a total of 13 second tumors (12 patients) seen in that group. Given the number of patient-years at risk, they expected a total of 1 SMN. Obviously, the treatment appeared to have a major impact on second tumors, although it is interesting that you cannot find in this analysis the outcome by treatment. One can see that 10 of the 12 neoplasms occurred before 1970, when the techniques presumably became somewhat improved in radiation therapy and a greater awareness of the problem was evolving. In any event, most of the neoplasms were associated with radiation, although of the 11 cases that had received radiation, 9 had received orthovoltage treatment, which is known to have a much greater absorption in bone. At least 1 case of leukemia occurred with chemotherapy and no radiation, but the bulk of the lesions appeared to be secondary to radiation.

This kind of retrospective study is obviously important; yet at the same time, because there are no controls, it is not easy to know exactly how to interpret it. Obviously, treatment has some side effects, and chemotherapy and radiation are both capable of inducing a tumor, largely because they both have the capability of scrambling the DNA. At the same time, it is important to understand that there are no data to describe what the incidence of a second cancer is in patients who do not undergo such treatment. It is presumably low and approaching zero, although if one has mutated cells that have ultimately become malignant, the question is, is the risk of a second cancer in that patient the same as in the normal population? I rather doubt it. This is the essential problem in making a conclusion in clinical medicine: exactly what is the control population for comparison?

E. Glatstein, MD

Subclinical Late Cardiomyopathy After Doxorubicin Therapy for Lymphoma in Adults

Hequet O, Le QH, Moullet I, et al (Centre Hospitalier Lyon-Sud, France)

J Clin Oncol 22:1864-1871, 2004 18–7

Background.—Doxorubicin is the most active agent for treating lymphoma. This anthracycline, however, is limited by severe cardiotoxicity, particularly at doses greater than 550 mg/m^2. The risk factors for high-dose, doxorubicin-induced congestive heart failure (CHF) are well documented, but risk factors for subclinical cardiac toxicity after lower-dose doxorubicin are less clear. Thus, the incidence and characteristics of cardiotoxicity in long-term survivors of non-Hodgkin's lymphoma (NHL) or Hodgkin's lymphoma (HL) were retrospectively examined.

Methods.—The medical records of 141 adults with HL or NHL (59% male; median age, 54 years) who had undergone doxorubicin-based chemotherapy (cumulative dose >250 mg/m^2) at least 5 years previously were reviewed. All patients agreed to undergo echocardiography, and all were in complete remission or had stable disease at the time of the cardiac evaluation. Echocardiography was used to evaluate the presence of CHF or subclinical cardiomyopathy (left ventricular fractional shortening <25% without clinical signs of CHF or other cardiomyopathy). The development of clinical or subclinical CHF was examined in light of the patients' clinical characteristics, including cardiovascular risk factors.

Results.—The median doxorubicin dose was 300 mg/m^2 (range, 250-550 mg/m^2). In the 5 years since treatment, only 1 patient (0.7%) had clinical cardiomyopathy develop. Thirty-nine patients (27.7%), however, had subclinical cardiomyopathy develop. Multivariate regression analyses identified 5 factors significantly and independently associated with an increased risk of subclinical cardiomyopathy: older age, male sex, higher cumulative dose of doxorubicin or receipt of an additional anthracycline, radiotherapy, and being overweight.

Conclusion.—Even with moderate doses of doxorubicin, cardiac abnormalities are common, occurring in approximately one fourth of these adult patients with NHL or HL. Risk factors for subclinical cardiotoxicity were similar to those for CHF in this population.

▶ The authors retrospectively assessed a cohort of 141 patients who had received anthracycline-based therapy for lymphoma a minimum of 5 years earlier for evidence of left ventricular dysfunction as evidenced by echocardiography. Of the 141 patients, only 1 had developed clinical symptoms of CHF, while an additional 39 patients demonstrated some evidence subclinical cardiomyopathy. The risk factors for left ventricular dysfunction included male sex, older age, and higher cumulative doses of doxorubicin. This study confirms that even in patients with cured lymphoma that a long-term effect on left ventricular function can be seen in up to 25% to 35% of patients and that further long-term evaluation of these patients is warranted to determine whether clinical symptoms of CHF develop as a survivorship issue.

M. S. Gordon, MD

Osteonecrosis of the Jaws Associated With the Use of Bisphosphonates: A Review of 63 Cases

Ruggiero SL, Mehrotra B, Rosenberg TJ, et al (Long Island Jewish Med Ctr, New Hyde Park, NY; Univ of Maryland, Baltimore)

J Oral Maxillofac Surg 62:527-534, 2004 18–8

Background.—Bisphosphonates are used widely to manage metastatic disease to the bone as well as osteoporosis. The authors recently encountered a group of patients with necrotic lesions of the jaw with 1 clinical feature in common: all had received chronic bisphosphonate treatment. This necrosis was otherwise typical of osteoradionecrosis, a condition rarely seen at the authors' center. A retrospective chart review was conducted.

Methods.—Records of patients presenting between February 2001 and November 2003 were searched to find those diagnosed as having refractory osteomyelitis and a history of chronic bisphosphonate treatment.

Findings.—Sixty-three patients with this diagnosis were identified. Fifty-six patients had received IV bispohosphonates for at least 1 year. Seven patients were receiving chronic oral bisphosphonate therapy. Typically, the lesions were a nonhealing extraction socket or an exposed jawbone. Both lesion types were refractory to conservative debridement and antibiotic therapy. Lesion biopsy specimens showed no evidence of metastatic disease. Most affected patients needed surgery to remove the involved bone.

Conclusions.—A risk of osteonecrosis of the jaw appears to be associated with the use of chronic bisphosphonate. Practitioners need to monitor patients for this previously unrecognized complication. Early diagnosis may prevent or decrease morbidity resulting from advanced destructive lesions of the jaw bone.

► As with many drugs in widespread use, new areas of potential usage as well as complications are recognized. This article outlines an unusual complication, osteonecrosis of the jaw, which is associated with the use of bisphosphonates. This recognition of this entity has prompted Novartis to send out an announcement[1] writing changes to the precautions and postmarketing experiences section for pamidronate disodium and zoledronic acid. The particular patient with this entity has been receiving intravenous bisphosphonates for at least a year including chronic bisphosphonate therapy and usually was a consequence of the nonhealing extraction socket of exposed jawbone after dental procedures. As a consequence, it is recommended that preventive dentistry be considered before bisphosphonate therapy especially in those who are going to receive concurrent chemotherapy and corticosteroids and for those patients with poor oral hygiene.

P. J. Loehrer, Sr, MD

Reference

1. Hohneker JA: September 24, 2004.

Subject Index

A

B

C

D

E

F

G

H

I

K

L

M

N

R

S

T

U

V

Author Index

A

B

C

D

J

K

L

M

N

O

P

Q

R

S

T

U

V

W

X

Y

Z